Hospital-Based Palliative Medicine

Hospital Medicine: Current Concepts

Scott A. Flanders and Sanjay Saint, Series Editors

Hospitalist's Guide to the Care of the Older Patient 1e
Brent C. Williams, Preeti N. Malani, David H. Wesorick, Editors, 2013

Inpatient Anticoagulation
Margaret C. Fang, Editor, 2011

Hospital Images: A Clinical Atlas
Paul B. Aronowitz, Editor, 2012

Becoming a Consummate Clinician: What Every Student, House Officer, and Hospital Practitioner Needs to Know
Ary L. Goldberger and Zachary D. Goldberger, Editors, 2012

Perioperative Medicine: Medical Consultation and Co-Management
Amir K. Jaffer and Paul J. Grant, Editors, 2012

Clinical Care Conundrums: Challenging Diagnoses in Hospital Medicine
James C. Pile, Thomas E. Baudendistel, and Brian J. Harte, Editors, 2013

Inpatient Cardiovascular Medicine
Brahmajee K. Nallamothu and Timir S. Baman, Editors 2013

Hospital-Based Palliative Medicine: A Practical, Evidence-Based Approach
Steven Pantilat, Wendy Anderson, Matthew Gonzales and Eric Widera, Editors, 2015

Hospital-Based Palliative Medicine

A Practical, Evidence-Based Approach

Edited by

Steven Pantilat, MD, FAAHPM, MHM
Palliative Care Program
Division of Hospital Medicine, Department of Medicine
UCSF School of Medicine
San Francisco, CA, USA

Wendy Anderson, MD, MS
Palliative Care Program
Division of Hospital Medicine, Department of Medicine
UCSF School of Medicine
San Francisco, CA, USA

Matthew Gonzales, MD
Division of Hospital Medicine, Department of Medicine
City of Hope National Medical Center
Duarte, CA, USA

Eric Widera, MD
Division of Geriatrics, Department of Medicine
University of California San Francisco
San Francisco, CA, USA

Series Editors

Scott A. Flanders, MD, MHM
Sanjay Saint, MD, MPH, FHM

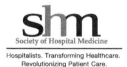

Hospitalists. Transforming Healthcare.
Revolutionizing Patient Care.

WILEY Blackwell

Published by John Wiley & Sons, Inc., Hoboken, New Jersey
Published simultaneously in Canada

The contents of this work are intended to further general scientific research, understanding, and
discussion only and are not intended and should not be relied upon as recommending or promoting
a specific method, diagnosis, or treatment by health science practitioners for any particular patient.
The publisher and the author make no representations or warranties with respect to the accuracy or
completeness of the contents of this work and specifically disclaim all warranties, including without
limitation any implied warranties of fitness for a particular purpose. In view of ongoing research,
equipment modifications, changes in governmental regulations, and the constant flow of information
relating to the use of medicines, equipment, and devices, the reader is urged to review and evaluate the
information provided in the package insert or instructions for each medicine, equipment, or device for,
among other things, any changes in the instructions or indication of usage and for added warnings and
precautions. Readers should consult with a specialist where appropriate. The fact that an organization or
Website is referred to in this work as a citation and/or a potential source of further information does not
mean that the author or the publisher endorses the information the organization or Website may provide
or recommendations it may make. Further, readers should be aware that Internet Websites listed in this
work may have changed or disappeared between when this work was written and when it is read. No
warranty may be created or extended by any promotional statements for this work. Neither the publisher
nor the author shall be liable for any damages arising herefrom.

For general information on our other products and services or for technical support, please contact our
Customer Care Department within the United States at (800) 762-2974, outside the United States at
(317) 572-3993 or fax (317) 572-4002.

Wiley also publishes its books in a variety of electronic formats. Some content that appears in print may
not be available in electronic formats. For more information about Wiley products, visit our web site at
www.wiley.com.

Library of Congress Cataloging-in-Publication Data:

Hospital-based palliative medicine : a practical, evidence-based approach / edited by Steven Pantilat,
Wendy Anderson, Matthew Gonzales, Eric Widera.
    p. ; cm. – (Hospital medicine, current concepts ; 8)
    Includes bibliographical references and index.
    ISBN 978-1-118-77257-7 (paperback)
I. Pantilat, Steven, editor.   II. Anderson, Wendy, editor.   III. Gonzales, Matthew,
editor.   IV. Widera, Eric, editor.   V. Series: Hospital medicine, current concepts; 8.
[DNLM: 1. Palliative Care–methods.   2. Evidence-Based Medicine–methods.   3. Hospitals.
WB 310]
    R726.8
    616.02′9–dc23
                                                                                    2014034458

Cover image: istockphoto-senior-17379381 / 08-09-11 © Syldavia;
istockphoto-doctor-using-digital-tablet-talking-with-senior-patient-24015116 / 04-24-13
© monkeybusinessimages; and
istockphoto.com-close-up-of-a-young-female-caring-doctor-3924891 / 08-03-07 © Yuri

Printed in the United States of America
10 9 8 7 6 5 4 3 2 1

Contents

Contributors   viii

1. **Hospital Care for Seriously Ill Patients and Their Families**   1

   Steven Z. Pantilat, Wendy G. Anderson, Matthew J. Gonzales, and Eric W. Widera

   Section 1   Symptom Management

2. **Pain Management: A Practical Approach for Hospital Clinicians**   11

   Solomon Liao, Kira Skavinski, Jamie Capasso, and Rosene D. Pirrello

3. **Dyspnea: Management in Seriously Ill Hospitalized Patients**   37

   Margaret L. Campbell and Michael A. Stellini

4. **Nausea and Vomiting: Evaluation and Management in Hospitalized Patients**   49

   Katherine Aragon and Matthew J. Gonzales

5. **Delirium: Identification and Management in Seriously Ill Hospitalized Patients**   61

   Marieberta Vidal and Eduardo Bruera

6. **Depression and Anxiety: Assessment and Management in Hospitalized Patients with Serious Illness**   71

   Nathan Fairman, Jeremy M. Hirst, and Scott A. Irwin

Section 2   Communication and Decision Making

7. **Effective Communication with Seriously Ill Patients in the Hospital: General Principles and Core Skills**   95

   Kristen A. Chasteen and Wendy G. Anderson

8. **Family Meetings and Caring for Family Members**   108

   Sara K. Johnson

9. **Assessing Goals of Care: A Case-Based Discussion**   121

   Elizabeth Lindenberger and Amy S. Kelley

10. **Documenting Goals of Care and Treatment Preferences in the Hospital: A Case-Based Discussion**   133

    Lynn A. Flint, Rebecca L. Sudore, and Brook Calton

11. **Prognostication: Estimating and Communicating Prognosis for Hospitalized Patients**   143

    Joshua R. Lakin and Eric W. Widera

12. **Managing Conflict over Treatment Decisions**   160

    Robert M. Arnold and Eva Reitschuler-Cross

Section 3   Practice

13. **Palliative Care Emergencies in Hospitalized Patients**   171

    Paul Glare, Yvona Griffo, Alberta Alickaj, and Barbara Egan

14. **Withdrawing Life-Sustaining Interventions**   195

    James M. Risser and Howard Epstein

15. **Artificial Nutrition and Hydration in Patients with Serious Illness**   206

    Thomas T. Reid

16. **Last Days of Life: Care for the Patient and Family**   223

    Jason Morrow

**17. Palliative Care after Discharge: Services for the Seriously
 Ill in the Home and Community**   237

Amy M. Corcoran, Neha J. Darrah, and Nina R. O'Connor

18. Interdisciplinary Team Care of Seriously Ill Hospitalized Patients   250

Dawn M. Gross and Jane Hawgood

19. Self-Care and Resilience for Hospital Clinicians   260

Sarah M. Piper, B.J. Miller, and Michael W. Rabow

Index   273

Contributors

Alberta Alickaj, MD, Urgent Care, Department of Medicine, Memorial Sloan Kettering Cancer Center, New York, NY, USA

Wendy G. Anderson, MD, MS, Division of Hospital Medicine and Palliative Care Program, Department of Medicine, UCSF School of Medicine, San Francisco, CA, USA

Katherine Aragon, MD, Palliative and Supportive Services, Lawrence General Hospital, Lawrence, MA, USA

Robert M. Arnold, MD, Leo H Criep Chair in Patient care, Section of Palliative Care and Medical Ethics, University of Pittsburgh, Palliative and Supportive Institute, UPMC Health System, Pittsburgh, PA, USA

Eduardo Bruera, MD, Palliative Care and Rehabilitation Medicine, F.T. McGraw Chair in the Treatment of Cancer, The University of Texas MD Anderson Cancer Center, Houston, TX, USA

Margaret L. Campbell, PhD, RN, FPCN, College of Nursing/Office of Health Research, Wayne State University, Detroit, MI, USA

Brook Calton, MD, MHS, Division of Geriatrics, Department of Medicine, University of California, San Francisco (UCSF), San Francisco, CA, USA

Jamie Capasso, DO, Division of Palliative Medicine, Hospitalist Department, University of California, Irvine, CA, USA

Kristen A. Chasteen, MD, Palliative Medicine, Henry Ford Hospital, Wayne State University School of Medicine, Detroit, MI, USA

Amy M. Corcoran, MD, CMD, FAAHPM, Center of Excellence in Palliative Medicine, Department of Medicine, Penn State Milton S. Hershey Medical Center, Penn State College of Medicine, Hershey, PA, USA

Neha J. Darrah, MD, Instructor of Clinical Medicine, Division of General Internal Medicine, Department of Medicine, Division of General Internal Medicine, Hospital of the University of Pennsylvania, Philadelphia, PA, USA

Barbara Egan, MD, SFHM, FACP, Hospital Medicine Service, Department of Medicine, Memorial Sloan Kettering Cancer Center, New York, NY, USA

Howard Epstein, MD, FHM, CHIE, Executive Vice President & Chief Medical Officer, PreferredOne® Health Plans, University of Minnesota Medical School, Twin Cities, MN, USA

Nathan Fairman, MD, MPH, Department of Psychiatry and Behavioral Sciences, UC Davis School of Medicine, Sacramento, CA, USA

Lynn A. Flint, MD, Division of Geriatrics, Department of Medicine, UCSF School of Medicine, San Francisco VA Medical Center, San Francisco, CA, USA

Paul Glare, MBBS, FRACP, FACP, Palliative Medicine Service, Memorial Sloan Kettering Cancer Center, New York, NY, USA

Matthew J. Gonzales, MD, Division of Supportive Medicine, Department of Supportive Care Medicine, City of Hope National Medical Center, Duarte, CA, USA

Yvona Griffo, MD, Palliative Medicine Service, Department of Medicine, Memorial Sloan Kettering Cancer Center, New York, NY, USA

Dawn M. Gross, MD, PhD, Division of Supportive Medicine, Department of Supportive Care Medicine, Sheri & Les Biller Patient and Family Resource Center, City of Hope National Medical Center, Duarte, CA, USA

Jane Hawgood, MSW, Palliative Care Program, Department of Medicine, University of California San Francisco, San Francisco, CA, USA

Jeremy M. Hirst, MD, Department of Psychiatry UC San Diego School of Medicine and Psychiatry & Psychosocial Services, UC San Diego Moores Cancer Center and Palliative Care Psychiatry, UC San Diego Health System, San Diego, CA, USA

Scott A. Irwin, MD, PhD, Psychiatry & Psychosocial Services, UC San Diego Moores Cancer Center; and Palliative Care Psychiatry, UC San Diego Health System; and Psychiatry, UC San Diego School of Medicine, San Diego, CA, USA

Sara K. Johnson, MD, Palliative Medicine, Hematology/Oncology Division, University of Wisconsin, Madison, WI, USA

Amy S. Kelley, MD, MSHS, Brookdale Department of Geriatrics and Palliative Medicine, Icahn School of Medicine at Mount Sinai, One Gustave L. Levy Place, New York, NY, USA

Joshua R. Lakin, MD, Department of Psychosocial Oncology and Palliative Care, Dana-Farber Cancer Institute, Boston, MA, USA

Solomon Liao, MD, FAAHPM, Palliative Care Service, Hospitalist Program, Department of Medicine, University of California, Irvine School of Medicine, Orange, CA, USA

Elizabeth Lindenberger, MD, Department of Geriatrics and Palliative Medicine, Icahn School of Medicine at Mount Sinai, New York, NY, USA

B. J. Miller, MD, Department of Medicine, University of California, San Francisco, CA, USA

Jason Morrow, MD, PhD, Division of Geriatrics, Gerontology, and Palliative Medicine, University of Texas Health Science Center at San Antonio and L.I.F.E Care/ Palliative Medicine Program, University Health System, San Antonio, TX, USA

Nina R. O'Connor, MD, Division of General Internal Medicine, University of Pennsylvania, Philadelphia, PA, USA

Steven Z. Pantilat, MD, FAAHPM, MHM, Division of Hospital Medicine, Department of Medicine, UCSF School of Medicine, San Francisco, CA, USA

Sarah M. Piper, MD, Department of Palliative Care, Kaiser Permanente Oakland Medical Center, Oakland, CA, USA

Rosene D. Pirrello, BPharm, RPh, Department of Pharmacy Services, University of California – UC Irvine Health, Orange, CA, USA

Michael W. Rabow, MD, Department of Medicine, University of California, San Francisco, San Francisco, CA, USA

Thomas T. Reid, MD, MA, Department of Medicine, University of California, San Francisco, CA, USA

Eva Reitschuler-Cross, MD, Division of General Internal Medicine, Section of Palliative Care and Medical Ethics, University of Pittsburgh Medical Center, Pittsburgh, PA, USA

James M. Risser, MD, Palliative Care and Hospital Medicine, Regions Hospital, Health Partners, St Paul, MN, USA

Kira Skavinski, DO, Palliative Care Service, Hospitalist Program, Department of Medicine, University of California, Irvine School of Medicine, Orange, CA, USA

Michael A. Stellini, MD, MS, FACP, Hospice and Palliative Medicine, John D. Dingell Veterans Administration Medical Center and Wayne State University School of Medicine, Detroit, MI, USA

Rebecca L. Sudore, MD, Medicine/Geriatrics, University of California, San Francisco, San Francisco, CA, USA

Marieberta Vidal, MD, Department of Palliative Care and Rehabilitation, The University of Texas, MD Anderson Cancer Center, Houston, TX, USA

Eric W. Widera, MD, Division of Geriatrics, Department of Medicine, University of California San Francisco, San Francisco, CA, USA

Chapter 1

Hospital Care for Seriously Ill Patients and Their Families

Steven Z. Pantilat, Wendy G. Anderson, Matthew J. Gonzales, and Eric W. Widera

Mrs Morton was an 82-year-old woman with ovarian cancer metastatic to the lung, liver, and peritoneum with massive ascites diagnosed 1 year ago. She had undergone many cycles of chemotherapy but stopped chemo several months ago due to progression of disease and increasing fatigue. Mrs Morton was living at home with her daughter, son-in-law, and three grandchildren. A few days earlier, she had stopped eating and drinking. She became sleepier and spent all of her time in bed. On the morning of admission, Mrs Morton's daughter awoke to find that her mother was not able to speak or even open her eyes and was moaning and breathing fast. Feeling panicked, her daughter called 911. The ambulance arrived within a few minutes. They found Mrs Morton hypotensive, tachypneic, tachycardic, hypoxic, and in respiratory distress. They asked about advance directives, but were told that Mrs Morton had not completed one. They started an IV, gave fluids, administered oxygen, and rushed Mrs Morton to the hospital.

On arrival in the emergency department, the emergency physician and nurse asked the family, "Would you like us to do everything possible?"

Her family responded, "Yes," as virtually anyone would to this question.

The emergency physician called the hospitalist on call STAT to the emergency department to admit Mrs Morton and notified the intensive care unit that she would soon be on her way up.

1.1 EPIDEMIOLOGY OF HOSPITAL CARE FOR THE SERIOUSLY ILL

For hospitalists, intensivists, emergency physicians, advance practice nurses, nurses, and all clinicians who practice in the hospital, the story of Mrs Morton is all too common. Overall, about one-third of Americans die in hospitals; many

Hospital-Based Palliative Medicine: A Practical, Evidence-Based Approach, First Edition.
Edited by Steven Pantilat, Wendy Anderson, Matthew Gonzales, and Eric Widera.
© 2015 John Wiley & Sons, Inc. Published 2015 by John Wiley & Sons, Inc.

more spend some time in a hospital in the last year of life [1]. Among Medicare beneficiaries, nearly 70% are hospitalized in the last 3 months of life, one-third receive ICU care in the last month of life, and over half die in a hospital or nursing home [2].

While it is arguable whether Mrs Morton needed hospital admission to receive quality care at the end of her life, as hospice or palliative care at home would likely have provided the care she needed, the reality is that for many people hospital care provides relief and recovery from exacerbations of chronic illness. People with acute shortness of breath from heart failure or chronic obstructive pulmonary disease (COPD), bowel obstruction from pancreatic cancer, altered mental status from liver failure, and pain from a pathologic fracture often experience rapid and dramatic improvement in symptoms and quality of life from hospital care. Even patients who prefer to avoid hospitalization may find that hospital care provides the quickest and best option for relief of symptoms. For example, Chapter 4 discusses options for treating patients with malignant bowel obstruction. In this clinical setting, hospitalization may offer the best option for relief of nausea, vomiting, and pain. At the same time, for a patient like Mrs Morton, there will likely come a time when hospitalization will not only fail to provide relief but may also impose additional burdens for her and her family. Although it can be difficult to predict which hospitalization will be the last one or whether hospitalization will provide more benefit than harm, each hospitalization for the seriously ill provides an opportunity to clarify goals of care to ensure that care is consistent with patient preferences, promotes benefit, and limits harm.

Studies of patients with serious illness have shown consistently what these patients need and want from the healthcare system: relief from pain and other symptoms; clear communication about their illness, prognosis, and treatment options; and psychosocial, spiritual, and practical support [3, 4]. Addressing these needs is critical for providing high-quality care to patients with serious illness, and as such provides the overarching organizational structure to this book. Further, it requires a team approach as no single clinician has expertise in all these domains. Hospitalists and other hospital-based physicians, nurses, social workers, and chaplains must collaborate to ensure that patient needs are attended to. Such collaboration can happen formally, as with a palliative care consultation team, or more informally through clinicians working together to share insights and develop and implement plans of care.

Increasingly, it is hospitalists and other hospital-based specialists who care for people with serious illness in the hospital like Mrs Morton [5]. Over time, hospitalists have come to care not only for people with classic medical conditions, such as pneumonia and COPD, but also for people with cancer and cardiac, neurologic, and surgical problems either as admitting physicians or through comanagement. The high frequency of hospitalization among the seriously ill and those approaching the end of life places the clinicians who work in these settings in an ideal position to promote optimal quality of life for these patients.

1.2 PALLIATIVE CARE

Palliative care is the field of medicine focused on providing the best possible quality of life to people with serious illness and those near the end of life. Palliative care is defined as follows:

> *...specialized medical care for people with serious illnesses. This type of care is focused on providing patients with relief from the symptoms, pain, and stress of a serious illness—whatever the diagnosis.*
>
> *The goal is to improve quality of life for both the patient and the family. Palliative care is provided by a team of doctors, nurses, and other specialists who work with a patient's other doctors to provide an extra layer of support. Palliative care is appropriate at any age and at any stage in a serious illness, and can be provided together with curative treatment.* [6]

There are several important parts of this definition that bear highlighting. First, palliative care is for people with *serious illnesses*. While palliative care is also about caring for people near and at the end of life such as Mrs Morton, fundamentally, palliative care is for people with serious illnesses such as heart disease, COPD, cirrhosis, cancer, and dementia and would have been appropriate for Mrs Morton from the time of diagnosis. The term *serious illness* is also helpful when talking with patients about the need for palliative care or the decision to involve palliative care specialists. Patients can easily relate to and understand that they have a serious illness and that additional care will be helpful to them. In the hospital, palliative care will also be appropriate for patients with fulminant acute illness such as massive intracranial hemorrhage and trauma. The important point for hospitalists to remember is that palliative care is not only for the terminally ill and also for those at the very end of life.

Palliative care is also *appropriate at any stage in a serious illness*, and patients can receive palliative care *while still pursuing curative intent treatment* such as chemotherapy, radiation therapy, percutaneous coronary interventions, surgery, and hemodialysis. Many patients and physicians harbor the misconception that receiving palliative care means that patients must forsake curative intent treatment. This misunderstanding is a common barrier that unnecessarily precludes patients from receiving palliative care. Patients admitted with exacerbations of heart failure or COPD, with complications of cancer or its treatment, and those with dementia all may benefit from symptom management, clarification of goals of care, and psychosocial support. One helpful question to ask for determining whether a patient would benefit from palliative care is, "Would I be surprised if this patient died in the next year?" This "surprise" question helps clinicians identify patients appropriate for palliative care [7]. If the question is difficult to apply to every patient, clinicians can also consider the types of patients who would be appropriate for palliative care (Table 1.1).

Consistent with what patients say they need from the healthcare system, palliative care seeks to *relieve the symptoms, pain, and stress of a serious illness.*

Table 1.1   Types of Patients Appropriate for Palliative Care

---

- Advanced heart failure, second readmission in a year
- Breast cancer and malignant pleural effusion
- Brain metastases
- Dementia and aspiration pneumonia
- New diagnosis of idiopathic pulmonary fibrosis
- Cirrhosis, second admission for altered mental status
- Awaiting solid organ transplant
- "Would I be surprised if this patient died in the next year?"
  - If the answer is "No," provide and/or refer for palliative care.

Relief of symptoms and pain is the first priority as patients can only focus on what is important to them and on having meaningful time when their symptoms are controlled. Control of symptoms allows patients to consider the issue that is at the heart and the ultimate goal of palliative care: *improving quality of life*. In fact, one helpful way to explain palliative care to patients and families is to state that the goal is to help patients "achieve the best possible quality of life for as long as possible." This focus on promoting quality of life and understanding that it is defined uniquely by each patient is at the crux of what palliative care is about. It is also helpful to explain to patients that palliative care provides an *extra layer of support*. Few hospitalized patients would decline extra support, and the more seriously ill the patient, the more attractive and necessary the extra support becomes.

Hospitalized patients fall along a continuum of an illness trajectory, and palliative care plays a significant role in the care of patients throughout this continuum. The needs of these patients with serious illness will vary over the course of illness, and as shown in Figure 1.1, the relative focus on palliative care and curative intent treatment may change. Similarly, the depth and intensity of involvement with palliative care concerns will change over time, but from diagnosis to death, patients with serious illness will encounter situations where they will need and benefit from palliative care.

As will be highlighted throughout this book, there is considerable evidence for the efficacy and effectiveness of palliative care. A review of the evidence shows that palliative care relieves symptoms such as pain and depression, improves quality of life, increases satisfaction with care, and reduces resource utilization including ICU length of stay and costs of care [8–11]. Such an impact is easy to imagine when thinking about Mrs Morton. In addition, palliative care and conversations between patients and physicians about goals and preferences for care not only improve quality of care and life for patients but also improve outcomes for loved ones of patients who die [12, 13]. Those loved ones are less likely to experience complicated grief and depression 6 months after their loved one died.

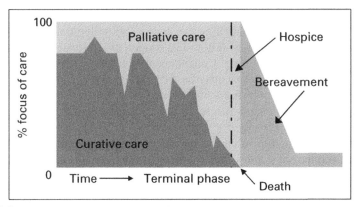

Figure 1.1   Concurrent model of palliative care. *Source*: © Steven Pantilat, MD and Regents of the University of California.

1.3   THE ROLE OF THE HOSPITAL-BASED CLINICIAN IN PALLIATIVE CARE

Hospitalists, intensivists, and other hospital-based clinicians frequently care for patients with serious illness and those approaching at the end of life like Mrs Morton. Hospitalists recognize the importance of palliative care to their practice and acknowledge a relative lack of education in pain management and palliative care during training [14]. Hospital-based clinicians can interact with palliative care in following four ways.

> *Refer to a Palliative Care Team*: At a basic level, these clinicians need to identify patients who need palliative care and make appropriate referrals. Mrs Morton would be just such a patient. Many patients, like her, who need palliative care have complex symptom management and communication needs that require an interdisciplinary team of palliative care experts. In addition, when hospitalists are too busy with other patients to have extended goals of care conversations and family meetings, palliative care teams can assist to ensure that patient needs are met.

> *Work as a Member of a Palliative Care Team*: Many hospitalists and other hospital-based clinicians will have extensive experience with palliative care and develop a strong interest in it. While currently the only path physicians in the US have to board certification in palliative medicine is through a 1-year clinical fellowship, many palliative care teams are challenged to find qualified physicians and advance practice nurses and would likely welcome experienced hospitalists dedicated to gaining continued education and experience in palliative care. Hospitalists, intensivists, and others can split their time between their primary specialty and working with a palliative care team, diversifying their professional responsibilities and income streams.

Become Board Certified in Palliative Care: Hospital-based clinicians who find palliative care compelling can pursue fellowship training in palliative care. The 1-year clinical fellowship is open to physicians from nearly all hospital-based disciplines. Understandably, taking a year away from practice to be a clinical fellow may be difficult financially. Some hospitals that have had difficulty hiring a board-certified palliative care physician have offered to supplement the salary of a hospital-based physician during fellowship in exchange for a guarantee of a certain number of years of work on the palliative care team. Given the shortage of palliative medicine-trained physicians, this arrangement can be a win–win for the hospital and the clinician and is often the fastest way of recruiting a board-certified palliative medicine physician. Nurses can also pursue board certification in palliative care. In addition, there are excellent educational courses for nurses in palliative care (End-of-Life Nursing Education Consortium (ELNEC) http://www.aacn.nche.edu/elnec), although there are few fellowships in palliative care for nurses.

Provide Primary Palliative Care: This option is the one that applies to all clinicians and could have the greatest impact on ensuring that all patients who need palliative care receive it [15]. For example, regardless of whether a hospital had a palliative care team, and many still do not [16], Mrs Morton needed to receive palliative care. All hospital-based clinicians should have a basic knowledge and facility with palliative care issues including pain and symptom management, discussing prognosis and goals of care, ensuring psychosocial and spiritual support to patients and families, and providing care that is culturally aware and sensitive. The tools, knowledge, and skills associated with palliative care—such as pain management and good communication—apply to the care of many, if not all, hospitalized patients. In addition to being able to address pain, hospital-based physicians should have facility with management of dyspnea, nausea, vomiting, bowel obstruction, depression, and anxiety. A thorough knowledge of good communication techniques including sharing bad news, running a family meeting, and discussing goals of care are critical activities for all hospital-based clinicians. Finally, addressing and attending to patients' psychological, social, emotional, and spiritual needs is important not only for patients nearing the end of life but also for many seriously and acutely ill patients. The fundamental goal of this book is to provide hospital-based clinicians with that knowledge base in an easy-to-use, evidence-based way with sufficient specificity and direction that will help guide care at the bedside.

Fortunately, there is large overlap in the knowledge, skills, and practice of hospital medicine, other hospital-based specialties, and palliative care. Clinical care in each realm includes interdisciplinary collaboration, seriously ill patients and those near the end of life, a wide range of clinical conditions, and a focus on improving quality of life and quality of care. This synergy across specialties can reinforce practice in each setting and help clinicians improve care overall.

1.4   THE STRUCTURE OF THIS BOOK

This book is divided into three parts that map the issues most important to seriously ill patients and their families and the major focus of palliative care: symptom management, clear communication, and psychosocial–spiritual support. The goal is to provide useful, practical, evidence-based information for busy hospital-based clinicians that forms the foundation of care for seriously ill patients and those near the end of life. This book also provides the science and the art of medicine and the science behind the art. In addition to evidence-based medicine, the authors share their clinical expertise and pearls of wisdom to put the evidence in context and offer guidance where evidence is lacking; akin to what they would impart in a consultation.

1.5   REWARDING PRACTICE

The care of seriously ill patients and those approaching the end of life can be challenging and richly rewarding [17]. Working with Mrs Morton and her family to help ease her respiratory distress; pausing the resuscitation long enough to understand her preferences for care; providing support, compassion, and empathy to her family; and implementing a plan consistent with her wishes allow the clinicians to use their heart as well as their head to provide the best possible care to patients and their families. In our technological age, it is easy to think that the only important aspects of medical care and the ones that patients value the most are the things we do to them. Such thinking grossly underestimates the importance that patients place in the human side of medicine and the caring that clinicians demonstrate by relieving symptoms and eliciting patient preferences carefully enough to really understand their goals and values and develop a plan to make those happen. In these cases, hospitalists and other hospital-based specialists can bring their humanism to bear on the care of the patient and can provide healing even, and especially, if cure is not possible.

1.6   CARING FOR MRS MORTON

A hospitalist or other hospital-based clinician well versed in palliative care can see the case of Mrs Morton as an opportunity to stop the onslaught of medical intervention for a patient who is dying and understand what her preferences would be to ensure she receives the care she and her family want. The hospitalist might start by asking, "How were you hoping we could help?" That question, much better in this situation than the one asked, could begin to elicit Mrs Morton's preferences as expressed by her family [18]. The hospitalist could order opioids for the tachypnea and respiratory distress. If the family expresses understanding that Mrs Morton is dying and states that her wish in this setting is to have her care focused on comfort and dignity, the hospitalist might recommend admission or explore the possibility of Mrs Morton returning home with hospice services. The hospitalist might also ask about spiritual and religious issues to ensure that these are addressed in case

Mrs Morton dies soon. The hospitalist could provide a best estimate of prognosis and explain about the dying process. Finally, the hospitalist could provide guidance to the family about what they can say and do at the bedside to promote comfort, dignity, and healing. The skills and knowledge essential for providing this type of care are the essence of this book.

REFERENCES

1. Hall M, Levant S, DeFrances C, *Trends in Inpatient Hospital Deaths: National Hospital Discharge Survey, 2000–2010*. NCHS data brief, no. 118. Huntsville, MD: National Center for Health Statistics, 2013.
2. Teno JM, Gozalo P, Mitchell SL, Tyler D, Mor V, Survival after multiple hospitalizations for infections and dehydration in nursing home residents with advanced cognitive impairment, *JAMA* 2013 Jul 17;**310**(3):319–320.
3. Steinhauser KE, Clipp EC, McNeilly M, Christakis NA, McIntyre LM, Tulsky JA, In search of a good death: observations of patients, families, and providers, *Ann Intern Med* 2000;**132**(10):825–832.
4. Singer PA, Martin DK, Kelner M, Quality end-of-life care: patients' perspectives, *JAMA* 1999; **281**(2):163–168.
5. Pantilat SZ, Palliative care and hospitalists: a partnership for hope, *J Hosp Med* 2006 Jan;**1**(1):5–6.
6. Care CtAP. *Get Palliative Care*. New York, 2013. [Cited 2014, February 23, 2014]. Available at http:// www.getpalliativecare.org/whatis/. Accessed on July 22, 2014.
7. Murray S, Boyd K, Using the "surprise question" can identify people with advanced heart failure and COPD who would benefit from a palliative care approach, *Palliat Med* 2011 Jun;**25**(4):382.
8. Aslakson R, Cheng J, Vollenweider D, Galusca D, Smith TJ, Pronovost PJ, Evidence-based palliative care in the intensive care unit: a systematic review of interventions, *J Palliat Med* 2014 Feb;**17**(2): 219–235.
9. El-Jawahri A, Greer JA, Temel JS, Does palliative care improve outcomes for patients with incurable illness? A review of the evidence. *J Support Oncol* 2011 May–Jun;**9**(3):87–94.
10. Gade G, Venohr I, Conner D, et al., Impact of an inpatient palliative care team: a randomized control trial, *J Palliat Med* 2008 Mar;**11**(2):180–190.
11. Temel JS, Greer JA, Muzikansky A, et al., Early palliative care for patients with metastatic non–small-cell lung cancer, *N Engl J Med* 2010;**363**(8):733–742.
12. Prigerson HG, Jacobs SC, Perspectives on care at the close of life. Caring for bereaved patients: "all the doctors just suddenly go", *JAMA* 2001;**286**(11):1369–1376.
13. Wright AA, Zhang B, Ray A, et al., Associations between end-of-life discussions, patient mental health, medical care near death, and caregiver bereavement adjustment, *JAMA* 2008 Oct 8;**300**(14): 1665–1673.
14. Plauth WH, 3rd, Pantilat SZ, Wachter RM, Fenton CL, Hospitalists' perceptions of their residency training needs: results of a national survey, *Am J Med* 2001;**111**(3):247–254.
15. Quill TE, Abernethy AP, Generalist plus specialist palliative care—creating a more sustainable model, *N Engl J Med* 2013 Mar 28;**368**(13):1173–1175.
16. Pantilat SZ, Kerr KM, Billings JA, Bruno KA, O'Riordan DL, Palliative care services in California hospitals: program prevalence and hospital characteristics, *J Pain Symptom Manage* 2012 Jan;**43**(1):39–46.
17. Chittenden EH, Clark ST, Pantilat SZ, Discussing resuscitation preferences with patients: challenges and rewards, *J Hosp Med* 2006;**1**(4):231–240.
18. Pantilat SZ, Communicating with seriously ill patients: better words to say, *JAMA* 2009 Mar 25;**301**(12):1279–1281.

Section 1

Symptom Management

Chapter 2

Pain Management: A Practical Approach for Hospital Clinicians

Solomon Liao, Kira Skavinski, Jamie Capasso, and Rosene D. Pirrello

2.1 ETIOLOGY AND TYPES OF PAIN

Pain is "localized physical suffering associated with a bodily disorder" or "acute mental or emotional distress or suffering" [1]. A comprehensive approach to diagnosing and understanding pain therefore requires evaluating not only the medical disorder causing the physical pain but also the psychosocial distress that contributes to the patient's overall suffering. Since every patient has a psychosocial aspect and a spiritual/existential component to their pain, the question is not whether the patient has nonphysical pain but how much. For example, a postoperative patient's pain may be 98% physical, 1.5% emotional, and 0.5% spiritual. A chronic cancer patient's pain, however, may be 45% physical, 35% psychosocial, and 20% existential. In reality, the different pain domains interact (as in Fig. 2.1), and separating them is both impractical and often impossible.

However, understanding the different pain domains allows for a structured approach to address all of the patient's sources of pain. Screening for depression and anxiety is important in all pain patients, but particularly in chronic pain patients. Generally when a patient rates their pain higher than a 10 out of a maximum 10 scale, they are saying they have more than just physical pain. The most important existential question to ask a pain patient is the meaning the patient gives to their pain. People are able to tolerate horrible pain, such as in childbirth, if they give the pain a positive meaning and see a purpose to their pain. However, if a patient gives a negative meaning to their pain, such as a cancer patient who interprets their pain as progression of their disease, then their ability to tolerate their pain worsens.

Hospital-Based Palliative Medicine: A Practical, Evidence-Based Approach, First Edition.
Edited by Steven Pantilat, Wendy Anderson, Matthew Gonzales, and Eric Widera.

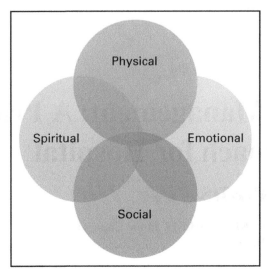

Figure 2.1   Biopsychosocial model of pain.

Even for physical pain, different categories have been suggested to divide the types of pain based upon etiologies and mechanisms. These categories include such terms as somatic, neuropathic, inflammatory, visceral, and nociceptive. However, the most useful or practical dichotomy of pain type is whether the pain is opioid responsive or opioid refractory. From a management standpoint, this distinction is the first point in the algorithm of treatment. If the patient's pain is opioid responsive, then the issue is finding the opioid dose needed to control the pain. If the patient's pain is opioid refractory, merely giving the patient more opioids gets the patient and the prescriber into more trouble, a phenomenon that occurs all too often.

The differential diagnosis for opioid refractory pain is relatively short. Neuropathic pain has an incomplete response to opioids, in that most patients with significant neuropathic pain say that opioids "take the edge" off the pain but do not relieve it [2]. The majority of patients with opioid refractory pain have some component of neuropathic pain. The second most common type of opioid refractory pain is inflammatory pain, such as metastatic bone pain, and the third is nonphysical pain. Less common but important causes of opioid refractory pain are complex regional pain syndrome (CRPS) and central pain syndrome. CRPS, previously called reflex sympathetic dystrophy, is an autonomic mediated pain from the sympathetic nervous system and thus presents with the classic triad of color and temperature changes, edema, and vague pain involving an entire limb. It occurs after trauma to a limb, particularly neurological or vascular trauma, regardless of severity. Central pain syndromes occur after damage to the central nervous system including spinal cord injury or strokes. Paradoxical pain occurs with opioids from accumulation of neurotoxic metabolites. This opioid-induced hyperalgesia typically occurs with chronic high-dose opioid use. Patients complain of escalating pain with increasing opioid doses.

Pain can also be divided by chronicity: acute, subacute, or chronic. Appreciating the chronicity of the pain allows for an appropriate response. In the hospital, clinicians often mistakenly respond to chronic pain with acute pain measures. Similarly, patients may have the erroneous expectation that their uncontrolled chronic pain will be controlled just because they are in the hospital. Overreacting to chronic pain with aggressive acute interventions can not only be nonbeneficial but also actually harmful to the patient and to the health system. On the other end of the spectrum, delays in diagnosing or treating a new or acute pain often occur, especially in patients who have chronic pain at baseline or those who are confused or nonverbal.

2.2 A PRACTICAL GENERAL APPROACH TO PAIN

Pain is the most common and important complaint for hospitalization and presentation to the emergency room. The consequences of pain include reduced quality of life, impaired physical function, extended recovery time, and high economic costs from hospital readmissions, longer lengths of stay, and repeated emergency room visits [3]. As patients' pain satisfaction scores become publicly reported, hospitals will be increasingly evaluated and ranked by their ability to manage pain. Improving pain management requires system changes in our hospitals. Fortunately acute care hospitals now have more resources to evaluate and address pain. Palliative care or pain consultations are increasingly available in hospitals for complex or refractory cases. Patients now have access to sophisticated pain therapies, such as ketamine or lidocaine infusions, epidural or intrathecal analgesia, and even surgical interventions for pain management.

The acute care setting poses challenges to good pain management. Acute illness not only increases the likelihood of pain but also increases the likelihood of complications from pain management. The ability of acutely ill patients to metabolize medications decreases when they develop acute kidney injury or acute hepatic failure. They are more sensitive to side effects of medications when they have exacerbations of their heart failure, COPD, or sleep apnea or when they have delirium or toxin-producing infectious colitis. Ironically when the patient most needs aggressive pain management, clinicians and hospital staff are the most fearful of giving them sufficient pain medications. The balance between the patient's comfort and an iatrogenic complication requires not only clinical skill but also an understanding of the patient's goals of care.

Management of acute pain requires a proactive, interdisciplinary approach. Frequent evaluation and adjustment of the treatment is more important than which initial therapy was started. The evaluation and treatment of pain in the hospital is everyone's responsibility, from the physician to nursing staff, case manager, pharmacist, social worker, occupational therapist, and physical therapist. Establishing expectations, an acceptable pain level, and functional goals for improvement are essential first steps for good pain management. While unidimensional pain scales, such as the visual analog or Wong–Baker FACES scale, are helpful in tracking the longitudinal severity of the patient's pain, multidimensional scales capture a fuller picture of the patient's pain and should be administered at least once during the hospitalization, preferably on admission or on onset of the pain. Links to different pain assessment scales are shown in Table 2.1. Attention should be given to the patient's peak pain score of the day rather than the average pain severity, since studies show that the peak pain score correlate best with clinical outcomes, such as function and patient satisfaction.

Table 2.1   Web Resources

Opioid Conversion Calculator at http://www.globalrph.com/opioidconverter2.htm.
Opioid Conversion Tables
   http://www.globalrph.com/narcotic.htm
   http://www.nhhpco.org/opioid.htm
   http://champ.bsd.uchicago.edu/documents/Pallpaincard2009update.pdf
Pain Guidelines
American Academy of Pain Medicine
   http://www.painmed.org/Library/Clinical_Guidelines.aspx
WHO treatment guidelines on chronic nonmalignant pain in adults
   http://www.who.int/medicines/areas/quality_safety/Scoping_WHOGuide_non-malignant_pain_adults.pdf
Management of persistent pain in older adults
   http://americangeriatrics.org/health_care_professionals/clinical_practice/clinical_guidelines_recommendations/2009/
Palliative Care Fast Facts
http://www.eperc.mcw.edu/EPERC/FastFactsandConcepts
Free Mobile Applications
   Pain Guide: Pain Management Quick
   NPC Opioid Guidelines
   PAIN Clinician
Pain Scales
Unidimensional
Wong–Baker FACES pain rating scale
   http://www.partnersagainstpain.com/printouts/A7012AS6.pdf
Visual analog (0 to 10) scale
   http://ergonomics.about.com/od/ergonomicbasics/ss/painscale.htm
Nonverbal or Observational
   Pain Assessment in Advanced Dementia Scale (PAINAD)
      http://www.healthcare.uiowa.edu/igec/tools/pain/PAINAD.pdf
   Revised nonverbal pain scale
      http://ccn.aacnjournals.org/content/29/1/59/T4.large.jpg
Multidimensional
McGill Pain Questionnaire
   http://www.ama-cmeonline.com/pain_mgmt/pdf/mcgill.pdf
Brief Pain Inventory
   http://www.partnersagainstpain.com/printouts/A7012AS8.pdf

Medication reconciliation is now required on admission to the hospital and is also part of good pain management. However, obtaining accurate medication reconciliation may be difficult in an acutely ill patient. Fortunately, most states now have electronic prescription drug monitoring programs (PDMP) that can help with the medication reconciliation process. These programs allow prescribers and pharmacists to look up an individual patient on the state's controlled substance database to see what pain medications they have received, when they received them, and from whom. Studies have shown that the use of PDMP actually increases (rather than inhibits) the prescribing of pain medications by reassuring the prescriber of the appropriate use of these medications [4]. PDMP can also help the care team identify patients who are at high risk for addiction or even pseudoaddiction (the appearance of drug-seeking behavior due to undertreatment of pain).

2.3 OPIOID ANALGESICS

2.3.1 Commonly Used Opioids (in the United States)

Table 2.2 summarizes the opioid medications that are commonly used in the United States. Morphine is the gold-standard opioid. It is available in short-acting and long-acting formulations. The benefits of morphine are that it is relatively inexpensive, is available in a liquid formulation, is ubiquitous, and is well known. Its familiarity translates to less medication errors in the hospital compared with other opioids. The liquid formulation is good for people who cannot swallow pills, have a tube feeding, or have poor bowel absorption (e.g., short bowel). Morphine is metabolized and glucuronidated in the liver to morphine-6-glucuronide and morphine-3-glucuronide. Both metabolites are renally excreted and are known neurotoxins. Accumulation of the metabolites leads to opioid-induced neurotoxicity which manifests as myoclonus, delirium, and then seizure. Morphine should be avoided in patients with moderate to severe renal impairment but can be used cautiously and for short term in patients with mild renal impairment.

Hydromorphone (Dilaudid) is more potent (mg to mg) than morphine but has no difference in efficacy. It is available in long-acting and short-acting formulations. However, the long-acting formulation is extremely expensive, not covered by insurance and cost prohibitive in most cases. Though not as neurotoxic as morphine, hydromorphone has toxic metabolites as well and is relatively contraindicated in patients with renal failure. The drawback of hydromorphone is its expense and the need to use a different opioid for long-acting pain relief.

Oxycodone is available in long-acting (OxyContin) and short-acting formulations. It is only available in oral formulations (pills and liquid) and not available in IV formulations. The disadvantage of long-acting oxycodone is its expense as it is not yet available in a generic formulation and therefore sometimes not covered by insurance. Additional drawbacks to long-acting oxycodone are its high potential for abuse and a high street value. Like hydromorphone, its metabolites are less neurotoxic than morphine's.

Table 2.2   Commonly Used Opioid Analgesics

Opioid	Dosage Form	Strength	Starting Doses of Short-Acting Opioids for Opioid-Naïve Patients
Morphine	Oral solution	2, 4, 20 mg/ml	5–10 mg PO q 60 min as needed
	Tablets ER (q 12 h)	15, 30, 60, 100, 200 mg	
	Tablets ER (q 24 h)	Kadian: 10, 20, 30, 50, 60, 80, 100, 150, 200 mg	
		Avinza: 30, 45, 60, 75, 90, 120 mg	
	Tablets IR	10, 15, 30 mg	
	Injectable SC, IV, infusion	Check hospital-specific concentrations	2–3 mg IV q 30 min as needed
Methadone	Oral solution	1, 2, 10 mg/ml	NA
	Tablets	5, 10 (for pain); 40 mg (methadone maintenance clinics only)	
	Injectable IV, infusion		
		Check hospital-specific concentrations	
Fentanyl	Transmucosal (buccal)	Actiq: 200, 400, 600, 800, 1200, 1600 mg	
	Transdermal	Patches: 12 (delivers 12.5), 25, 50, 75, 100 mcg/hr	
	Injectable SC, IV, infusion	Check hospital-specific concentrations	25–50 IV mcg q 30 min as needed
Hydromorphone	Oral solution	1 mg/ml	2 mg PO q 60 min as needed
	Tablets ER (q 24 h)	8, 12, 12, 32 mg	
	Tablets IR	2, 4, 8 mg	
	Injectable SC, IV, infusion	Check hospital-specific concentrations	0.5 mg IV q 30 min as needed
Oxycodone	Oral solution	1, 20 mg/ml	5 mg PO q 60 min as needed
	Tablets ER (q 12 h)	10, 15, 20, 30, 40, 60, 80 mg	
	Tablets IR	5, 10, 15 mg	
Oxymorphone	Tablets ER (q 12 h)	7.5, 10, 15, 20, 30, 40 mg	5 mg PO q 60 min as needed
	Tablets IR	5, 10 mg	

The oral solutions of morphine, oxycodone, and hydromorphone are useful for enteral tube administration, and because they are short-acting, they are usually dosed every 4 h around the clock and/or as needed.

Methadone (in consultation with a palliative care specialist), because of its long duration of action, is an ideal "long-acting" opioid for enteral tube administration and is usually administered every 8 h.

Table 2.3   Advantages and Disadvantages of Transdermal Fentanyl Compared to Oral or IV/SC Opioids

Transdermal Fentanyl versus Oral Opioid	
Advantages of Transdermal Fentanyl	Disadvantages of Transdermal Fentanyl
Convenience	High cost
Continuous administration	Slower onset of action
Longer duration of action	More difficult to reverse side effects
Greater patient adherence	Slow titration
Avoids PO in patients with nausea/vomiting	Possible adhesive sensitivity
Transdermal Fentanyl versus Continuous IV/SC Opioid Infusion	
Advantages of Transdermal Fentanyl	Disadvantages of Transdermal Fentanyl
Less expensive	Slower onset of action
Easier for caregiver	More difficult to reverse side effects
Less invasive (no needles, no pumps)	Separate intermittent medication required for breakthrough pain

Fentanyl comes in many formulations including intravenous, transdermal (TD), intranasal, sublingual, and buccal. It is estimated to be 80 times more potent than morphine as an analgesic. Its lipid solubility, high potency, and low molecular weight make it ideal for administration systemically through a relatively small area of the skin or mucosa. One of the biggest advantages of fentanyl is that its metabolites appear to be inactive, conferring neither analgesia nor toxicity. Therefore, fentanyl does not have the neurotoxicity in the setting of renal impairment as seen in the other opioids listed earlier. Table 2.3 summarizes the advantages and disadvantages of TD fentanyl compared to orally and IV or SC administered opioids. A major disadvantage of fentanyl is its expense. Its absorption is unpredictable in cachectic patients and should not be used in this population. The Food and Drug Administration (FDA) black box warns that *the TD patch is not intended for opioid-naïve patients.* Absorption into serum begins approximately 4–8 h after application; however, therapeutic blood levels are not achieved for 12 to 16 h with mean time to maximum concentration between 29 and 36 h. At steady state TD fentanyl produces drug levels similar to those produced by intravenous or subcutaneous infusion with the same infusion rate. Levels vary between patients based on individual differences in skin absorption characteristics and fentanyl clearance rates. Patients with elevated body temperature (especially > 102°F) must be carefully monitored and may need to be switched to an alternate oral or parenteral opioid. Fentanyl patches causing less constipation than other opioids is a myth. All opioids cause the same side effects.

2.3.2   Methadone Friend or Foe?

Methadone has several advantages but should be used in consultation with a palliative care or pain specialist. An important advantage is that it is very inexpensive, $20–$30 a month. Most patients can afford methadone even if it is not covered by their insurance. Methadone has no known active metabolites and only needs to be dose adjusted when renal function drops below 10%. It is the only long-acting opioid that comes in a liquid formulation and can therefore be given through feeding tubes or to patients with dysphagia who cannot swallow pills. In addition to its opioid activity, methadone also antagonizes the N-methyl-d-aspartate (NMDA) receptors, giving it a second analgesic effect. Because of its very low potential for abuse and hence, low street value, Methadone is the safest option in patients with a history of drug abuse or at risk for opioid diversion.

Methadone metabolism differs from other opioids in that it *does not* follow first order pharmacokinetics. Methadone has a biphasic pharmacokinetics: its opioid (first phase or plasma) effects peak in 2–3 h; its NMDA receptor antagonism (second phase or tissue) effect has an individually variable and long half-life and resultant peak. Therefore, methadone can be used both as a long-acting analgesic and a short-acting analgesic. Because methadone is long acting, it is usually prescribed every 8 h in younger patients and every 12 h in older patients, when used as a maintenance analgesic. As an as-needed, short-acting analgesic, it is used similar to other short-acting opioids. Although methadone quickly binds to the mu-opioid receptors, methadone takes 3–5 days to antagonize the NMDA receptors and become maximally effective. Because of this, methadone must be titrated slowly. *Increasing methadone doses more frequently than every 3–5 days is strongly discouraged given the possibility for overdose when the methadone reaches steady state.*

Opioid equivalency has only been established between oral morphine and methadone and uses a sliding scale that depends on the total amount of oral morphine equivalents required in 24 h (Table 2.4). This sliding scale is needed to account for its NMDA receptor blocking analgesic effect. As with all other opioids, there are variations of conversion tables in textbooks and online. The conversion ratio of oral to IV methadone is 2:1. Therefore, the IV methadone dose is half of the oral dose.

If overdosed, methadone requires a naloxone infusion to reverse. A negative side effect more common with methadone than other opioids is the risk for QTc prolongation.

Table 2.4   Morphine to Methadone Conversion

24 h Oral Morphine Dose	Oral Morphine–Oral Methadone
<100 mg	3:1
101–300 mg	5:1
301–600 mg	10:1
601–800 mg	12:1
801–1000 mg	15:1
>1001 mg	20:1

Please note that unlike the opioid equianalgesic equivalency chart above, given the variable metabolism of methadone, this chart can only be used left to right. Methadone should not be converted back to oral morphine equivalents using this chart. In the event the patient must stop methadone, retitration with an immediate-release opioid is recommended.

This risk is heightened with the addition of other QTc-prolonging medications. Although the documented cases of methadone-induced QTc prolongation have occurred only in patients taking more than 150 mg a day, electrocardiogram (EKG) monitoring of patients on lower doses of methadone is prudent if they are taking other QTc-prolonging medications or if they will be taking methadone for more than 6 months. QTc prolongation with methadone is more likely in the presence of hypokalemia and hypomagnesemia.

2.3.3 Opioid Adverse Effects

Since every medication has side effects, the goal of opioid therapy is to titrate to analgesia while minimizing these adverse effects as much as possible. These effects can be addressed with the following approaches: (1) dose reduction of the prescribed opioid, (2) rotation to an equianalgesic dose of a different opioid, or (3) treatment of the side effect (e.g., constipation). Table 2.5 lists the most common and clinically relevant opioid side effects. They can range from bothersome but benign to serious

Table 2.5 Side Effects of Opioids

Adverse Effect	Management
Gastrointestinal	
• Constipation	• Prophylactic bowel regimen
	• PRN suppository or enema
• Nausea/vomiting	• Antiemetics, promotility agents
Delayed gastric emptying	
• Ileus	• Opioid antagonists (methylnaltrexone)
	• Opioid minimizing with or without adjuvant medications
Central Nervous System	
• Somnolence	• Psychostimulants, opioid reduction or rotation
Cognitive impairment	
• Delirium	• Careful medication review and evaluation of medical scenario (for infection, neurologic or cardiac event)
	• Antipsychotic medication (Haldol frequently used)
• Hyperalgesia	• Opioid reduction or rotation
Respiratory Depression	• Frequent assessment and reevaluation of patient
	• Prescreen patients for predisposing comorbidities and medications
	• Supplemental oxygen or noninvasive positive pressure ventilation as appropriate
	• Pulse oximetry
	• Cautious use of dilute (1:10) naloxone if hypoxemia or respiratory rate is less than or equal to 6
Cutaneous	
• Pruritus	• Trial of antihistamine
• Perspiration	• Icepacks

and fatal. Though rare, the most feared adverse effects are respiratory depression and death. Respiratory depression is more likely to occur in patients with impaired ventilation such as chronic lung disease, sleep apnea, or obesity. Patients with concomitantly administered sedating medications such as benzodiazepines are also at higher risk for respiratory depression. Pulse oximetry monitoring though reassuring on the surface does not reduce the risk of respiratory depression. Supplemental oxygen is not helpful as hypoxemia typically occur after hypercapnia.

2.3.4   Opioid Titration

Opioid titration is usually necessary in the management of pain in the hospital. There is no theoretical dose ceiling as long as opioids are titrated safely. However, practically speaking, most opioids are limited in their dose by the neurotoxic effect of their metabolites.

The use of an intravenous opioid is the most rapid way to provide pain relief for a patient who has poorly controlled acute pain. All IV opioids are short acting with the exception of methadone. If a patient is still in severe pain 30 min after administration of IV pain medication, the dose can be doubled and given again. This can be repeated until the patient is comfortable or until the patient begins to experience side effects from the medication. For patients in severe pain, titration is best achieved with PCA (see following section).

To control a pain exacerbation, the short-acting oral formulation of an opioid can be used in patients who are able to take oral medications. Long-acting formulations are useful once initial pain control is achieved and the 24 h opioid requirement is known. Long-acting formulations should not be used for rapid titration of pain medications during a pain exacerbation. For patients in severe pain, oral opioid doses can be given every 60 min to control pain. If a patient is still in severe pain 60 min after administration of oral pain medication, the dose can be doubled and given again. This can be repeated until the patient is comfortable or until the patient begins to experience side effects from the medication.

Long-acting opioids are preferred over short-acting opioids for the management of chronic pain, based on the principle that "an ounce of prevention is better than a pound of cure." The use of long-acting opioids allows a patient to sleep through the night without waking up to take their pain medication. Long-acting medications should be prescribed as scheduled medications as they require consistent dosing to maintain steady state. An effective starting dose of long-acting opioid is based on the total amount of opioid required in 24 h to make a patient comfortable. By using the total 24 h dose to establish a long-acting regimen, the patient receives what they have already tolerated in 24 h, thus reducing the potential for overdose while providing pain relief for the patient. Most long-acting opioids are dosed every 12 h. However, for patients who are fast metabolizers of the opioid, they may experience end of dose failure and require every 8 h dosing. If an opioid-tolerant patient presents with a pain exacerbation, an appropriate initial titration would be to increase their usual long-acting opioid by 50–100%, for example, for a patient taking ER morphine 30 mg orally every 12 h, an initial titration would be to 45 mg orally every 12 h for mild pain or 60 mg orally every 12 h for moderate or severe pain. Extended-release medications cannot be crushed and given via feeding tubes. For patients who have chronic pain, short-acting opioids can be given regularly every 4 h, in addition to as-needed doses, to provide around-the-clock coverage.

An ideal opioid regimen for a patient with chronic pain consists of a long-acting opioid to cover continuous pain and a short-acting opioid prescribed for as-needed use to cover breakthrough, incidental, or acute pain. Short-acting opioids are usually dosed every 2–4 h. A good rule of thumb for the breakthrough medication dose is 10% of the 24 h maintenance dose for each as-needed dose. If a patient is consistently requiring more than 3 doses in 24 h, they will need an increase in their long-acting medication.

2.3.5 Opioid Conversion

An opioid can be safely and effectively converted to another opioid using the concept of equal analgesia (i.e., opioids are equally effective but have different potencies). Multiple equal analgesic conversion tables are available (Table 2.1). Table 2.6 presents an easy-to-use set of conversions. The variations between conversion tables come from the fact that the conversions are actually a range and not a single number as the tables suggest. The range comes from the normal distribution of metabolism of the opioids in a population. While the tables may give the median or the mean of that normal distribution, the user of the tables should keep in mind that a particular patient may be a fast metabolizer of one opioid and a slow metabolizer of another. Since the prescriber cannot yet tell which patients are fast or slow metabolizers, a clinically more useful approach is direction of the patient's pain control. For example, if the patient's pain is uncontrolled or anticipated to get worse, a more aggressive conversion should be used to achieve a higher dose. If the patient's pain is expected to get better, then a

Table 2.6 Easy-to-Use Equal Analgesic Conversions between Opioids

	Oral Dose (mg)	IV/SC Dose (mg)
Morphine	15	5
Hydromorphone	3	1
Oxycodone	10	Not available
Hydrocodone	15	Not available
Oxymorphone	5	Not available
Codeine	150	50
Levorphanol	2	1

Source: Adapted from Ferris and Pirrello: *Improving Equianalgesic Dosing for Chronic Pain Management*, American Association for Cancer Education Annual Meeting Presentation, Cincinnati, OH, Sept 2005.

This table is a *guideline sample* which attempts to account for the limitations of published tables, simplify mathematical relationships, and promote consistency across practitioners. Several equianalgesic tables have been published, all of which are approximations, derived from single-dose studies with small sample size and do not address cross-tolerance. The "calculated number" result should always be carefully considered in the context of the patient's clinical circumstances.

conversion should be used to achieve a dose on the lower end of the range. Similarly, if a nonopioid analgesic is being added, a lower conversion dose should be used.

Another variation to the equal analgesic conversion is the concept of incomplete cross-tolerance. A patient who is taking one type of opioid may have an increased or decreased analgesia when switched to a different opioid at the "equivalent" dose. To adjust for this phenomenon and to avoid oversedation when starting a new medication, the dose can be reduced 20–30% based on the patient's pain control (Table 2.7). The text box illustrates case examples of conversion between different opioid routes and drugs.

Multiple methods are available to switch patients from another opioid to TD fentanyl [5]. All the methods require conversion to an oral morphine equivalent and

Table 2.7 Incomplete Cross-Tolerance Adjustment When Converting between Opioids

Severe pain (7–10 on pain scale)	Give 100% of equivalent dose
Moderate pain (4–6 on pain scale)	Give 80% of equivalent dose
Mild pain (0–3 on pain scale)	Give 70% of equivalent dose

Case Examples Illustrating Conversions between Opioid Routes and Drugs

Case Example #1: Escalation of Long-Acting PO Morphine Based on IV PRN Use

A 64-year-old gentleman with known pancreatic cancer presents with severe, acute worsening of his chronic abdominal and midback pain. He rates his pain severity as 8 out of 10. At home he takes sustained-released morphine 60 mg twice a day. In the emergency room he is given 2 mg of IV morphine with no relief. Thirty minutes later he is given 4 mg of IV Morphine with minimal improvement. Forty minutes after that, he is given 8 mg of morphine and reports a decrease of his pain level to 3 out of 10, which is tolerable for this patient. On admission to the medical ward, his sustained-released morphine 60 mg is continued twice a day, and an order is written for 8 mg IV Morphine q 2 h PRN pain. The patient uses a total of four more doses in the next 24 h with good control of his pain, in addition to the sustained-released morphine.

Step 1: Sum total IV PRN morphine used in 24 h: 2 mg + 4 mg + 8 mg × 5 = 2 + 4 + 40 = 46 mg IV morphine.

Step 2: Conversion. Convert 24 h IV morphine into oral equivalents: 46 mg × 3 = 138 mg oral morphine (note that we multiply by 3 because in many opioid conversions, 1 mg IV morphine = 3 mg oral morphine).

Step 3: Divide 24 h long-acting dose to recommended dosing frequency: since sustained-released morphine should be given every 12 h, the total dose of opioid required by this patient should be divided by 2 to find the amount needed every 12 h, 138 mg/2 = 69 mg every 12 h. Therefore, his long-acting dose of morphine should be increased to 120 mg twice a day (rounded down because long-acting morphine comes in 60 mg tabs). Some palliative care specialists recommend starting the new opioid at 75% of the calculated dose to account for interindividual variation in first-pass effect (e.g., 90 mg twice a day).

Case Example #2: Conversion of IV Hydromorphone (Dilaudid) to Oral Morphine

A patient's pain has been well controlled on a hydromorphone PCA with a bolus of 0.2 mg IV q 10 min PRN pain without a basal. She has required 40 bolus doses in 24 h. She is being discharged home with oral medications.

Step 1:   Sum total IV PRN morphine used in 24 h: 0.2 mg × 40 doses = 8 mg IV hydromorphone.

Step 2:   Conversion. 1 mg IV hydromorphone = 20 mg oral morphine. Use the ratio to cross multiply: 8 mg × 20 = 160 mg oral morphine = 80 mg q 12 h.

Step 3:   Reduce for incomplete cross-tolerance (because we are converting between different opioid drugs). To reduce for incomplete cross-tolerance, a good choice would be to start a long-acting morphine at a lower dose of 120 mg/2 doses = 60 mg long-acting morphine q12 h (75% dose of calculated in Step 2).

Step 4:   Calculate breakthrough. Each breakthrough dose should be about 10% of the daily long acting, so 12 mg. Tabs are 10 mg so breakthrough dose is 10 mg of short-acting morphine every 3 h as needed for pain.

---

calculating the patient's 24 h oral morphine requirement. Patients who are receiving a stable dose of IV fentanyl as a continuous infusion or patient-controlled analgesia (PCA) can be switched directly to TD fentanyl using a 1:1 (IV infusion–TD) conversion ratio [6]. The manufacturer's recommendation for converting from morphine to TD fentanyl is listed in Table 2.8; this table should not be used to convert from a fentanyl patch to another opioid. Conversion from fentanyl patch to other opioids can be complicated and is one of the areas where specialist pain or palliative care assistance may be helpful.

2.3.6   DEFINE PATIENT CONTROLLED ANALGESIA (PCA)

PCA is a technique allowing patients to self-administer parenteral analgesics. The primary advantage of PCA is to shorten the time of patient-identified need for pain relief to the time of actual drug administration. PCA achieves better acute pain control with less medication and less side effects. It takes the titration principle of using a smaller amount of medication more frequently to the ultimate degree. In addition to immediate relief of pain, PCA may give patients a greater sense of control over their pain and decrease the often-associated anxiety. Monitoring includes the patient's subjective report of pain, the clinician's observation of the patient's progress, and objective monitoring of respiratory rate including assessment of respiratory depth and quality and level of alertness or sedation. In hospital settings pulse oximetry and/or capnography may be monitored in patients with sleep apnea. In a severe pain crisis, the loading dose may be repeated every 4 h through the PCA by clinician "override" dosing until the patient is comfortable. After 24 h the total dose received should be evaluated and the parameters for PCA may be reset based on the patient's comfort level, presence of undesirable side effects, if any, and goals of care. Patients recovering from surgery may need downward dosing adjustment as they recover.

Table 2.8 FDA-Approved Manufacturer's Conversion from Oral Morphine to Fentanyl Patch [7]

Step 1: Sum total opioid received in 24 h and convert to oral morphine equivalents using equianalgesic table (e.g., Table 2.6).
Step 2: Using the table below, select the fentanyl patch dose that corresponds to the morphine equivalent dose range that the patient is receiving.

Daily Morphine Equivalent Dose 24 h PO Morphine (mg/day) Equivalent	FDA-Approved Manufacturer's Conversion TD Fentanyl Dose (mcg/h)
60–134	25
135–224	50
225–314	75
315–404	100
405–494	125
495–584	150
585–674	175
675–764	200
765–854	225
855–944	250
945–1034	275
1035–1124	300

Notes:
- The fentanyl patch should only be used in opioid-tolerant patients, that is, those receiving a stable dose of at least 60 mg oral morphine equivalent per day.
- This table should not be used to convert from a fentanyl patch to another opioid, as it will result in too high a dose of the new opioid.
- Because this table gives conservative doses for the fentanyl patch, many patients will require additional breakthrough opioids dosed as needed, which can be used to further titrate the fentanyl patch dose.
- For a patient receiving a stable dose of a fentanyl IV infusion or PCA, the IV fentanyl of the patient should be converted to the fentanyl patch at the equivalent dose, rounding down to the nearest available fentanyl patch dose, for example, a stable infusion of 60 mcg/h of fentanyl in a patient receiving it should be converted to a 50 mcg/h fentanyl patch.

The patients who benefit most from PCA use are those:

1. Whose analgesic requirement is unknown or changes day to day, including postoperative patients
2. Whose pain is intermittent or episodic
3. Who are cognitively capable of using a PCA
4. Who are sufficiently motivated

Please see the accompanying tables for the indications and contraindications for PCA use (Table 2.9), basic parameters needed for a PCA, and recommended staring doses (Table 2.10). Opioid-tolerant patients and those with increasing

Table 2.9 Indications and Contraindications for PCA Use

PCA Indications	PCA Relative Contraindications	Risk Factors for Oversedation and Respiratory Depression
Severe pain	Anticipated opioid need < 24 h	Opioid-naïve status
Rapid dose titration and "dose finding" for acute pain	Patient lacks cognitive ability to understand how to use a PCA device	Advanced age
Oral, transdermal, rectal route not available	The patient does not wish to participate	Obesity
Relief of "air hunger," dyspnea		Altered mental status
		Intrinsic lung disease
		Obstructive sleep apnea
		Renal and hepatic impairment
		"PCA by proxy"[a]

[a]PCA by proxy is when family members or unauthorized clinicians press the PCA button. Hospital policies prohibit this practice. The PCA process has inherent safety because patients will stop pushing the button when they are sedated. If unauthorized others press the button, the patient is at risk for oversedation and respiratory depression.

Table 2.10 Recommended Opioid Starting Doses for Intravenous Patient-Controlled Analgesia [8]

Parameter	Most Opioid-Naïve Patients	Patients > 64 Years Old or with Sleep Apnea	Opioid-Tolerant[a] Patients
Morphine			
Loading dose	3 mg	2 mg	4 mg
PCA dose	1 mg	0.7 mg	1.2 mg
PCA lockout interval	10 min	10 min	10 min
Continuous dose	None	None	≤2 mg/h
Max limit in 4 h	20 mg	15 mg	30 mg
Hydromorphone			
Loading dose	0.6 mg	0.4 mg	1 mg
PCA dose	0.3 mg	0.2 mg	0.4 mg
PCA lockout interval	10 min	10 min	10 min
Continuous dose	None	None	≤0.3 mg/h
Max limit in 4 h	4 mg	3 mg	6 mg

[a]Opioid-tolerant patients are those using at least 60 mg of oral morphine/day, 30 mg of oral oxycodone/day, 8 mg of oral hydromorphone/day, or an equianalgesic dose of another opioid for a week or longer. Doses may need to be higher based on previous opioid dose and may be calculated based on patient's previous opioid use.

pain may benefit from a continuous infusion administered with the PCA. For opioid-tolerant patients, the PCA and continuous infusion doses should be calculated based on the patient's opioid usage.

2.4   NONOPIOID CLASSES OF MEDICATIONS

Nearly any class of medications can be used to treat pain. For example, nitrates are used to treat angina and proton pump inhibitors (PPI) are used to treat many causes of epigastric pain. The most commonly used analgesic is the opioid class. Because this class is what most physicians tend to want to go to first, it actually should be the last class the physicians think of. Medications that treat inflammation and neuropathic pain are often called adjuvants or coanalgesics because they can be useful additions to opioids, resulting in improved pain control at lower opioid doses. Frequently used coanalgesics are summarized in Table 2.11.

2.4.1   Anti-inflammatory Drugs

Many drug classes have direct or indirect anti-inflammatory effect. For example, antibiotics are effective anti-inflammatory medications by reducing the underlying infection while some antibiotics have direct anti-inflammatory effects as well. The most commonly used anti-inflammatory drugs are steroids and nonsteroidal anti-inflammatory drugs (NSAIDs). They are generally thought of for musculoskeletal pain but are also effective for inflammatory visceral pain and some cancer pain, especially metastatic bone pain.

Due to their strong anti-inflammatory properties, glucocorticoids are one of the best and first-line choices. The analgesic effect of steroids begins within 24–48 h and reaches its peak in 3–4 days. After 5 days the analgesic benefit diminishes and the risks of side effect increases. Palliative care patients generally tolerate steroids better than NSAIDs. Steroids also have beneficial side effects for palliative care patients, such as increased appetite, weight gain, increased energy, decreased nausea, and decreased shortness of breath. They can reduce the effects of brain metastases and bowel obstruction. Dexamethasone is the steroid of choice for most palliative care patients, because it has a high anti-inflammatory potency compared to other steroids. Dexamethasone also has little mineralocorticoid effects and thus does not cause or increase edema/fluid retention. Since the analgesic effect is related to the dose and side effects are generally associated with duration, a short-course, high-dose burst of steroids is recommended for pain management. Typical doses range from 12 to 20 mg/day. Even when given for only 4 or 5 days, the analgesic effect of steroids can last up to 2 weeks.

For the best results, NSAIDs should be given scheduled or around the clock. In the hospital, short-acting NSAIDs such as ibuprofen are preferred, in case of adverse effects. Long-acting NSAIDs, such as naproxen, are easier for patients to take as an outpatient. For patients who are unable to take oral NSAIDs, intravenous ketorolac (Toradol) can be given. A PPI should be given with high-dose NSAIDs for gastric protection. NSAIDs are contraindicated in patients with increased risk of bleeding, renal impairment, heart failure, and/or uncontrolled hypertension.

Table 2.11 Commonly Used Coanalgesic Medications

Adrenergic/ Serotonergic Agonist Action	NMDA Antagonist Action	Calcium Channel Modulation	Sodium Channel Modulation	Alpha-2 Adrenergic Agonist	Muscle Relaxants
Amitriptyline Start: 25 mg/day Max: 200 mg/day	Methadone[a]	Gabapentin Start: 300 mg/day Max: 3600 mg/day *Caution*: adjustment for renal function required	Carbamazepine Start: 200 mg/day Max: 1200 mg/day *Caution*: requires therapeutic blood level and periodic lab test monitoring	Clonidine Usually combined with an opioid in intraspinal infusions for severe pain	Baclofen Start: 15–30 mg/day Max: 80 mg/day
Imipramine Start: 10 mg/day Max: 150 mg/day	Ketamine[b]				Diazepam Start: 6–40 mg/day Max: ~100 mg/day
Nortriptyline Start: 10 mg/day Max: 100 mg/day	**Consult palliative care specialist**	Pregabalin Start: 75–150 mg/day Max: 600 mg/day *Caution*: adjustment for renal function required	Lidocaine **Consult palliative care specialist** *Caution*: requires therapeutic blood level monitoring	**Consult palliative care specialist**	*Note*: No max dose in the literature; however, additional muscle relaxation is unlikely >100 mg
Desipramine Start: 10 mg/day Max: 150 mg/day			Mexiletine Start: 200 mg/day Max: 10 mg/kg/day		Tizanidine Start: 6–12 mg/day Max: 36 mg/day
Venlafaxine Start: 37.5–75 mg/day Max: 225 mg/day			Topiramate[c,d] Start: 50 mg/day Max: 400 mg/day *Caution*: adjustment for renal function required		
Duloxetine Start: 20–60 mg/day Max: 120 mg/day			Valproic acid[a] Start: 500–1000 mg/day Max: 60 mg/kg/day *Caution*: requires therapeutic blood level and periodic lab test monitoring		

Medications in this table require titrating to effect often in divided doses per day and tapering to prevent withdrawal symptoms.

[a]Opioid agonist.
[b]Weak opioid agonist.
[c]May inhibit glutamate release.
[d]May augment GABA activity.

Bisphosphonates reduce bone inflammation through inhibition of osteoclast function. They are particularly effective in patients with bone pain secondary to bone metastases. They are given via the intravenous route and therefore must be given in the inpatient or at an outpatient infusion center. These doses should be repeated monthly for continued effect and adjusted for renal function.

2.4.2 Neuropathic Pain Agents

Neuropathic pain is often described as a burning, tingling, or electrical pain. It frequently has hyperalgesia and allodynia. Common causes of neuropathic pain include nerve trauma (phantom limb, postsurgical), direct nerve impingement (tumor, discopathy, edema/inflammation), and toxins (diabetes, chemotherapeutics, opioid metabolites).

Tricyclic Antidepressants (TCAs). The exact mechanism of the TCAs for treatment of neuropathic pain is unknown. Some theories include serotonin and norepinephrine reuptake inhibition, alpha-adrenergic blockage, sodium channel effect, and NMDA receptor antagonism.

TCAs should be dosed at night due to their sedative effects. Desipramine and nortriptyline have less anticholinergic side effects than amitriptyline and imipramine. The other major dose limiting side effect is orthostatic hypotension. Their cardiac side effects limit their use in patients with major cardiac problems. Their multiple drug interactions also limit their use in patients on multiple medications, as most palliative care patients tend to be. All TCAs should be started at a low dose and titrated up to maximum effect as tolerated.

Serotonin–Norepinephrine Reuptake Inhibitors (SNRIs). SNRIs are often effective adjuvants for neuropathic pain. They are good choices for patients who also require treatment for depression but cannot take a TCA. The doses effective for pain are often lower than those effective for depression. Just as these medications often need 2–6 weeks to reach full effect in the treatment for depression, they also require 1–2 weeks to reach full effect in the treatment of pain. SNRIs tend to be activating and are better dosed in the morning to prevent insomnia.

Duloxetine is approved by the FDA for treatment of both pain and depression. It is not yet generic and therefore is expensive and often not covered by insurance companies as a first-line treatment for neuropathic pain. Venlafaxine has the same mechanism as duloxetine and is equally effective for both pain and depression [9]. Venlafaxine is generic and therefore less expensive and more likely to be covered by insurance.

Anticonvulsants. Gabapentin was originally developed as an antiepileptic drug. It was found to have weak antiepileptic properties but works very well as a treatment for neuropathic pain. While built from the GABA molecule, its mechanism is not related to the GABA receptor, but instead, it binds to the alpha-2-delta ligand receptor of the calcium channel on the cell membrane of neurons. Gabapentin is started at a low and often subtherapeutic dose because of its sedating side effect. It should be titrated over time to maximum effect. Because of its sedating effect, gabapentin is a good choice for patients who have insomnia, a common complaint in pain patients. Gabapentin is usually dosed every 8 h for seizures, but should be dosed predominately at night and at bedtime (twice daily) for pain to avoid daytime sedation. For example, 25% of the daily dose can be given in the morning, 25–50% of the daily dose around 5–6 PM, and 50% or more of the daily dose at bedtime. Gabapentin is 90% renally excreted and therefore requires dosing adjustment in patients with renal impairment.

Pregabalin is structurally similar to gabapentin and is thought to work in the same way for the treatment of neuropathic pain. It is not yet generic and tends to be more expensive than gabapentin. Often, insurance companies will not cover pregabalin unless the patient has failed gabapentin treatment. A small subset of patients will respond to pregabalin when they have not responded to gabapentin. The side effect profile of pregabalin is the same as gabapentin. Like gabapentin, pregabalin requires titration to an effective dose and should be given mostly in the evening and at bedtime.

Valproic acid is another antiepileptic medication that also can be used for treatment of neuropathic pain. Due to its side effect profile including black box warnings for hepatotoxicity, teratogenicity, and pancreatitis, it is not a first-line treatment for neuropathic pain, unless the patient concomitantly needs treatment for bipolar disorder or seizure. Doses can be increased as needed for pain effect; however, serum valproic acid levels must be monitored. Liver function tests, platelet count, and coagulation tests should be monitored frequently. Valproic acid should be avoided in women with pregnancy potential given the risk of teratogenicity.

Carbamazepine, like valproic acid, can also be used for the treatment of neuropathic pain; however, due to its side effect profile, it should not be a first-line treatment for neuropathic pain. It should only be considered for use in neuropathic pain if a patient also needs bipolar or seizure treatment and cannot take valproic acid. Carbamazepine levels should be monitored. A complete blood count, reticulocyte count, iron level, complete metabolic profile, urinalysis, and an ophthalmologic exam should be done at baseline, before starting the medication, and should continue to be periodically monitored while the patient takes this medication.

In patients with refractory neuropathic pain or opioid-induced hyperalgesia, infusions of lidocaine, a sodium channel blocker, or ketamine, an NMDA receptor antagonist, can be used for pain management, often with very good results. Ketamine can also be given orally, and the oral equivalent of lidocaine is mexiletine. A palliative care or pain management consultation is strongly recommended for use of these medications for pain management.

2.5 NONPHARMACOLOGICAL INTERVENTIONS

Nonpharmacological interventions should be considered before pharmacological therapies. Because clinicians tend to want to jump to pharmacological therapies right away, a best practice is to stop, "take a time out" before writing the prescription or order, and consider nonpharmacological therapies. Since nonphysical sources of pain usually do not respond well to medications, a comprehensive pain approach requires the use of nonpharmacological interventions to address the psychosocial and existential/spiritual components of pain. Finally, nonpharmacological interventions generally have fewer side effects than medications. They should be considered especially for those patients who are the most sensitive to side effects of medications, such as the elderly, patients with multiorgan failure, and those with polypharmacy.

Acupuncture has been shown to be effective for pain relief in several studies [10]. It has gained increasing acceptance and popularity in American society. However, it has several drawbacks. The analgesic effect of acupuncture is short lived. Even for those patients who do respond, most require therapy three to four times a week to maintain adequate effect. Long-term use of acupuncture can be quite costly, especially since most medical insurance will not cover it. A 30 min session of acupuncture can cost between $80 and $160, depending on the extent and quality of the service. The absence of quality measures and regulations leads to significant variability in the quality of the acupuncture. Barriers to acupuncture in the hospital include the lack of a reimbursement mechanism, since it is considered an ancillary service that is lumped into the overall room cost, and credentialing difficulties for the acupuncturist to obtain hospital privileges.

Several distraction techniques have been used and studied in pain management. The most popular of these are music therapy and guided imagery. Music therapy has been shown in studies to help with pain and relaxation. It has been effective in reducing anxiety and the need for medications in critically ill patients on ventilators [11]. Unfortunately, few hospitals have trained music therapist available. Guided imagery involves the generation or recall of different mental images, such as perception of objects or events, and engages mechanisms used in cognition, memory, and emotional and motor control [12]. The images are typically visualized within a state of relaxation. All the senses should be used, because the more detail with which the image is sensed, the more potential for pain relief it has. A trained staff can show the patient how to use guided imagery. Thereafter, patients and families can self-direct the therapy.

Rehabilitation techniques have been shown to help relieve pain in many studies [13]. Physical therapy, occupational therapy, speech therapy, respiratory therapy, and kinesiology all can reduce pain and improve or maintain function, which is the goal of chronic pain management. Exercise programs, such as Tai Chi, have been shown in studies to reduce chronic pain [14]. Massage can also relief pain, though the effect is temporary. In the hospital, massage therapy can be performed by occupational therapists or physical therapists.

Spiritual care is needed to address the existential element of the patient's pain. In addition to exploring the meaning of their pain, patients need to put their pain into their worldview or religious context. Questions from patients such as "Why is God doing this to me?" should prompt a chaplain referral. A patient or family's spiritual beliefs can be a barrier to their pain management. For example, if a patient believes their pain is a punishment from God, they may refuse medications, in order to "earn" approval from God. Counseling from their trusted spiritual leader is usually needed to overcome such barriers.

Many psychosocial dynamics contribute to the patient's pain. Counseling, evaluation, and intervention by clinical social workers and psychologists can reduce the psychosocial components of their pain. Pain psychologist can help chronic pain patients and their families adapt to the consequences of their pain, learn to cope with their pain exacerbations, and minimize the impact of their pain on themselves and others. At the extreme, when a family or caregiver interferes with the patient's pain management, such as stealing or withholding medications, a report of abuse or neglect should be called into adult protective services [15].

2.6 TRANSITION TO OUTPATIENT

Pain management should be part of discharge planning. Good pain management consists of establishing a system of care for the patient's pain. This system requires monitoring of the pain at home, monitoring the pain medications (including adherence and side effects), and providing education and contingency plans for exacerbations and crises. Discharge planning for pain management includes education about medications, teaching about their pain therapy, and ensuring good follow-up. A follow-up phone call a few days after discharge can not only answer questions and address problems but can also potentially prevent rehospitalization or a visit to the emergency room.

Home health care is frequently needed for palliative care patients with pain or other symptoms. Unfortunately, home health care is underutilized. Home palliative care programs have been shown to improve patient care outcomes and reduce cost, hospital readmissions, and emergency room visits [16, 17]. The Center for Medicare and Medicaid Services has designated pain and symptom management as a skilled need for both home care and for facilities. Rehabilitative services are also covered under Medicare while on home palliative care. The ultimate home pain management program is hospice care, which provides the most extensive coverage of pain management in the home.

Transition from intravenous opioids to oral or long-acting opioids for discharge home should ideally occur 24 h in advance. The home opioid regiment should be started in the hospital the day before discharge to ensure adequate pain control and to allow overlap coverage of their inpatient regiment and their outpatient regiment. However, on those occasions when an immediate transition is needed for same day discharge, doses of different onset formulations can be given simultaneously or back to back. For example, an intravenous dose of morphine can be given along with an oral dose of short-acting morphine and a dose of long-acting morphine all at the time of discharge (Table 2.12). As one formulation wanes, the next kicks in, covering the patient's transition home and allowing the family time to fill their outpatient prescriptions.

Home PCAs are rarely needed. However, some patients with high opioid needs or inability to take oral medications and have a contraindication to Fentanyl

Table 2.12 Morphine Dosing Pharmacokinetics

	Onset	Peak	Duration
Intravenous bolus	8–10 min	45–60 min	2–3 h
Oral short acting	30–40 min	60–90 min	4 h
Sustained release	2 h	4 h	Over 12 h

may need a PCA at home to keep them out of the hospital. Home PCA can be infused subcutaneously or through a permanent or semipermanent indwelling intravenous catheter.

While opioids are the first-line analgesic therapy in the hospital and for cancer patients, they should not be the mainstay therapy for chronic, nonmalignant pain in the outpatient setting. Nonopioid therapies, particularly nonpharmacological therapies, should be the focus. Other analgesic medications classes should be optimized. However, opioids can be part of the global pain approach.

2.7 OPIOID RISK EVALUATION AND MITIGATION STRATEGIES

The FDA Amendment Act of 2007 granted the FDA new powers to enhance drug safety by requiring the pharmaceutical industry to develop Risk Evaluation and Mitigation Strategies (REMS) [18]. The intent is to provide a strategy to manage known or potential serious risks associated with a drug. The FDA has required a REMS for sublingual and transmucosal fentanyl dosage forms and extended-release and long-acting (ER/LA) opioid analgesics by identifying risks of life-threatening respiratory depression and abuse potential (Table 2.13) [19].

Under REMS conditions, prescribers of these opioids are strongly encouraged to complete a REMS-compliant prescriber education program (Table 2.14) [20]. There is no deadline or requirement for prescribers to complete this training. Efforts are underway to amend the controlled substances act so that completion of REMS-compliant training becomes a prerequisite for registration to prescribe ER/LA opioid analgesics. Prescribers should encourage patients and caregivers regarding the importance of reading the "medication guide" they will receive from their pharmacist each time a prescription for an ER/LA opioid is dispensed to them (Fig. 2.2) [21]. These guides are unique for each drug and are mainly intended for prescription medications used in the outpatient setting. The guides emphasize that the drug is important to the patient's health and that patient adherence to directions for use is crucial for the effectiveness and safety of the drug.

Table 2.13   Products Subject to Risk Evaluation and Mitigation Strategies (REMS)

- Extended-release, oral dosage forms containing:
  - Hydromorphone
  - Morphine
  - Oxycodone
  - Oxymorphone
  - Tapentadol
- Transdermal delivery systems
  - Fentanyl
  - Buprenorphine
- Fentanyl sublingual and transmucosal
- Methadone tablets and solutions

Table 2.14   Risk Evaluation and Mitigation Strategies (REMS) Resources

- A current list of REMS-compliant training activities from accredited CE providers may be found by accessing the following link:
  - https://search.er-la-opioidrems.com/Guest/GuestPageExternal.aspx
- Educate your patients using the REMS "Patient Counseling Document" (Fig. 2.2):
  - This form may be accessed for copying at the following link: http://www.er-la-opioidrems.com/IwgUI/rems/pdf/patient_counseling_document.pdf
  - Copies of this form may be ordered by accessing: http://www.minneapolis.cenveo.com/pcd/SubmitOrders.aspx
- Medication guides and U.S. prescribing information may be viewed by accessing the following link: http://www.er-la-opioidrems.com/IwgUI/rems/products.action

Patient counseling document on extended-release/long-acting opioid analgesics	Patient counseling document on extended-release/long-acting opioid analgesics
Patient Name:	Patient Name:
The DOs and DON'Ts of Extended-release/long-acting opioid analgesics	**Patient specific information**
DO: • Read the medication guide • Take your medicine exactly as prescribed • Store your medicine away from children and in a safe place • Flush unused medicine down the toilet • Call your healthcare provider for medical advice about side effects. You may report side effects to FDA at 1-800-FDA-1088.	
Call 911 or your local emergency service right away if: • You take too much medicine • You have trouble breathing, or shortness of breath • A child has taken this medicine	
Talk to your healthcare provider: • If the dose you are taking does not control your pain • About any side effects you may be having • About all the medicines you take, including over-the-counter medicines, vitamins, and dietary supplements	
DON'T: • Do not give your medicine to others • Do not take medicine unless it was prescribed for you • Do not stop taking your medicine without talking to your healthcare provider • Do not break, chew, crush, dissolve, or inject your medicine. If you cannot swallow your medicine whole, talk to your healthcare provider. • Do not drink alcohol while taking this medicine	Take this card with you every time you see your healthcare provider and tell him/her: • Your complete medical and family history, including any history of substance abuse or mental illness • The cause, severity, and nature of your pain • Your treatment goals • All the medicines you take, including over-the-counter (non-prescription) medicines, vitamins, and dietary supplements • Any side effects you may be having
For additional information on your medicine go to: dailymed.nlm.nih.gov	Take your opioid pain medicine exactly as prescribed by your healthcare provider.

Figure 2.2   Sample opioid medication guide for patients and caregivers.

2.8 ADDICTION AND DIVERSION

With the increase in opioid usage among the general American population came a concomitant increase in opioid overdoses and opioid-related deaths [22]. The highly publicized opioid-related deaths of celebrities, such as Anna Nicole Smith, highlight the problem of prescription drug addiction in the United States. However, the benefit of using opioids for people with serious and life-threatening illnesses still outweighs the risk. Several studies have shown that the use of even high-dose opioids does not shorten the survival of hospice and palliative care patients [23]. Concerns about opioid addiction still remain a barrier to adequate pain management for the palliative care patient. A multiprong approach is needed to address these concerns about addiction. Use of drug contracts is inappropriate and ineffective in palliative care patients, since stopping services and care would constitute abandonment. Even patients with active substance addiction deserve and are ethically entitled to good palliative care and appropriate pain management.

A multiprong approach to addiction concerns should include screening for addiction risk, education about opioids and addiction, establishing a drug monitoring system, optimizing nonopioid medications, selection of low-risk opioids, and addressing psychosocial problems. (The following discussion about opioids applies equally well to other controlled substance used for analgesia, such as ketamine.) All pain patients should be screened for their addiction risk, either formally or informally. Such screening has benefit for both the high- and low-risk patients. For low-risk patients, the screening can be reassuring to the prescriber and to the patient and family. For high-risk patients, the screening validates the need to implement a preventive plan. Patients with depression, anxiety, and personality disorders are at higher risk for addictive behaviors. People with past addictions to substances, including nonopioids and especially alcohol, are also at high risk. A screening discussion should extend beyond the patient to those around the patient, such as family and friends. A discussion about the risk of diversion can lead to a plan to prevent diversion of the opioid.

Education is a key intervention to prevent addiction and diversion and to reduce the barrier to pain management. The interdisciplinary team should educate the patient and family about the difference between true addiction and pseudoaddiction. This education will require defining the difference between appropriate physical dependency on medications and addiction as harmful psychological dependency to meet ulterior needs. The prescriber should reassure the patient and family that if and when the patient's pain improves, their opioid will be weaned off or to the lowest dose needed. Education can then transition to a discussion about setting up an appropriate drug monitoring system, in which the family participates in the storage, administration, and tracking of medications. Home health programs can help with drug monitoring and education. PDMP is another tool for prescription drug monitoring. For high-risk patients, the conversation should be nonjudgmental and nonconfrontational. Instead, the education and discussion should focus on addiction as an illness and positive practical ways to improving the overall care of patient. Understanding and addressing the underlying psychosocial problems gets to the root of the addictive behaviors. Discussing their psychosocial needs also demonstrates to the patient and family the genuine concern of the treating team and helps to alleviate the sense of discrimination they frequently feel.

Selection of medications can minimize the risk for opioid addiction. For high-risk patients, methadone is the preferred opioid, because it provides good analgesia while reducing the risk for diversion and abuse. For patients who refuse methadone, long-acting morphine is an alternative that also has low street value. Nonopioid analgesic medications should be optimized, particularly antidepressants and anxiolytics. For example, SNRIs have been shown to reduce opioid usage [24].

In conclusion, the same treatment principles apply to high-risk addiction patients as to all palliative care patients. These pain principles as discussed in this chapter are (1) an interdisciplinary, comprehensive approach to address all aspects of the patient's pain, (2) optimizing nonpharmacological therapy and nonopioid therapy, (3) establishing an overall system of care and discussing goals of pain management, and (4) a tailored, individualized therapy based upon the mechanism of their pain.

REFERENCES

1. *Definition of Pain.* Available at http://www.merriam-webster.com/dictionary/pain. Accessed on September 5, 2013.
2. *Opioid Resistant Pain.* Available at http://learn.chm.msu.edu/painmanagement/opioidresist.asp. Accessed on September 6, 2013.
3. Sinatra R, Causes and consequences of inadequate management of acute pain, *Pain Med* 2010;**11**: 1859–1871.
4. Simoni-Wastila L, Qian J, Influence of prescription monitoring programs on analgesic utilization by an insured retiree population, *Pharmacoepidemiol Drug Saf* 2012;**21**(12):1261–1268.
5. Breitbart W, Chandler S, Eagel B, et al., An alternative algorithm for dosing transdermal fentanyl for cancer-related pain, *Oncology* 2000;**14**:695–705.
6. Kornick CA, Santiago-Palma J, Schulman G, et al., A safe and effective method of converting cancer patients from intravenous to transdermal fentanyl, *J Pain* 2001;**2**(Suppl 1):S35.
7. Janssen Pharmaceutica Products: Duragesic (Fentanyl Transdermal System) [drug summary information]. Titusville, NJ. Available at www.jansseen.com. Accessed on July 26, 2014.
8. Institute for Safe Medication Practices, Beware of basal opioid infusions with PCA therapy. *ISMP Medication Safety Alert!* March 12, 2009. Available at http://www.ismp.org/Newsletters/acutecare/articles/20090312.asp. Accessed on August 13, 2013.
9. Attal N, Cruccu G, Baron R, et al., EFNS guidelines on the pharmacological treatment of neuropathic pain: 2010 revision, *Eur J Neurol* 2010 Sep; **17**(9):1113–e88.
10. Franconi G, Manni L, Schröder S, Marchetti P, Robinson N, A systematic review of experimental and clinical acupuncture in chemotherapy-induced peripheral neuropathy, *Evid Based Complement Alternat Med* 2013;**2013**:516916.
11. Chlan LL, Weinert CR, Heiderscheit A, et al., Effects of patient-directed music intervention on anxiety and sedative exposure in critically ill patients receiving mechanical ventilatory support: a randomized clinical trial, *JAMA* 2013 Jun 12;**309**(22):2335–2344.
12. Posadzki P, Lewandowski W, Terry R, Ernst E, Stearns A, Guided imagery for non-musculoskeletal pain: a systematic review of randomized clinical trials, *J Pain Symptom Manage* 2012 Jul;**44**(1): 95–104.
13. Barawid EL, Covarrubias N, Tribuzio B, Perret-Karimi D, Liao S, Rehabilitation modalities in palliative care, *Crit Rev Phys Rehabil Med.* 2013 Oct;**25**:77–100.
14. Lauche R, Langhorst J, Dobos G, Cramer H, A systematic review and meta-analysis of Tai Chi for osteoarthritis of the knee, *Complement Ther Med* 2013 Aug;**21**(4):396–406.

15. Jayawardena KM, Liao S, Elder abuse at the end of life, *J Palliat Med* 2006;**9**(1):127–136.
16. Ranganathan A, Dougherty M, Waite D, Casarett D, Can palliative home care reduce 30-day readmissions? Results of a propensity score matched cohort study, *J Palliat Med* 2013 Sep 5;**16**(10):1290–1293 [Epub ahead of print].
17. Ornstein K, Wajnberg A, Kaye-Kauderer H, et al., Reduction in symptoms for homebound patients receiving home-based primary and palliative care, *J Palliat Med* 2013 Jun 8;**16**(9):1048–1054 [Epub ahead of print].
18. Meyer BM, The food and drug administration amendments act of 2007: drug safety and health-system implications, *Am J Health-Syst Pharm* 2009; **66**(Suppl 7):S3–S5.
19. ER/LA Opioid Analgesics REMS Website. Available at http://www.er-la-opioidrems.com. Accessed on July 29, 2013.
20. Nicholson SC, Petereson J, Yektashenas B, Risk evaluation and mitigation strategies (REMS): educating the prescriber, *Drug Safety* 2012;**35**(2):91–104.
21. Shane R. Risk evaluation and mitigations strategies: impact on patients, health care providers, and health systems. *Am J Health-Syst Pharm* 2009;**66**(Suppl 7):S6–S12.
22. Paulozzi LJ, Centers for Disease Control and Prevention (CDC), Drug-induced deaths—United States, 2003–2007, *MMWR Surveill Summ* 2011 Jan 14;**60**(Suppl):60–61.
23. Azoulay D, Jacobs JM, Cialic R, Mor EE, Stessman J, Opioids, survival, and advanced cancer in the hospice setting, *J Am Med Dir Assoc* 2011 Feb;**12**(2):129–134.
24. Wu N, Chen SY, Hallett LA, et al., Opioid utilization and health-care costs among patients with diabetic peripheral neuropathic pain treated with duloxetine vs. other therapies, *Pain Pract* 2011 Jan–Feb;**11**(1):48–56.

Chapter 3

Dyspnea: Management in Seriously Ill Hospitalized Patients

Margaret L. Campbell and Michael A. Stellini

3.1 DEFINITIONS, PREVALENCE, AND TRAJECTORIES

Dyspnea is "a subjective experience of breathing discomfort that consists of qualitatively distinct sensations that vary in intensity" [1]. Dyspnea, also referred to as breathlessness, shortness of breath, or difficulty in breathing, is akin to suffocation and one of the most frightening symptom experiences. Dyspnea prompts visits to the emergency department and subsequent hospital admissions for three to four million patients per year in the United States [2]. Dyspnea predicts imminent respiratory failure and warrants rapid clinical responsiveness consistent with the patient's treatment goals.

As many as 50% of patients admitted to hospitals complain of dyspnea. Patients at greatest risk include those with heart failure (HF), chronic obstructive pulmonary disease (COPD), primary and secondary lung cancer, and pneumonia, which is commonly seen at the end of life in patients dying from any cause. Patients with advanced COPD typically have high levels of dyspnea throughout disease progression contrasted with patients with lung cancer who develop dyspnea in the last weeks of life [3]. HF patients experience dyspnea during a pulmonary edema exacerbation and at the end of life secondary to respiratory muscle wasting [4]. Of critically ill patients, including those mechanically ventilated, dyspnea is the most distressing reported symptom [5].

Hospital-Based Palliative Medicine: A Practical, Evidence-Based Approach, First Edition.
Edited by Steven Pantilat, Wendy Anderson, Matthew Gonzales, and Eric Widera.
© 2015 John Wiley & Sons, Inc. Published 2015 by John Wiley & Sons, Inc.

3.2   ASSESSMENT

High-quality palliative care for dyspnea requires comprehensive, valid, and reliable measurement. The simplest assessment in patients who are able to self-report symptoms is to ask "Are you short of breath?" or "Are you getting enough air?" The numeric rating scale, for those able to report, is an appropriate palliative care tool, although limited since only presence and intensity are identified [6]. A typical numeric rating scale is anchored at 0 for "no shortness of breath" to 10 representing "the worst possible shortness of breath." Patients may have familiarity with a 0–10 scale since most hospitals use this medium for routine pain assessment.

Seriously or critically ill and patients near death are often temporarily or permanently cognitively impaired or unconscious and limited in their abilities to provide a symptom self-report [7]. The Respiratory Distress Observation Scale (RDOS) is a valid and reliable tool for measuring signs consistent with dyspnea presence, intensity, and response to treatment for patients unable to use a self-report measure. The RDOS is an eight-item ordinal tool with eight behavioral variables (see Table 3.1). Each item is scored from zero to two points and the points are summed. Higher scores suggest higher intensity respiratory distress [8]. The RDOS has application for all patients at risk for respiratory distress who are unable to reliably report dyspnea, including those undergoing invasive and noninvasive mechanical ventilation. This tool is in use in some hospital systems. In the absence of the RDOS, physical signs can be observed to indicate distress, including tachycardia, tachypnea, restlessness, accessory muscle use, paradoxical breathing pattern, grunting at end expiration, and a fearful facial display [9].

3.3   DIFFERENTIAL DIAGNOSIS

When the patient is not near death it is prudent to consider the etiology of dyspnea in the event a disease-modifying intervention is indicated. When the patient is near death, the burden of a workup may be out of proportion to the benefit. The patient's treatment goals will determine when a workup is indicated. In the case of advanced and terminal illness, the least invasive test that yields the most information is helpful.

For patients with known chronic illnesses causing dyspnea, aggressive treatment of the underlying disease is the first approach. For example, the "palliative" treatment of HF is the treatment of HF. When dyspnea is refractory to aggressive usual treatments, the use of specific symptom control measures, global dyspnea treatment, described below is indicated.

Specific Conditions Which Cause Dyspnea to Consider

- Pulmonary infection (bacterial or viral pneumonia, empyema)
- Pulmonary edema
- Abdominal ascites—can be due to malignant ascites or portal hypertension and exacerbated by low serum albumin, which is common in many advanced and terminal illnesses.
- Anemia
- Pleural effusion (CHF, pneumonia, hypoalbuminemia, malignancy)

Table 3.1   Respiratory Distress Observation Scale

Variable	0 Points	1 Point	2 Points	Total
Heart rate per minute	<90 beats	90–109 beats	≥110 beats	
Respiratory rate per minute	≤18 breaths	19–30 breaths	>30 breaths	
Restlessness: nonpurposeful movements	None	Occasional, slight movements	Frequent movements	
Paradoxical breathing pattern: abdomen moves in on inspiration	None		Present	
Accessory muscle use: rise in clavicle during inspiration	None	Slight rise	Pronounced rise	
Grunting at end expiration: guttural sound	None		Present	
Nasal flaring: involuntary movement of nares	None		Present	
Look of fear	None		Eyes wide open, facial muscles tense, brow furrowed, mouth open, teeth together	
Total				

Source: Figures courtesy of Ursula Hess, University of Quebec at Montreal.
Instruction for use:

1. RDOS is not a substitute for patient self-report if able.
2. RDOS is an adult assessment tool.
3. RDOS cannot be used when the patient is paralyzed with a neuromuscular blocking agent.
4. Count respiratory and heart rates for 1 min; auscultate if necessary.
5. Grunting may be audible with intubated patients on auscultation.
6. Fearful facial expressions.

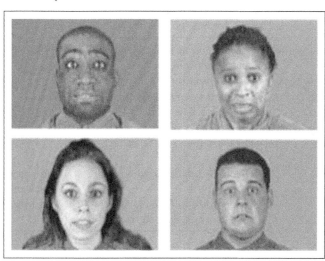

- Radiation pneumonitis—consider the patient's history in conjunction with radiographic findings.
- Pulmonary embolism—increased risk in many cancers
- Progression of primary or secondary pulmonary tumors
- Lymphangitic carcinomatosis—can occur with any cancer and is most common in breast, gastric, and lung primary (radiographic findings may mimic those of sarcoidosis)
- Amyotrophic lateral sclerosis
- Pneumothorax (spontaneous, postprocedure)

3.4 DIAGNOSTIC PROCEDURES

3.4.1 Physical Exam

Physical examination is a foundation of diagnostic efforts. Following and during history taking (in the verbal patient), *observe* for facial signs of distress ("fear face," nasal flaring, pursed lip breathing), how long the patient can talk without stopping, respiratory effort, respiratory rate, intercostal retractions, abdominal breathing, and end-expiratory grunting. (You can observe a lot just by looking—Yogi Berra.)

Auscultation and percussion are also useful in helping to determine diagnosis and guiding use of imaging studies. In addition to lung findings summarized in the following, listen to the heart for rate, murmurs, and gallops. Also, evaluate the neck for venous distension and the abdomen for evidence of ascites (Table 3.2).

Table 3.2 Chest Auscultation and Percussion Summary

Condition	Findings on Auscultation	Findings on Percussion
Infection/consolidation	Bronchial breath sounds, rhonchi, increased fremitus	Dullness
Pulmonary edema	Basilar crackles	
Pleural effusion	Diminished sounds over effusion; *no* increased fremitus	Dullness
Pneumonitis and fibrosis	Diffuse "dry" crackles	
Lymphangitic carcinomatosis	Possible diffuse "dry" crackles	
Pneumothorax	Diminished/absent breath sounds	Hyperresonance over area of pneumothorax
Emphysema	Diminished sounds, prolonged expiratory phase, wheezes	Diffuse hyperresonance

3.4.2   Imaging Studies

Chest X-Ray. A great deal can be determined from a simple upright chest film, for example, detection of pulmonary edema, infection, pleural effusion, or pneumothorax.

Computed Tomography. This can be used for detection of pulmonary embolism, pneumonitis, fibrosis, or carcinomatosis. Use should be guided by the stage of known underlying disease and goals of treatment.

Ultrasound. Occasionally, symptomatic effusions not detected with chest X-ray can be found with ultrasound.

3.4.3   Laboratory Tests

Arterial Blood Gases. Blood gases are painful and of little value in terminal illness and when the patient is near death unless mechanical ventilation use is consistent with the patient's treatment goals and hypercarbic respiratory failure is suspected. If determining hypercarbia is important, capnography (where available) to measure exhaled carbon dioxide or venous blood gases [10] can be used with less burden to the patient. Hypoxemia can be reliably measured with oximetry.

Hemoglobin. Severe anemia will produce dyspnea and other symptoms. Consider the potential cause, for example, blood loss, hemolysis, and marrow failure/infiltration, and whether investigation is warranted based on the invasiveness of the diagnostic tests and likelihood of reversibility. Transfusion provides symptomatic relief, but at some point, benefit wanes as the patient's overall condition deteriorates.

3.5   TREATMENT

Treatment of dyspnea will depend on the patient's treatment goals, nearness to death, and likelihood of a positive response.

3.5.1   Disease-Modifying Treatments

Disease-modifying treatments such as antibiotics or chemotherapy may be considered based on the stage of underlying disease, prognosis, and treatment goals. These, as well as interventions such as mechanical ventilation, often can be more burdensome than beneficial for patients near death. The availability of an intervention does not mandate its use, when the burden/benefit ratio is not favorable. We are not obligated, nor should we provide interventions that are useless. This "withholding of care" often requires detailed, empathic discussion with patients and families. However, supportive treatments such as bronchodilators and anticholinergics, where indicated, should be maintained. These agents can be transitioned from metered-dose inhalers to aerosol (nebulized) treatments as the patient becomes cognitively impaired.

3.5.2 Supportive Interventions for Symptom Relief

Thoracentesis. Draining pleural effusions can provide significant relief of dyspnea. If the effusion is recurring, consider placement of a permanent catheter. A simple pigtail catheter or a tunneled device can be used; the latter has potential for decreased risk of infection. Some of the equipment needed for ongoing, repeated drainage can be quite expensive depending on the brand. If life expectancy is short, for example, weeks, the simple pigtail catheter, equipped with a stopcock, is both convenient and inexpensive, and infection risk is not high or of great concern. Case management assistance will be needed to plan for home or facility discharge when a tube is left in place. While the management of these tubes is not generally difficult, they can induce initial anxiety in family caregivers who will need teaching prior to home discharge.

While the insertion of permanent drainage catheters is generally simple, quick, and not uncomfortable, the alternative approach of pleurodesis may be considered. Recent published guidelines for initial management of malignant pleural effusions recommend pleurodesis. However, good evidence is available about the equivalence of pleurodesis and catheter management in relieving dyspnea in the short term, with some advantage of catheters at 6 months or greater. About half of catheter treated patients had spontaneous pleurodesis and many had the catheter subsequently removed. Patients receiving catheters had significantly shorter initial and follow-up hospital lengths of stay [11]. For patients with an expected very short life-expectancy, the length of stay issue may be very important—favoring catheters. Overall, comfort of the patient and caregivers with an ability to handle the catheter care and use and length of hospital stay are the major considerations in choosing therapy.

Paracentesis. Removal of ascites can provide great relief of dyspnea as well as abdominal symptoms such as pain, constipation, and urinary urgency. Removal of 2–4 l is generally safe and does not require the use of albumin administration. For recurrent accumulation, a permanent catheter can be placed with the same considerations as for thoracentesis.

Others. Interventions such as transfusions and diuretics should be given if they provide symptom relief without causing other complications. For transfusions in particular, consider the burden of repeated use and the overall picture of the patient's condition. Glucocorticoids can be useful in the treatment of COPD as well as other pulmonary conditions. In addition to relief of dyspnea, other effects such as a feeling of increased energy, increased appetite, and overall feeling of enhanced well-being may be achieved. In the palliative setting, consideration of long-term effects of steroids may be less of a concern. Do be mindful of short-term adverse effects such as hyperglycemia and confusion/psychosis.

3.5.3   Global Dyspnea Treatment

Refractory dyspnea is understood to be present when the patient's underlying condition has been optimized. Treatment for refractory dyspnea is also known as "global dyspnea treatment" (Table 3.3).

Positioning. An upright position with the head of the bed as high as possible is generally useful, particularly in COPD [12]. Arms elevated and resting on a pillow on the overbed table with the head of the bed elevated increases vital capacity and may foster dyspnea relief. In some patients with unilateral disease, a side-lying position with the "good" lung up or down improves ventilation or perfusion. Trial-and-error approaches using the individual patient as his/her own control will yield the ideal position. Nurses need to be aware of the "ideal" position for respiratory comfort so other imperatives such as "turn q2" can be overridden.

Oxygen. Oxygen is useful to treat dyspnea when the patient is hypoxemic ($SpO_2 \leq 85\%$). Oxygen is better tolerated delivered by nasal cannula; a face mask induces a feeling of suffocation and is aesthetically less desirable as well. Humidification should be added if flow rates exceed 4 l/min to minimize the risk of

Table 3.3   Summary of Global Dyspnea Interventions

Intervention	Dose	Mode of Action
Optimal positioning, usually upright with arms elevated and supported [12, 13]	Whenever patient reports dyspnea or displays respiratory distress	Increased pulmonary volume capacity
Oxygen as indicated by goals of therapy; no evidence for use in terminal illness unless patient is hypoxemic [14–16].	Variable, guided by goals of therapy and patient characteristics	Improves the partial pressure of oxygen, reduces lactic acidemia
Cold cloth on face [17]	As needed	Trigeminal nerve stimulation, action on dyspnea unknown
Opioids, such as morphine or fentanyl [18]	Low doses titrated to the patient's report of dyspnea or display of dyspnea behaviors is effective; oral or parenteral; no evidence to support inhaled; no evidence on dosing regimens	Uncertain direct effect, reduced brainstem sensitivity to oxygen and carbon dioxide, altered central nervous perception
Benzodiazepines, such as lorazepam or midazolam [19, 20]	Low doses titrated to the patient's report of dyspnea or display of dyspnea behaviors, no evidence for benzodiazepine regimens	Anxiolysis

nasal drying and/or nosebleed. High-flow oxygen (where available) delivers up to 40 l/min; as of this writing, clinical trials are underway to determine if there is a role for high-flow oxygen in the palliation of refractory dyspnea [21].

If the patient is being discharged to home, an oxygen assessment must be performed for insurance to cover the cost of oxygen. The patient must desaturate at rest or with activity to a PaO_2 of less than 55mmHg or SpO_2 of less than 88%. NOTE that if the patient is being discharged with hospice care, this assessment is not usually required, as the hospice agency is the payer and will provide the oxygen based on its own criteria. Oxygen has not been found to be useful in nonhypoxemic dyspnea; no significant or clinically important differences were found when oxygen was compared to medical air [14, 22]. Relief may be achieved from cool air flowing toward the patient's face. A bedside fan may be useful but is sometimes difficult to operationalize in the hospital due to bioengineering constraints [23, 24].

When the patient is near death and is hypersomnolent or unconscious, with no signs of respiratory distress, oxygen need not be initiated, and if flowing, it can usually be withdrawn, regardless of oxygenation [25]. Withdrawing oxygen during last hours permits a natural death trajectory; continued oxygen in the absence of patient distress may merely prolong dying.

Removing a visible intervention such as oxygen may be disconcerting to the family; alternatively removing oxygen produces an aesthetically pleasing, natural patient appearance. Tactfully explain the rationale for removing this nonbeneficial and burdensome intervention to the family as well as the nursing and respiratory therapy staff. An added benefit of removing oxygen is a quieter environment for the dying patient and family, particularly when humidifiers or masks were in use. Close bedside observation for signs of respiratory distress for several minutes after oxygen withdrawal is indicated. There is no benefit to measuring peripheral oxygen saturation as this is a measure of pulmonary function and not a measure of dyspnea or respiratory distress.

Opioids. Opioids, morphine, and fentanyl, in oral or parenteral preparations, are the only medications supported by evidence to reduce dyspnea as primary agents [18]. Opioids reduce the effect of hypoxemia or hypercarbia on ventilation [1, 26]. Optimal dosing for dyspnea has not been established, and pharmacovigilance studies are underway [27, 28]. Typical doses of opioids for dyspnea relief are smaller than those used for pain control. Most of the opioid research for treating dyspnea has been conducted with morphine or fentanyl; similar effectiveness with other classes of opioids such as hydromorphone or methadone has not been established. Morphine is the drug of choice for dyspnea relief; fentanyl is safer when the patient has renal impairment.

Severe, unrelieved dyspnea is a palliative care emergency that warrants frequent assessment and rapid titration of opioids (morphine or fentanyl). A recommended titration plan follows. In general, the onset of action of intravenously administered morphine is at 5–10 min with peak effect usually at 15–30 min. Fentanyl has an onset of 1–5 min with a peak effect at 3–5 min. As always in the palliative setting, goals and expected outcomes should be considered when deciding on how quickly to repeat doses. The other consideration is the degree of discomfort displayed by the patient. So, for a patient who is actively dying and in severe distress, a more rapid readministration, for instance, at 5–10 min, may be acceptable and the best approach. For a patient with less severe distress and whose life expectancy is *not* just minutes to hours, a more conservative approach of redosing at 15–30 min would be prudent. The general pharmacokinetic principle here is that redosing before steady state has been achieved can lead to overdosing. While we never intentionally overdose patients, even in the palliative setting, a high degree of suffering and nearness to death will permit a more "aggressive titration" which is acceptable.

SAMPLE MORPHINE TITRATION PLAN: PATIENT IN SEVERE DISTRESS. Administer an initial intravenous (2 mg) dose of morphine. Wait for 10–15 min for an IV peak effect. Standing by waiting for the peak effect can be difficult; reassure the patient that you are not leaving until they have relief. Relief is indicated by the patient's report or RDOS or reduction in signs of respiratory distress (decreased use of accessory muscles, less tachypnea, etc.). If dyspnea persists, administer another dose that is 50–100% greater than the original dose (3–4 mg); continue administration every 5–15 min until relief is obtained. Maintain relief with an around-the-clock dose every 4 h that corresponds to the total amount of medication given during rapid titration; a continuous morphine infusion at 50% of the bolus dosing alternatively may be useful. Thus, if 5 mg of intravenous morphine produced respiratory comfort then 5 mg every 4 h or 2.5 mg/h as a continuous infusion is indicated. Breakthrough dyspnea will require an as needed dose of morphine. When respiratory comfort is established using intravenous morphine, conversion to an oral immediate-release formulation is indicated, particularly if the patient is not near death and/or is going home or to a facility. The effectiveness of long-acting formulations has not been established; thus, it may be most prudent to maintain respiratory comfort with immediate-release formulations.

When the patient is near death, the ability to swallow becomes impaired. Maintain an IV access, if possible, for rapid onset and ease of administration. When there is no IV access, concentrated immediate-release morphine (20 mg/ml) can be effective when instilled into the buccal space (cheek) with eventual trickling down the pharynx into the esophagus. Constipation remains a problem with opioid use and a laxative bowel regimen should be initiated with the opioid regimen and continued as long as the patient can swallow. Respiratory depression in the dying patient is difficult to detect since respiratory slowing typifies the last hours; respiratory depression was not evident in previous opioid studies [18, 27].

Benzodiazepines. Benzodiazepines as primary agents for dyspnea were not effective [29]; they may be useful as an adjunct to opioids [19]. Consider adding a benzodiazepine to the dyspnea opioid regimen when the patient requires frequent doses, when the doses are escalating, or when the patient reports or displays anxiety or fear. Starting with lorazepam 1 mg orally or parenterally every 6 h as needed is a reasonable approach. Alprazolam can also be used but is only available orally. Lorazepam tablets easily dissolve and are quite reliably absorbed sublingually and are a good option when there is no IV access and the patient cannot swallow pills easily.

Noninvasive Ventilation. Noninvasive ventilation (NIV) is an effective treatment for acute respiratory failure [30]. Effectiveness to palliate dyspnea is less well established [31]. In the case of refractory dyspnea with no expectations for disease modification, NIV becomes a relatively permanent treatment; end points need to be determined with the patient. When the patient is near death, and conscious, NIV may be useful to provide some additional time for life closure. When the patient is near death and hypersomnolent or unconscious, there is no patient role for NIV; families may request prolongation to meet the family needs. Stopping points when the patient no longer benefits need to be diplomatically negotiated with the family.

An NIV task force of the Society of Critical Care Medicine made recommendations regarding three categories of patients: (1) NIV with no limits on advanced life support, (2) NIV with "do not intubate" limitations, and (3) NIV with comfort measures only. In Category 1 the expectation is a return to baseline and unassisted breathing; the patient may deteriorate in spite of NIV and accept mechanical ventilation or improve. In Category 2 the goal is also a return to baseline but in this case if the patient declines with NIV or finds NIV intolerable than other palliative treatments for dyspnea are indicated, such as opioids. In Category 3, for which there is little evidence, the goal of NIV is to reduce dyspnea. The end point is improved symptoms; failure to improve symptoms or worsening discomfort from the NIV warrants discontinuation [32].

Useful Online Resources

Palliative Care Fast Facts: http://www.eperc.mcw.edu/EPERC/FastFactsandConcepts
COPD Foundation: http://www.copdfoundation.org/What-is-COPD/Living-with-COPD/Breathing-Techniques.aspx

---

REFERENCES

1. Parshall MB, Schwartzstein RM, Adams L, et al., An official American Thoracic Society statement: update on the mechanisms, assessment, and management of dyspnea, *Am J Respir Crit Care Med* 2012;**185**:435–452.
2. Nawar EW, Niska RW, Xu J, National Hospital Ambulatory Medical Care Survey: 2005 emergency department summary, *Adv Data* 2007;**386**:1–32.
3. Currow DC, Smith J, Davidson PM, Newton PJ, Agar MR, Abernethy AP, Do the trajectories of dyspnea differ in prevalence and intensity by diagnosis at the end of life? A consecutive cohort study, *J Pain Symptom Manage* 2010;**39**:680–690.
4. Goodlin SJ, Palliative care in congestive heart failure, *J Am Coll Cardiol* 2009;**54**:386–396.
5. Puntillo KA, Arai S, Cohen NH, et al., Symptoms experienced by intensive care unit patients at high risk of dying, *Crit Care Med* 2010;**38**:2155–2160.
6. Mularski RA, Campbell ML, Asch SM, et al., A review of quality of care evaluation for the palliation of dyspnea, *Am J Respir Crit Care Med* 2010;**181**:534–538.
7. Campbell ML, Templin T, Walch J, Patients who are near death are frequently unable to self-report dyspnea, *J Palliat Med* 2009;**12**:881–884.

8. Campbell ML, Templin T, Walch J. A Respiratory distress observation scale for patients unable to self-report dyspnea, *J Palliat Med* 2010;**13**:285–290.
9. Campbell ML. Fear and pulmonary stress behaviors to an asphyxial threat across cognitive states. *Res Nurs Health* 2007;**30**:572–583.
10. Malatesha G, Singh NK, Bharija A, Rehani B, Goel A, Comparison of arterial and venous pH, bicarbonate, PCO2 and PO2 in initial emergency department assessment, *Emerg Med J* 2007;**24**:569–571.
11. Davies HE, Mishra EK, Kahan BC, et al., Effect of an indwelling pleural catheter vs chest tube and talc pleurodesis for relieving dyspnea in patients with malignant pleural effusion: the TIME2 randomized controlled trial, *JAMA* 2012;**307**:2383–2389.
12. Barach AL, Chronic obstructive lung disease: postural relief of dyspnea, *Arch Phys Med Rehabil* 1974;**55**:494–504.
13. Sharp JT, Drutz WS, Moisan T, Foster J, Machnach W. Postural relief of dyspnea in severe chronic obstructive lung disease, *Am Rev Respir Dis* 1980;**122**:201–211.
14. Abernethy AP, McDonald CF, Frith PA, et al., Effect of palliative oxygen versus room air in relief of breathlessness in patients with refractory dyspnoea: a double-blind, randomised controlled trial, *Lancet* 2010;**376**:784–793.
15. Campbell ML, Yarandi H, Dove-Medows E, Oxygen is non-beneficial for most patients who are near death, *J Pain Symptom Manage* 2013;**45**:517–523.
16. Mahler DA, Selecky PA, Harrod CG. Management of dyspnea in patients with advanced lung or heart disease: practical guidance from the American college of chest physicians consensus statement, *Pol Arch Med Wewn* 2010;**120**:160–166.
17. Schwartzstein RM, Lahive K, Pope A, Weinberger SE, Weiss JW, Cold facial stimulation reduces breathlessness induced in normal subjects, *Am Rev Respir Dis* 1987;**136**:58–61.
18. Jennings AL, Davies AN, Higgins JP, Gibbs JS, Broadley KE, A systematic review of the use of opioids in the management of dyspnoea, *Thorax* 2002;**57**:939–944.
19. Navigante AH, Cerchietti LC, Castro MA, Lutteral MA, Cabalar ME, Midazolam as adjunct therapy to morphine in the alleviation of severe dyspnea perception in patients with advanced cancer, *J Pain Symptom Manage* 2006;**31**:38–47.
20. Sironi O, Sbanotto A, Banfi MG, Beltrami C, Midazolam as adjunct therapy to morphine to relieve dyspnea? *J Pain Symptom Manage* 2007;**33**:233–4; author reply 4–6.
21. Hui D, Morgado M, Chisholm G, et al., High-flow oxygen and bilevel positive airway pressure for persistent dyspnea in patients with advanced cancer: a phase II randomized trial, *J Pain Symptom Manage* 2013;**46**:463–473.
22. Uronis H, McCrory DC, Samsa G, Currow D, Abernethy A, Symptomatic oxygen for non-hypoxaemic chronic obstructive pulmonary disease, *Cochrane Database Syst Rev* 2011;**6**:CD006429.
23. Bausewein C, Booth S, Gysels M, Higginson IJ, Non-pharmacological interventions for breathlessness in advanced stages of malignant and non-malignant diseases, *Cochrane Database Syst Rev* 2011;2(CD005623):1–27.
24. Bausewein C, Booth S, Gysels M, Kuhnbach R, Higginson IJ, Effectiveness of a hand-held fan for breathlessness: a randomised phase II trial, *BMC Palliat Care* 2010;**9**:22.
25. Campbell ML, Yarandi H, Dove-Medows E, Oxygen is nonbeneficial for most patients who are near death. *J Pain Symptom Manage* 2013;**45**:517–523.
26. Banzett RB, Adams L, O'Donnell CR, Gilman SA, Lansing RW, Schwartzstein RM, Using laboratory models to test treatment: morphine reduces dyspnea and hypercapnic ventilatory response, *Am J Respir Crit Care Med* 2011;**184**:920–927.
27. Currow DC, McDonald C, Oaten S, et al., Once-daily opioids for chronic dyspnea: a dose increment and pharmacovigilance study, *J Pain Symptom Manage* 2011;**42**:388–399.
28. Currow DC, Quinn S, Greene A, Bull J, Johnson MJ, Abernethy AP, The longitudinal pattern of response when morphine is used to treat chronic refractory dyspnea, *J Palliat Med* 2013;**16**:881–886.
29. Simon ST, Higginson IJ, Booth S, Harding R, Bausewein C, Benzodiazepines for the relief of breathlessness in advanced malignant and non-malignant diseases in adults, *Cochrane Database Syst Rev* 2010;1(CD007354). doi:10.1002/14651858.CD007354.pub2

30. Azoulay E, Kouatchet A, Jaber S, et al., Noninvasive mechanical ventilation in patients having declined tracheal intubation, *Intensive Care Med* 2013;**39**:292–301.
31. Nava S, Ferrer M, Esquinas A, et al., Palliative use of non-invasive ventilation in end-of-life patients with solid tumours: a randomised feasibility trial, *Lancet Oncol* 2013;**14**:219–227.
32. Curtis JR, Cook DJ, Sinuff T, et al., Noninvasive positive pressure ventilation in critical and palliative care settings: understanding the goals of therapy. *Crit Care Med* 2007;**35**:932–939.

Chapter 4

Nausea and Vomiting: Evaluation and Management in Hospitalized Patients

Katherine Aragon and Matthew J. Gonzales

Nausea is an unpleasant sensation that usually precedes vomiting. Nausea and vomiting are common in patients with serious illness, with almost three-quarters of patients admitted to a palliative care unit reporting it [1]. It is common in many end-stage diseases: 60% of advanced cancer patients, 43% of AIDS patients, 30% of end-stage renal disease patients, and 17% of heart failure patients [1, 2]. These symptoms are distressing for patients and families. Nausea and vomiting can lead to dehydration, electrolyte imbalances, and weight loss. Quick diagnosis and treatment can greatly improve these symptoms. In this chapter, we will detail a mechanism-based approach to the evaluation and management of nausea and vomiting.

4.1 PATHOPHYSIOLOGY

When exposed to a noxious stimulus, neuroreceptors activate one or more of the following four pathways: the cortex, the vestibular system, the chemoreceptor trigger zone (CTZ), or the receptors located in gastrointestinal (GI) tract. These pathways trigger the vomiting center located in the brain stem, which activates parasympathetic and motor-efferent nerves inducing vomiting [1, 3].

4.2 MANAGEMENT

While research in this area is limited, small studies have shown a mechanism-based approach, where the initial antiemetic agent is selected according to the most likely causative pathway, to be 80–90% effective in the palliative care population [4, 5]. An

Hospital-Based Palliative Medicine: A Practical, Evidence-Based Approach, First Edition.
Edited by Steven Pantilat, Wendy Anderson, Matthew Gonzales, and Eric Widera.

Table 4.1 Mechanism-Based Approach to Initial Management of Nausea and Vomiting

1. Thorough evaluation: history and examination to narrow differential diagnosis
2. Determine underlying pathway and associated neuroreceptor involved
3. Choose antiemetic targeted against activated neuroreceptor
4. Initiate IV antiemetic on an around-the-clock basis
5. Titrate antiemetic to maximum recommended dose if symptoms not resolved
6. Add an additional antiemetic aimed at a different neurotransmitter for persistent symptoms
7. Evaluate for additional mechanisms that may be reversible and treat accordingly

alternative strategy is an empiric approach starting with a dopamine antagonist regardless of the underlying etiology [6]. We prefer a mechanism-based approach as it allows for systematic workup and targeted management and minimizes polypharmacy. Table 4.1 summarizes this approach, which is described in detail later.

4.2.1 Evaluation

A thorough history and examination is essential in elucidating the cause of nausea and/or vomiting. In over two-thirds of seriously ill patients, one or more causes will be determined [2]. History should focus on onset, frequency, and severity of nausea, recent medications, underlying medical illnesses, and associated symptoms. Ask about recent initiation or titration of opioids as commonly associated with nausea. Inquire about gastritis, reflux disease, and constipation as appropriate treatment may relieve symptoms. For cancer patients, find out the type of cancer, location of tumor(s), and any recent chemotherapy or radiotherapy. Key questions can help lead to determining the activated pathway. Early satiety, bloating, and relief of nausea with small-volume emesis are suggestive of gastric stasis. Alternatively, gastric obstruction is associated with colicky abdominal pain and large-volume bilious emesis. Nausea associated with certain smells or the sight of food suggests activation of the CTZ in the brain. Motion-induced nausea, often associated with vertigo indicates vestibular activation. Increased intracranial pressure typically causes early morning nausea and is associated with headaches and impaired cognition. Finally, anxiety or emotionally induced nausea suggests a cortical component [2, 7].

Physical examination should be attuned to confirming the pathway identified in the history. GI causes can be confirmed by evidence of ascites, enlarged liver, palpable abdominal mass, or impacted stool on rectal exam. Look for fever, confusion, asterixis, or neurological signs. Evidence of dehydration or weight loss may suggest symptom severity.

Laboratory tests may not be necessary on all patients with nausea and vomiting. A basic metabolic panel may show evidence of a reversible cause as detailed in Table 4.2 requiring appropriate medical management. A plain abdominal radiograph

Table 4.2 Reversible Causes of Nausea and Vomiting

Causes	Management
• Hypercalcemia	• IV fluids
• Hyponatremia	• Determine underlying cause and treat accordingly
• Infection	• Antibiotics
• Constipation	• Bowel regimen
• Gastric irritation from anti-inflammatory medications	• Stop anti-inflammatory; initiate PPI or H2 antagonist
• Medications	• Choose alternative agent

can help distinguish between constipation and obstruction. For patients near the end of life, it may be appropriate to treat symptomatically without additional laboratory or radiological testing depending on the goals of care.

4.2.2   Treatment

According to a mechanism-based model, initial antiemetic should be effective against the most likely neuroreceptor involved. In the hospital setting, severe nausea and vomiting require initiation of an IV antiemetic. The chosen antiemetic should be prescribed around the clock and titrated to the maximum recommended dose until relief is achieved. If symptoms persist, add another agent directed against a different receptor [1, 3, 8]. Once nausea is controlled, transition patients to an oral formulation. Many patients will require antiemetics on discharge for chronic symptoms.

4.2.3   Alternative Treatments

Nonpharmacological approaches to nausea and vomiting may be of benefit in addition to antiemetics. For chemotherapy-induced nausea, acupuncture and acupressure are beneficial [9]. More feasible options in the hospital setting include small meals, carbonated drinks, and avoidance of strong odors [8].

4.3   APPROACH TO COMMON CAUSES

A small study of an inpatient palliative care unit found that the majority of nausea symptoms were caused by gastric stasis/outlet obstruction (35%) and chemical/metabolic disturbances (30%), primarily opioids [5]. A study of causes of nausea in hospice patients was similar: 44% were caused by impaired gastric emptying, 33% by chemical disturbance, and 19% by bowel obstruction [4]. In both studies, anxiety, increased intracranial pressure, and vestibular conditions made up only a few cases. Table 4.3 reviews common syndromes causing nausea/vomiting in seriously ill

Table 4.3 Common Causes of Nausea/Vomiting in Seriously Ill Patients

Clinical Syndrome	History and Exam Findings	Specific Causes	Associated Pathway	Antiemetics of Choice
Gastric stasis/impaired gastric emptying	History • Early satiety • Postprandial fullness • Small-volume emesis • Nausea relieved by vomiting Exam • Abdominal distension • Ascites	• Abdominal malignancy • Ascites • Autonomic dysfunction • Malnutrition • Chemotherapy • Radiotherapy • Gastritis • Drugs (e.g., opioids)	• Gastrointestinal stretch activating mechanoreceptors in the gut • Stimulation of D2 receptors in the gut	1. Metoclopramide 2. Haloperidol 3. Prochlorperazine
Chemical/metabolic disturbances	History • Persistent nauseas despite vomiting • Worsened by certain smells Exam • Signs of infection • Signs of renal failure and liver failure	• Hypercalcemia • Infection • Uremia • Chemotherapy • Drugs (e.g., opioids, antibiotics)	• Activation of CTZ (D2, 5HT3 receptors) • Stimulation of D2 receptors in the gut • Stimulation of 5HT3 receptors in the gut	1. Haloperidol 2. Metoclopramide 3. Prochlorperazine
Malignant bowel obstruction	History • Colicky abdominal pain • Nausea relieved by vomiting • Bilious emesis • Constipation Exam • Abdominal distension • Pain with palpation • Hyperactive bowel sounds	• Malignancy (primary and metastatic) • Hepatomegaly • Ascites • Adhesions	• Gastrointestinal stretch activating mechanoreceptors in the gut • Activation of CTZ (D2, 5HT3 receptors)	1. Haloperidol 2. Octreotide 3. Dexamethasone

Vestibular	History • Nausea associated with movement • Vertigo	• Vestibular disorders • Motion sickness • Drugs (e.g., opioids)	• Activation of the vestibular center (H1, Achm receptors) via vestibulocochlear nerve	1. Scopolamine 2. Promethazine
Increased intracranial pressure	History • Early morning vomiting • Headaches • Impaired cognition Exam • Papilledema • Neurological signs	• Brain tumor • Meningeal disease	• Elevated intracranial pressure • Meningeal irritation activating the vomiting center (Achm, H1 receptors)	1. Dexamethasone
Cortical	• Associated with anxiety	• Anxiety • Prechemotherapy		1. Benzodiazepine

5HT3, serotonin receptor; Achm, muscarinic acetylcholine receptor; CTZ, chemoreceptor trigger zone; D2, dopamine receptor; H1, histamine receptor.

patients and their associated history and exam findings, specific causes, mechanism, and recommended treatment. These are detailed later (Table 4.4).

4.3.1 Impaired Gastric Motility

Autonomic dysfunction is common in advanced cancer leading to gastroparesis [6]. Causes for autonomic dysfunction include malnutrition, cachexia, chemotherapy, radiation therapy, and medications [1]. Nausea in this case is often described as intermittent, associated with early satiety and bloating, and improves after small-volume emesis [2, 5]. Stretching of the GI tract stimulates mechanoreceptors, which via peripheral afferent nerve fibers activates the vomiting center. An antiemetic with prokinetic effects like metoclopramide is the agent of choice. If a patient is unable to tolerate or needs an additional agent, an antiemetic against the dopamine (D2) receptor such as haloperidol or prochlorperazine is next choice.

4.3.2 Opioid-Induced Nausea and Vomiting

The prevalence of opioid-induced nausea and vomiting in seriously ill patients is 6–30% [10, 11]. Symptoms usually begin with initiation or dose escalation of an opioid and subside within a week of regular use [1]. Some patients may continue to experience nausea despite prolonged opioid use. Opioid-induced nausea is triggered through several pathways. Opioids stimulate D2 receptors in both the CTZ and the gut. They also decrease gastric motility and cause constipation stimulating gut mechanoreceptors. Finally, opioids directly act on the vestibular system [11]. A D2 antagonist is the first choice for opioid-induced nausea and vomiting. These include haloperidol, chlorpromazine, prochlorperazine, and metoclopramide. All have proven efficacy and the choice is largely dependent on considerations of the side effect profile. If a patient has significant nausea with opioids, schedule an antiemetic for 7 days during initiation or titration of an opioid. If nausea persists, decreasing the opioid dose by 10–20% is often effective without changing analgesic effect [1]. If this does not work, switching to a different opioid may be necessary.

4.3.3 Chemotherapy-Induced Nausea and Vomiting

Nausea associated with chemotherapy is defined as acute, delayed, or anticipatory. Acute nausea occurs in the first 24 h. Delayed nausea happens more than 24 h after chemotherapy. Anticipatory nausea is a conditioned response that often happens prior to administration of chemotherapy [10]. Chemotherapeutic drugs are categorized based on emetogenic risk, from high (>90%) to minimal (<10%) risk. For highly emetogenic chemotherapies, ondansetron, dexamethasone, and aprepitant are prescribed for prophylaxis [12]. Despite prophylaxis, up to 30% of patients will still have acute or delayed emesis [13].

Table 4.4 Properties of Antiemetics

Antiemetic	Neuroreceptor Targeted (Bold = Highest Affinity Receptor)	Dosing	Dose Reduction	Side Effects	Cost (Based on epocrates.com)
Metoclopramide	Prokinetic agent, **D2**	5–20 mg PO/IV/SQ before meals and at bedtime	Cr Cl 10–40 ml/min 50% reduction Cr Cl <10 ml/min 75% reduction	Dystonia, tardive dyskinesia, restlessness	$0.31/10 mg pill
Haloperidol	**D2**	0.5–5 mg PO 2–3 times/day 0.5–2 mg IV every 8 h	Caution in hepatic impairment	Extrapyramidal symptoms	$0.40/1 mg pill
Prochlorperazine	**D2**, H1, Achm, and 5HT3	5–10 mg PO/IV every 6 h 25 mg PR 1–2 times/day	None	Extrapyramidal symptoms, agranulocytosis, sedation	$1.04/10 mg pill
Chlorpromazine	**D2**, H1, Achm, and 5HT3	10–25 mg PO every 6 h	None	Extrapyramidal symptoms, agranulocytosis, sedation	$1.03/10 mg pill
Ondansetron	**5HT3**	4–8 mg PO/SL/IV every 6–8 h	Severe hepatic impairment—max dose 8 mg/24 h	Headache, constipation, QTc prolongation	$31.49/4 mg IV dose $3.57/4 mg pill $44.39/8 mg pill
Promethazine	**H1**, Achm, D2	12.5–25 mg PO/IV every 6 h	Caution advised in hepatic impairment and elderly population	Extravasation/tissue damage with IV use, sedation, urinary retention	$0.66/25 mg pill
Scopolamine	**Achm**	1.5 mg TD every 3 days	Caution advised in renal and hepatic impairment	Sedation, dizziness, urinary retention	$15.88/1.5 mg patch
Olanzapine	**D2**, 5HT3, H1, Achm	5–10 mg SL/PO at bedtime	Caution advised in hepatic impairment	Extrapyramidal symptoms, sedation, weight gain	$14/5 mg oral-dissolving tablet $11.33/5 mg pill

(Continued)

Table 4.4 (*Continued*)

Antiemetic	Neuroreceptor Targeted (Bold = Highest Affinity Receptor)	Dosing	Dose Reduction	Side Effects	Cost (Based on epocrates.com)
Mirtazapine	5HT3	15–45 mg PO at bedtime	Caution advised renal and hepatic impairment	Agranulocytosis, sedation, weight gain, dry mouth	$3.25/15 mg oral-dissolving tablet $2.92/15 mg pill
Dexamethasone	Unknown	4–16 mg PO/IV per day, divide 1–2 times per day	None	Dyspepsia, insomnia, mood changes, edema	$1.75/4 mg pill

Achm = muscarinic acetylcholine receptor, H1 = histamine receptor, D2 = dopamine receptor, 5HT3 = serotonin receptor.

Chemotherapy directly stimulates the CTZ through serotonin 5HT3 receptor, D2 receptor, and NK1 receptor. It can also injure GI epithelial cells, triggering 5HT3 receptors in the gut. Ondansetron was the first widely used selective 5HT3-receptor antagonist. Numerous studies show its benefit for acute chemotherapy-induced nausea [12–14]. However, the same benefit has not been consistently shown for refractory nausea in the palliative care population [2]. Given the high expense, if ondansetron has been ineffective in the past or if it is not clearly chemotherapy-induced nausea, another agent should be considered. Benzodiazepines, such as lorazepam, are commonly prescribed for anticipatory nausea. Their anxiolytic and sedative effects likely potentiate the effectiveness of an antiemetic regimen, but we discourage routine use for nausea.

4.3.4 Malignant Bowel Obstruction

Malignant bowel obstruction is a serious condition and affects many patients with advanced cancer. Symptoms often begin insidiously over several weeks. Common symptoms include colicky abdominal pain, nausea, bilious vomiting, distension, constipation, and eventually obstipation. Obstruction can occur from a mass within the GI tract, from a mass compressing the GI tract externally, or by tumor infiltration in the wall of the stomach or intestines. As the bowel contracts against the obstruction, GI hormones are released leading to inflammation and edema of the bowel, further causing obstruction.

Management of an obstruction often includes multiple modalities. Surgery may be beneficial for some patients; however, studies suggest variable symptom response, with 42–80% of patients having symptom improvement, and a significant chance of reobstruction (10–50%) [15]. Symptom improvement in most of these studies was either the ability to eat a full meal or survival time after surgery [15]. Complication rates postsurgery are also high, even for patients considered good candidates [16, 17]. Factors which indicate poor candidacy for surgery include age over 70 years, presence of ascites, palpable abdominal masses, metastatic disease, prior radiation to the abdomen or pelvis, prior combination chemotherapy, and evidence of multiple obstructions [3].

Often for the palliative care population medical management is the only option. Several medications have shown to offer symptomatic benefit in bowel obstruction (Table 4.5).

Antiemetics that inhibit the D2 receptor at the CTZ or H2 receptor directly at the vomiting center are most effective in malignant bowel obstruction. In partial obstruction, metoclopramide can be used. It should not be given for a complete obstruction as it may worsen abdominal pain. Parenteral haloperidol is recommended for complete obstruction [16]. Corticosteroids, such as dexamethasone, may be added. Corticosteroids may help relieve an obstruction by reducing inflammatory edema in the gut [18]. A recent systematic review reported benefit with corticosteroids, though the effect was not statistically significant [18]. However, a follow-up analysis challenged the methodology used in some of the studies reviewed [19]. While we await

Table 4.5   Nonsurgical Management of Small Bowel Obstruction

---

- Analgesia with IV opioid
- Initiation of IV antiemetic
  - Haloperidol 5–10 mg/24 h, divided in three doses or continuous infusion
- Addition of antisecretory agent for persistent pain and/or vomiting
  - Octreotide 100–300 mcg SQ/IV TID or as a continuous infusion
  - Hyoscine butylbromide 60–300 mg SQ/IV per 24 h
  - Glycopyrrolate 0.2 mg SQ/IV q 6 h
- Trial of dexamethasone for added antiemetic effect
  - Dose 6–16 mg/day
- Consideration of venting gastrostomy for long-term management in select patients

---

better research, clinical experience supports using corticosteroids in individual situations, as they may be beneficial in relieving nausea with little harm when used for a short period of time.

Antisecretory agents are added for persistent pain and vomiting. Octreotide is a somatostatin analogue. It inhibits the release of GI hormones which leads to decreased fluid production, increased absorption of fluids and electrolytes, and decreased GI motility [16]. Hyoscine butylbromide and glycopyrrolate are anticholinergic agents that are also used to minimize secretions. While octreotide and hyoscine butylbromide are both effective, several comparative studies have concluded that octreotide may offer superior symptom relief [19]. Recent studies have shown ranitidine to be effective in reducing gut secretions although a clear role in small bowel obstruction has not been defined [20]. For many patients the combination of an analgesic, antiemetic, and antisecretory agent will lead to relief of symptoms and allow patients to take in small amounts of liquids and food.

Patients with gastric outlet obstruction may respond poorly to medical management alone [3]. In these patients, suction via a silicone nasogastric (NG) tube may provide temporary relief. Silicone NG tubes are slightly more expensive than vinyl tubes but are more pliable and more comfortable. For long-term management, placement of a percutaneous endoscopic gastrostomy (PEG) tube used as a venting gastrostomy should be considered. Studies on patients with gynecological malignancies have shown these tubes to be successful in improving symptoms in 94–98% of patients, even in the presence of ascites and tumor infiltration, with 84% having complete resolution of symptoms [16].

4.4 INTRACTABLE NAUSEA AND VOMITING

Despite utilizing a mechanism-based approach, some patients will not have sufficient symptom relief. In these cases, alternative agents may be required in order to relieve suffering. Although there is limited data from clinical trials to support the use of the following drugs in the management of refractory nausea, clinical experience in these difficult cases supports consideration as treatment options.

4.4.1 Corticosteroids

Corticosteroids are used frequently in palliative care for intractable nausea. The antiemetic mechanism of steroids is unknown. The efficacy of steroids for alleviating nausea and vomiting due to chemotherapy is well established [12, 14]. Dexamethasone is commonly used as it comes in multiple formulations. Benefit should be seen by 1 week. If no benefit is noted, then steroids should be discontinued.

4.4.2 Nontraditional Antiemetics

Olanzapine and mirtazapine, although commonly thought of as psychiatric medications, have been shown in case reports to be effective for the management of nausea [21–23]. Table 4.4 describes mechanism and dosing.

4.5 CONCLUSION

A mechanism-based approach to the management of nausea and vomiting is an effective way to treat these symptoms in the hospitalized patient. A thorough history and examination will often get to the underlying cause with limited need for laboratory and radiological investigation. A single antiemetic should be chosen that is tailored to the patient's clinical situation and titrated until symptoms resolve or the maximum dose is reached. If symptoms persist, an antiemetic targeted against a different pathway should be added.

In the palliative care population, impaired gastric motility and chemical/metabolic disturbances are common causes of nausea and vomiting. Malignant bowel obstructions can be challenging to manage, but with a combination of analgesia, antiemetics, and antisecretory agents, most patients will have relief of symptoms without the need for surgery or a gastric tube. In some cases, nausea will not improve despite following the aforementioned approach. For these patients, considering alternative agents is warranted.

REFERENCES

1. Wood GJ, Shega JW, Lynch B, Von Roenn JH, Management of intractable nausea and vomiting in patients at the end of life, *JAMA* 2007;**298**(10):1196–1207.
2. Glare P, Miller J, Nikolova T, Tickoo R, Treating nausea and vomiting in palliative care: a review, *Clin Interv Aging* 2011;**6**:243–259.
3. Baines MJ, ABC of palliative care. Nausea, vomiting, and intestinal obstruction, *BMJ* 1997 Nov 1;**315**(7116):1148–1150.

4. Stephenson J, Davies A, An assessment of aetiology-based guidelines for the management of nausea and vomiting in patients with advanced cancer, *Support Care Cancer* 2006 Apr;**14**(4):348–353.
5. Bentley A, Boyd K, Use of clinical pictures in the management of nausea and vomiting: a prospective audit, *Palliat Med* 2001 May;**15**(3):247–253.
6. Bruera E, Belzile M, Neumann C, Harsanyi Z, Babul N, Darke A, A double-blind, crossover study of controlled-release metoclopramide and placebo for the chronic nausea and dyspepsia of advanced cancer, *J Pain Symptom Manage* 2000 Jun;**19**(6):427–435.
7. Davis MP, Walsh D, Treatment of nausea and vomiting in advanced cancer, *Support Care Cancer* 2000 Nov;**8**(6):444–452.
8. Gonzales MJ, Widera E, Nausea and other nonpain symptoms in long-term care, *Clin Geriatr Med* 2011 May;**27**(2):213–228.
9. Ezzo JM, Richardson MA, Vickers A, et al., Acupuncture-point stimulation for chemotherapy-induced nausea or vomiting, *Cochrane Database Syst Rev* 2006(**2**):CD002285.
10. Cheung WY, Zimmermann C, Pharmacologic management of cancer-related pain, dyspnea, and nausea, *Semin Oncol* 2011 Jun;**38**(3):450–459.
11. Herndon CM, Jackson KC, 2nd, Hallin PA, Management of opioid-induced gastrointestinal effects in patients receiving palliative care, *Pharmacotherapy* 2002 Feb;**22**(2):240–250.
12. Kris MG, Hesketh PJ, Somerfield MR, et al., American Society of Clinical Oncology guideline for antiemetics in oncology: update 2006, *J Clin Oncol* 2006 Jun 20;**24**(18):2932–2947.
13. Naeim A, Dy SM, Lorenz KA, Sanati H, Walling A, Asch SM, Evidence-based recommendations for cancer nausea and vomiting, *J Clin Oncol* 2008 Aug 10;**26**(23):3903–3910.
14. Ioannidis JP, Hesketh PJ, Lau J, Contribution of dexamethasone to control of chemotherapy-induced nausea and vomiting: a meta-analysis of randomized evidence, *J Clin Oncol* 2000 Oct 1;**18**(19):3409–3422.
15. Feuer DJ, Broadley KE, Shepherd JH, Barton DP, Surgery for the resolution of symptoms in malignant bowel obstruction in advanced gynaecological and gastrointestinal cancer, *Cochrane Database Syst Rev* 2000(**4**):CD002764.
16. Ripamonti CI, Easson AM, Gerdes H, Management of malignant bowel obstruction, *Eur J Cancer* 2008 May;**44**(8):1105–1115.
17. Helyer LK, Law CH, Butler M, Last LD, Smith AJ, Wright FC, Surgery as a bridge to palliative chemotherapy in patients with malignant bowel obstruction from colorectal cancer, *Ann Surg Oncol* 2007 Apr;**14**(4):1264–1271.
18. Feuer DJ, Broadley KE, Corticosteroids for the resolution of malignant bowel obstruction in advanced gynaecological and gastrointestinal cancer, *Cochrane Database Syst Rev* 2000(2):CD001219.
19. Mercadante S, Casuccio A, Mangione S, Medical treatment for inoperable malignant bowel obstruction: a qualitative systematic review, *J Pain Symptom Manage* 2007 Feb;**33**(2):217–223.
20. Clark K, Lam L, Currow D, Reducing gastric secretions—a role for histamine 2 antagonists or proton pump inhibitors in malignant bowel obstruction? *Support Care Cancer* 2009 Dec;**17**(12): 1463–1468.
21. Passik SD, Lundberg J, Kirsh KL, et al., A pilot exploration of the antiemetic activity of olanzapine for the relief of nausea in patients with advanced cancer and pain, *J Pain Symptom Manage* 2002 Jun;**23**(6):526–532.
22. Theobald DE, Kirsh KL, Holtsclaw E, Donaghy K, Passik SD, An open-label, crossover trial of mirtazapine (15 and 30 mg) in cancer patients with pain and other distressing symptoms, *J Pain Symptom Manage* 2002 May;**23**(5):442–447.
23. Jackson WC, Tavernier L, Olanzapine for intractable nausea in palliative care patients, *J Palliat Med* 2003 Apr;**6**(2):251–255.

ADDITIONAL RESOURCES

- End of Life/Palliative Education Resource Center
  - http://www.eperc.mcw.edu/EPERC/FastFactsIndex/ff_005.htm
  - http://www.eperc.mcw.edu/EPERC/FastFactsIndex/ff_025.htm
- NCCN Guidelines Antiemesis
  - http://www.nccn.org/professionals/physician_gls/f_guidelines.asp#antiemesis

Chapter 5

Delirium: Identification and Management in Seriously Ill Hospitalized Patients

Marieberta Vidal and Eduardo Bruera

Delirium is a multifactorial syndrome that occurs due to a global organic brain dysfunction. It is a serious medical condition that affects consciousness, perception, attention, thought, memory, and sleep and wake cycles of the individual [1]. Delirium is one of the most common neuropsychiatric complications in general hospital practice. Delirium occurs in approximately 30% of hospitalized patients and 51% of postsurgical patients. It is associated with increased mortality and morbidity [2]. The prevalence of delirium is even higher in patients with advanced disease, like AIDS and cancer, at the last weeks of life, ranging from 25 to 85%.

Delirium is such a common event in patients with serious illness that it makes the assessment of pain and symptoms difficult and is a major cause of distress among patients, family members, and health-care providers. Approximately 50% of delirium episodes are reversible (Fig. 5.1). Diagnosis of delirium is commonly missed, and its early symptoms, such as anxiety, insomnia, and mood changes, may be treated with anxiolytics and antidepressants, which may worsen the delirium [3, 4].

5.1 CLINICAL FEATURES OF DELIRIUM

The symptoms of delirium tend to fluctuate during the day and develop acutely, usually from hours to days. Its main diagnostic criteria, based on DSM-IV-TR criteria, are:

- Disturbance of consciousness (i.e., reduced clarity of awareness of the environment) with reduced ability to focus, sustain, or shift attention
- A change in cognition (such as deficit, disorientation, language disturbance) or the development of a perceptual disturbance that is not better accounted for by a preexisting, established, or evolving dementia [1]

Hospital-Based Palliative Medicine: A Practical, Evidence-Based Approach, First Edition.
Edited by Steven Pantilat, Wendy Anderson, Matthew Gonzales, and Eric Widera.

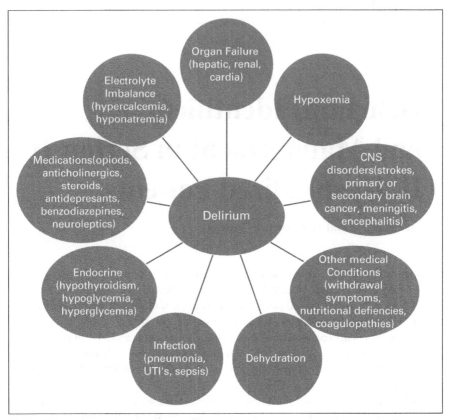

Figure 5.1   Causes of Delirium

Three clinical subtypes of delirium have been described based on the type of arousal disturbance. Hyperactive delirium is characterized by confusion, agitation, hallucinations, delusions, myoclonus, and/or hyperalgesia. Hyperactive delirium is commonly mistaken as anxiety or extrapyramidal symptom. Hypoactive delirium is characterized by confusion, somnolence, and/or withdrawal, which might simulate depression. Mixed delirium presents as alternating symptoms of both hyperactive and hypoactive delirium [3–5].

Terminal delirium is the term used for the approximately 80% of patients who develop delirium in the last hours to days of life. Bruera et al. have shown in a study of 52 hospitalized patients that 88% of patients died with delirium and 83% with cognitive failure, occurring on average 16 days before death [6]. In the last 24–48 h of life, the delirium is most likely not reversible. This is due to the irreversibility of the common process that occurs at final hours of life, like multiorgan failure [6].

5.2   DIFFERENTIAL DIAGNOSIS OF DELIRIUM

The symptoms of delirium can also been associated with other psychiatric disorders like depression, anxiety, mania, psychosis, and dementia. Patients with hypoactive delirium are frequently diagnosed with depression or even overlooked completely.

Table 5.1   Main Differential Diagnosis of Delirium

Clinical Features	Delirium	Dementia	Psychosis	Depression
Onset	Acute	Chronic	Acute	Chronic
Level of consciousness	Altered	Spared (except in advance stage)	Spared	Spared
Attention	Impaired	Spared (except in advance stage)	Can be impaired	Can be impaired
Cognition	Impaired	Impaired	Can be impaired	Can be mildly impaired
Hallucinations	Present (visual or tactile)	Often absent	Present (usually auditory)	Absent
Psychomotor activity	Increased, reduced, or mixed	Often normal	Often increased	Normal or reduced
Involuntary movements	Myoclonus, tremors, or asterixis in some cases	Usually absent	Absent	Absent

However, while delirium is common in palliative care patients at the advance stage of their disease, depression occurs less frequently. On the other hand, patients with mild delirium often have depressive symptoms. To differentiate between delirium and depression, the important factors to consider are the following: the abrupt onset, severity of cognitive symptoms, and characteristic fluctuating arousal or consciousness, which is the most predominant symptom of delirium [7]. Another confounding diagnosis to be considered is dementia, as it shares some clinical features with delirium, but differs in that there is little or no clouding of consciousness and has an insidious onset. Patients with dementia may also develop superimposed delirium, acutely exacerbating their usual symptoms [8] (please see Table 5.1 for clinical features of delirium, dementia, psychosis, and depression).

5.3 CAUSES FOR DELIRIUM

The pathophysiology of delirium is still not fully understood, but many neurotransmitters are thought to play a role on it. The most important hypothesized mediators are an excess of dopamine and a deficiency of acetylcholine. Circulating cytokines and other neurotransmitters have also been implicated [8].

The etiology of delirium is often multifactorial [9, 10]. Inouye et al. describe the interaction between predisposing or vulnerability factors and precipitating or incident factors [11, 12]. Patients with baseline cognitive impairment, poor functional status, advanced age, as well as increased severity of illness and multiple comorbidities are at higher risk of developing delirium (Table 5.2). Precipitating factors include medications, acute illness, underlying neurologic disease, surgery sleep deprivation, and certain environmental conditions [11–13]. Delirium in the palliative care setting is

Table 5.2   Risk Factors for Delirium in Hospitalized Patients

- Advanced age
- Severe illness
- Preexisting cognitive impairment
- Sensory impairment
- Elevated BUN/creatinine ratio >18
- Recent surgery
- Precipitating factors
    3 new medications during hospitalization
    Use of bladder catheters
    Immobilization (including physical restraints)
    Infection

almost always multifactorial and in most cases a specific cause often remains unidentified. However, this should not deter the health-care professional from investigating for underlying causes as some of them might be reversible if treated adequately.

Delirium is a common complication near the end of life. Symptoms and signs of delirium—including confusion, restlessness, agitation, and/or day–night reversal—occurring in the last days of life are referred to as terminal delirium. It is not reversible and usually is accompanied by other clinical signs of the dying process like increased pharyngeal secretions, moaning, groaning, and grimacing that, in combination with agitation and restlessness, may be misinterpreted as physical pain. A hypoactive form of delirium may occur with less psychomotor activity. Delirium can be distressing to family members and interpreted as an "uncontrolled pain or traumatic death" unless it is recognized and treated appropriately [14–16].

5.4   DELIRIUM ASSESSMENT

Delirium is frequently missed but more often misdiagnosed, because the symptoms might mimic other entities. A detailed history and physical exam, including listening to the observations of caregivers, are key to the early diagnosis of delirium. All the possible reversible causes should be investigated since the treatment will depend on correction of the cause. All medications should be revised, particularly opioids, benzodiazepines, antiemetics, and steroids, as they are frequent causes of delirium.

The health provider should maintain a high index of suspicion and use a scale or instrument to rapidly screen for delirium.

Screening tools such as the Memorial Delirium Assessment Scale (MDAS) and the Confusion Assessment Method (CAM) have been validated in the diagnosis of delirium. These screening tools should be used even in patients with no overt signs of delirium to make an early diagnosis. The selection of the tool is not as important as to maintain a high suspicion for delirium and screen for it. Most of the time, the clinician will choose a tool that is easy to use and that is familiar to him. MDAS is a reliable tool for screening and assessing delirium severity among medically ill population. It is a screening tool with 10 items that give a score range from 0–30, with score higher than or equal to 7 being recommended as a cutoff for delirium. Scale items assess disturbances in arousal and level of consciousness, as well as several areas of cognitive functioning (memory, attention, orientation, and disturbances in thinking) and psychomotor activity [17].

The CAM is a diagnostic scale that uses the DSM-III-R criteria for delirium. It includes an algorithm of four items that requires the presence of acute onset or fluctuating course, inattention, disorganized thinking, and altered level of consciousness. The CAM-ICU has been validated for identification of delirium in intensive care unit as it can be used in patients unable to communicate due to mechanical ventilation.

The Delirium Rating Scale (DRS) is a 10-item tool designed to identify delirium and distinguish it from dementia and other neuropsychiatry disorders. A score of 12 or greater is considered diagnostic of delirium [18].

In the palliative care setting, we used the MDAS more frequently as it is very well validated on hospitalized patients with advanced cancer and AIDS. It is also a diagnostic tool that measures the severity of delirium and can be used to reevaluate the patients after an intervention. For nonverbal mechanical ventilated patients, the CAM-ICU is the tool of choice. Our recommendation is to use a diagnostic tool to screen for delirium as it can very easily be missed or misdiagnosed.

It is important to ask the patient and caregivers specifically about hallucinations (they are more often tactile than visual) and delusional thoughts. Look for clinical signs of sepsis, opioid toxicity, dehydration, metabolic abnormalities, or other potential causes of delirium. Order appropriate tests, such as a complete blood count, electrolytes, calcium, renal and liver function, chest X-ray, O_2 saturation, neuroimaging, and others as indicated.

5.5   PHARMACOLOGIC TREATMENT OF DELIRIUM

The appropriate management of delirium includes identifying and treating the underlying causes. Discontinue any possibly inciting medication, especially benzodiazepines, anticholinergic, corticosteroids, antidepressants, certain antiemetics and antivirals, antibiotics (quinolones), cimetidine, and ranitidine. In the palliative care, patient pain is a common symptom, and delirium can sometimes be caused either by uncontrolled pain or pain medications. It can be challenging to distinguish between these two because delirium also affects the pain expression. If opioids are suspected to be the cause, opioid rotation or dose reduction should be attempted. Short-acting opioids should be considered as a test dose to treat pain. Treating infection, hydrating the patient, and correcting electrolyte abnormalities might be enough to correct the symptoms. Supplement oxygen if hypoxia and add steroids if intracranial lesions with edema are present. Caregivers and staff should be educated on the etiology and clinical course of delirium as their involvement is necessary to guarantee patient safety.

Symptomatic treatment of the agitation is achieved by using neuroleptics. Haloperidol is the drug of choice for treatment of delirium due to its high potency, low incidence of side effects, and alternate routes of administration. Haloperidol is a dopamine blocker with useful sedatives effects and low incidence of cardiovascular and anticholinergic side effects [19]. Starting dose is usually 1–2 mg PO/SC/IV every 6 h and as needed for agitation, paranoia, and hallucinations. Occasionally acute dystonias and extrapyramidal symptoms can be seen with haloperidol, in which case benztropine can be administered. If symptoms are not controlled with a 24 h dose of 20 mg of haloperidol, switching to a more sedating neuroleptic such as chlorpromazine might be necessary. Methotrimeprazine, a phenothiazine neuroleptic, is sometimes used effectively to control agitated delirium, and it has also been shown to provide analgesia.

Sometimes a combination of a haloperidol and a benzodiazepine is useful. In a study by Brietbart, lorazepam alone was ineffective in the treatment of the delirium and instead contributed to worsening of the cognitive impairment [19]. The atypical antipsychotics, such as olanzapine, risperidone, and quetiapine, are also used in the treatment of delirium. Olanzapine has been shown to be effective in the treatment of delirium without significant incidence of extrapyramidal symptoms [20]. The usual starting dose is from 2.5 to 5 mg every 8 h. Unfortunately, the newer generations of antipsychotics are more costly than haloperidol (please see Table 5.3 for a guide on antipsychotics doses range, route, and side effects).

For symptomatic management of acute delirium, we recommend initiating haloperidol at 2 mg orally or 1 mg subcutaneously/IV every 2 h until settled and then every 6 or 8 h as needed. A 50% dose reduction is recommended for the elderly. If delirium symptoms are not controlled, haloperidol may be more rapidly titrated or

Table 5.3   Neuroleptics Used to Treat Delirium

Drug	Dose	Route	Side Effects
Haloperidol	0.5–5 mg every 2–4 h	PO/SC/IM/IV	EPS, QTc prolongation, anticholinergic
Droperidol	0.625–2.5 mg every 4–6 h	IM/IV	EPS, QTc prolongation, sedation, anticholinergic
Methotrimeprazine	12.5–50 mg every 4–8 h	PO/SC/IV	Sedation, hypotension, rare QTc prolongation, anticholinergic
Chlorpromazine	12.5–50 mg every 4–8 h	PO/IM/IV	Highly sedating, hypotension, QTc prolongation, EPS, anticholinergic
Olanzapine	2.5–15 mg every 8–12 h	PO	Sedation, anticholinergic, EPS
Risperidone	0.5–3 mg every 12–24 h	PO	Sedation, hypotension
Quetiapine	50–200 mg every 12–24 h	PO	Sedation, anticholinergic, QTc prolongation, EPS, suicidal ideation
Ziprasidone	10–80 mg every 12–24 h	PO/IM	QTc prolongation, sedation

changed to chlorpromazine. For terminal delirium, the addition of a benzodiazepine to an antipsychotic is reasonable to achieve needed sedation and comfort. It is important to bring agitated delirium under control as rapidly as possible to prevent patient, family, and staff distress. Once symptoms are under control, start reducing the dose to the minimal effective dose as soon as possible. In terminal conditions that present with severe agitated delirium, palliative sedation should be considered preferable under the care of a palliative care specialist [21, 22].

5.5.1   Palliative Sedation

Palliative sedation (PS) is the monitored use of sedative medication to decrease patients' awareness of intractable and refractory symptoms near the end of life. PS should be performed in consultation with a palliative care specialist. Many hospitals have protocols for determining whether it is appropriate and initiating and titrating mediations. In the case of delirium, it is used when conventional treatments like antipsychotics and nonpharmacological therapies have failed in controlling the symptoms. Studies have shown that delirium is a common symptom for which PS is used [22]. In a study by Carceni, delirium was present in 31% of patients who underwent PS [23]. In a systematic review by Mercadante et al., they reported that delirium was a common problem requiring PS in advanced cancer patients in the home setting [24]. The goal for PS is to control distressing symptom and not to hasten death. Reasons and goals of PS should be discussed with the patient and/or the family and documented in the medical records. Midazolam is the drug of first choice for PS. The starting dose of midazolam is 1 mg/h and titrated according to clinical response. The lowest dose possible to provide comfort should be used. It is recommended to use a clinical instrument to monitor the degree of agitation or sedation such as the Richmond Agitation Sedation Scale (RASS) to guide therapy [22]. Frequent reassessment of the necessity to continue PS is important as there might be cases where the condition might be improving. For these patients, reduction of PS or discontinuation is recommended.

5.5.2   Hydration for Treatment of Delirium

Hydration in the terminally ill patient is still controversial. Bruera et al. have shown that careful hydration can decrease the incidence of delirium in patients admitted to the palliative care unit, though their recent randomized controlled trial revealed only a trend toward less deterioration in mental status in the hydration group compared with placebo [25, 26]. In patients who could present with adverse side effects due to inability of the body to clear toxic drug metabolites, the risk might be overcome by the benefits. Palliative care patients often present with symptoms like hallucinations, myoclonus, and excessive sedation that could improve with hydration. In patients with difficulty swallowing, hypodermolysis or subcutaneous infusion of fluids may be a good option. Goals of care should be clearly discussed with the family when continuation of hydration is considered.

5.6 NONPHARMACOLOGIC TREATMENT OF DELIRIUM

Nonpharmacologic measures that help reduce the disorientation are helpful [3]. Provide a safe and quiet environment without excessive light. Other nonpharmacologic measures include ensuring the presence of familiar objects to the patient, a visible clock, or a calendar and the presence of family. Educate family members and caregivers to assist with reorientation. Frequent reassurances, touch, and verbal orientation from a familiar person might decrease disruptive behaviors. Avoid physical restraints and noxious environmental stimuli [12, 13].

Family members and caregivers need to be counseled about the symptoms of delirium as it can be a cause of significant distress [3]. Families sometimes interpret the typical confusion, agitation, and verbal expression of the patients as signs of suffering [15, 16, 27]. Disinhibiting is commonly seen in delirium and may result in

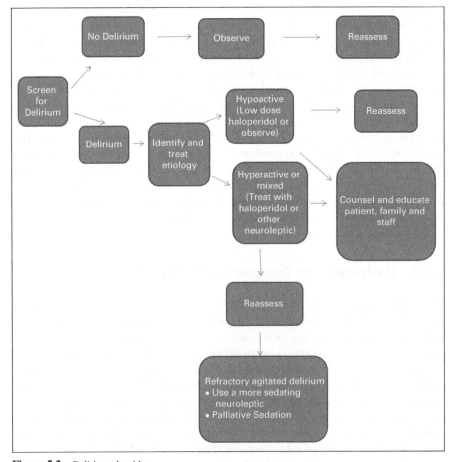

Figure 5.2   Delirium algorithm.

an exaggerated expression of physical symptoms that were well controlled previously. Unfortunately with the observer distress, this can lead to the patient's excessive use of opioids and/or adjuvant drugs and the accompanying potential for exacerbation of delirium. Providing information about the pathology of delirium, explaining the expected course, being present with the family, providing appropriate psychosocial support, and respecting the patient's dignity and values are important factors to decrease the distress on the patients and their families [15, 16, 27]. A simple clinical algorithm for assessing and treating delirium is shown in Figure 5.2.

REFERENCES

1. American Psychiatric Association, *Diagnostic and Statistical Manual of Mental Illness*. Washington, DC: APA, 1994.
2. Inouye, SK, Rushing JT, Foreman MD, Palmer RM, Pompei P, Does delirium contribute to poor hospital outcomes? A three-site epidemiologic study, *J Gen Intern Med* 1998;**13**(4):234–242.
3. Centeno C, Sanz A, Bruera E, Delirium in advanced cancer patients, *Palliat Med* 2004;**18**(3):184–194.
4. Lawlor PG, Bruera E, Delirium in patients with advanced cancer, *Hematol Oncol Clin North Am* 2002;**16**(3):701–714.
5. Lawlor PG, Gagnon B, Mancini IL, et al., Occurrence, causes, and outcome of delirium in patients with advanced cancer: a prospective study, *Arch Intern Med* 2000;**160**(6):786–794.
6. Bruera E, Miller L, McCallion J, Macmillan K, Krefting L, Hanson J, Cognitive failure in cancer patients in clinical trials, *Lancet* 1993;**341**(8839):247–248.
7. Breitbart W, Alici Y, Agitation and delirium at the end of life: "We couldn't manage him," *JAMA* 2008;**300**(24):2898–910, E1.
8. Breitbart W, Psycho-oncology: depression, anxiety, delirium, *Semin Oncol* 1994;**21**(6):754–769.
9. Fick DM, Agostini JV, Inouye SK, Delirium superimposed on dementia: a systematic review, *J Am Geriatr Soc* 2002;**50**(10):1723–1732.
10. Fang CK, Chen HW, Liu SI, Lin CJ, Tsai LY, Lai YL, Prevalence, detection and treatment of delirium in terminal cancer inpatients: a prospective survey, *Jpn J Clin Oncol* 2008;**38**(1):56–63.
11. Inouye SK, Predisposing and precipitating factors for delirium in hospitalized older patients, *Dement Geriatr Cogn Disord* 1999;**10**(5):393–400
12. Inouye SK, Delirium in older persons, *N Engl J Med* 2006;**354**(11):1157–1165.
13. Fong, TG, Tulebaev SR, Inouye SK, Delirium in elderly adults: diagnosis, prevention and treatment, *Nat Rev Neurol* 2009;**5**(4):210–220.
14. Breitbart W, Gibson C, Tremblay A, The delirium experience: delirium recall and delirium-related distress in hospitalized patients with cancer, their spouses/caregivers, and their nurses, *Psychosomatics* 2002;**43**(3):183–194.
15. Bruera E, Bush SH, Willey J, et al., Impact of delirium and recall on the level of distress in patients with advanced cancer and their family caregivers, *Cancer* 2009;**115**(9):2004–2012.
16. Cohen MZ, Pace EA, Kaur G, Bruera E, Delirium in advanced cancer leading to distress in patients and family caregivers, *J Palliat Care* 2009;**25**(3):164–171.
17. Breitbart W, Rosenfeld B, Roth A, Smith MJ, Cohen K, Passik S, The memorial delirium assessment scale, *J Pain Symptom Manage* 1997;**13**(3):128–137.
18. Inouye SK, The recognition of delirium, *Hosp Pract (Off Ed)* 1991;**26**(4A):61–62.
19. Breitbart W, Marotta R, Platt MM, et al., A double-blind trial of haloperidol, chlorpromazine, and lorazepam in the treatment of delirium in hospitalized AIDS patients, *Am J Psychiatry* 1996;**153**(2):231–237.
20. Boettger S, Breitbart W, Atypical antipsychotics in the management of delirium: a review of the empirical literature, *Palliat Support Care* 2005;**3**(3):227–237.
21. Alonso-Babarro A, Varela-Cedeira M, Torres-Vigil I, Rodriguez-Barrientos R, Bruera E, At-home palliative sedation for end-of-life cancer patients, *Palliat Med* 2010;**24**(5):486–492.

22. Elsayem A, Curry Iii E, Boohene J, et al., Use of palliative sedation for intractable symptoms in the palliative care unit of a comprehensive cancer center, *Support Care Cancer* 2009;**17**(1):53–59.

23. Caraceni A, Zecca E, Martini C, et al., Palliative sedation at the end of life at a tertiary cancer center, *Support Care Cancer* 2012;**20**(6):1299–1307.

24. Mercadante S, Porzio G, Valle A, Fusco F, Aielli F, Costanzo V, Palliative sedation in advanced cancer patients followed at home: a retrospective analysis, *J Pain Symptom Manage* 2012;**43**(6):1126–1130.

25. Bruera E, Sala R, Rico MA, et al., Effects of parenteral hydration in terminally ill cancer patients: a preliminary study, *J Clin Oncol* 2005;**23**(10):2366–2371.

26. Bruera E, Hui D, Dalal S, Torres-Vigil I, et al., Parental hydration in patients with advanced cancer: a multicenter, double blind, placebo-controlled randomized trial, *J Clin Oncol* 2013 Jan 1;**31**(1):111–118.

27. Delgado-Guay MO, Yennurajalingam S, Bruera E, Delirium with severe symptom expression related to hypercalcemia in a patient with advanced cancer: an interdisciplinary approach to treatment, *J Pain Symptom Manage* 2008;**36**(4):442–449.

ONLINE RESOURCES

Confusion Assessment Method: Training Manual: http://hospitalelderlifeprogram.org/private/cam-disclaimer. php?pageid=01.08.00

MedCalc app includes CAM-ICU calculator: http://www.appannie.com/apps/ios/app/medcalc-medical-calculator/

Palliative Care Fast Facts: http://www.eperc.mcw.edu/EPERC/FastFactsandConcepts

Up to date: http://www.uptodate.com and mobile application

Chapter 6

Depression and Anxiety: Assessment and Management in Hospitalized Patients with Serious Illness

Nathan Fairman, Jeremy M. Hirst, and Scott A. Irwin

6.1 INTRODUCTION

Symptoms of depression and anxiety are a common source of suffering in patients with advanced, life-threatening medical illness. In the palliative care setting, and particularly near the end of life, clinicians and caregivers may overlook the impact of these psychological symptoms, assuming that they are normal or expected experiences. However, addressing symptoms of depression and anxiety is an important therapeutic aim, for a variety of reasons. When unrecognized, or ineffectively treated, depression and anxiety can contribute to significant morbidity and mortality. High levels of psychological distress can negatively impact physical health and quality of life, complicate management of a primary illness, and contribute to significant distress in the patient, loved ones, and clinicians. Depression, for example, is a well-known risk factor for suicide, and it also independently predicts mortality in cancer [1], and it is a significant predictor of caregiver stress [2]. Similarly, anxiety symptoms in patients with advanced illness undermine quality of life and can erode patients' trust in their physicians [3].

Fortunately, even among seriously ill patients, these symptoms can often be effectively treated. For these reasons, there is a great need for generalist competency in the identification, diagnosis, and management of depression and anxiety in palliative care patients in the acute care setting. These competencies include:

1. Recognizing symptoms of depression and anxiety in seriously ill patients
2. Differentiating among a variety of conditions marked by the symptoms of depression and anxiety

Hospital-Based Palliative Medicine: A Practical, Evidence-Based Approach, First Edition.
Edited by Steven Pantilat, Wendy Anderson, Matthew Gonzales, and Eric Widera.

3. Initiating evidence-based treatments, both pharmacological and nonphar-macological

4. Knowing when and how to consult with other specialists in order to comprehensively address psychological distress

This chapter is aimed at helping hospital clinicians to acquire these competencies.

Several caveats warrant mention: first, for the most part, the focus of this chapter is on patients who *do not* have preexisting psychiatric illness (psychotic disorders, affective disorders, personality disorders, etc.). When these conditions are present, management often requires consultation with a psychiatrist, preferably with expertise/experience in psychosomatics or palliative medicine. The fourth competency—knowing when and how to consult—addresses this issue in more detail at the end of the chapter.

Second, depression and anxiety both exist on continua. "Depression" can range from transient feelings of sadness to the pathological condition of unrelenting and debilitating impairments in mood and cognition that are observed in major depressive disorder (MDD). Similarly, although anxiety and worry may be part of the normal response to the stress of a serious medical problem, high levels of persistent and disabling anxiety are *not* an inevitable part of the illness experience for patients with an advanced medical illness [4]. MDD and anxiety disorders are psychiatric illnesses, which account for an enormous burden of suffering; yet, they are treatable. An important challenge for hospital clinicians is to be able to distinguish the normal experiences of sadness and worry from the disorders of depression and anxiety, so that these symptoms may be effectively addressed.

Finally, the general approach to addressing psychiatric distress in seriously ill patients, including in the acute hospital setting, is rooted in basic palliative care principles: optimal care is provided by an interdisciplinary team, interventions need to be informed by knowledge of prognosis and goals of care, physical symptoms and other dimensions of distress need to be addressed, nonpharmacologic interventions should be optimized, and drug treatments should be provided in time-limited therapeutic trials.

6.2 RECOGNIZING SYMPTOMS OF DEPRESSION AND ANXIETY IN SERIOUSLY ILL PATIENTS

6.2.1 Prevalence of Depression and Anxiety in Palliative Care

Symptoms of depression and anxiety are common in patients with serious medical illnesses, and prevalence estimates range widely, depending on the definitions used and populations studied. Symptoms of depression have been reported in up to 42% of patients in palliative medicine settings [5], and significant anxiety may occur in up to 70% of patients with serious medical illness [6]. In terms of psychiatric disorders, prevalence estimates have not been systematically investigated in palliative care populations, though many studies suggest that MDD and anxiety disorders—beyond just symptoms—are present at higher levels than among healthy individuals. For example, recent data indicates that 20.7% of patients with advanced cancer may meet criteria for major or minor depression, and 13.9% meet the diagnostic threshold for an anxiety disorder [6].

6.2.2 Assessment of Depression and Anxiety

As in the vast majority of psychiatric illnesses, disorders of depression and anxiety are established based on a *clinical diagnosis*; there are no diagnostic tests to confirm a hunch, though some screening tools may be helpful. Diagnosis relies on the patient's subjective history, collateral information from reliable sources, and careful observation by the clinician—coupled with knowledge of the distinguishing characteristics of the different conditions marked by depression and/ or anxiety.

Depression may manifest with obvious changes in mood (feeling sad, down, deflated, etc.) or with disinterest in enjoyable activities. In the hospital setting, such changes are frequently accompanied by disengagement during visits by loved ones or apathy and low motivation to participate in hospital treatments. Depression frequently affects patients in behavioral, cognitive, and somatic domains as well, which will be described in more detail later. The emergence of any of these changes may raise suspicion for depression.

The experience of anxiety, too, may occur in several different domains—emotional, physical, behavioral, and cognitive—each associated with unique signs and symptoms. Patients frequently use words such as "concerned," "scared," "worried," and "nervous" to convey the psychological experience of anxiety or fear. Attention to these keywords can aid the clinician in pinpointing the presence of anxiety [7]. In palliative care settings, anxiety is frequently described as a feeling of helplessness or fear, often generated by illness-related factors. Fear of uncontrolled symptoms, or losing independence, may even result in a desire for death. Patients with a short prognosis often worry about the dying process. They frequently voice concerns about religious beliefs, spiritual issues, existential matters, or how to achieve a good death.

Several simple, clinically useful screening instruments have been shown to improve the detection of depression and anxiety, though the reliability and validity of these measures in the palliative care population have not been systematically examined [8]. With respect to depression, the Patient Health Questionnaire (PHQ-9), the Hospital Anxiety and Depression Scale (HADS), and the CES-D Boston Short Form are perhaps the most widely used, and useful, screening tools in a clinical setting for these issues. Even the simple query "Are you depressed?" has been shown to have high validity in diagnosing depression [9]. The Profile of Mood States and the Generalized Anxiety Disorder Screener (GAD–7) are commonly used, in addition to the HADS, to identify and characterize symptoms of anxiety.

6.3   DIFFERENTIATING AMONG CONDITIONS MARKED BY SYMPTOMS OF DEPRESSION AND ANXIETY

6.3.1   Differential Diagnosis: Major Depression and Its Look-Alikes

Perhaps the most challenging task in addressing depression and anxiety in seriously ill patients is to be able to distinguish among the many different conditions that are marked by these symptoms. For example, while depressed mood is the hallmark of MDD, this symptom may also characterize a variety of other conditions, including adjustment disorder, dysthymia, grief, and demoralization syndrome. The features that distinguish these conditions are described in detail later and summarized in Table 6.1. Since treatment approaches may differ, it can be important to distinguish one condition from another.

Major depression is the condition against which others are compared [10]. The disorder is characterized by the presence of a major depressive episode,[1] which occurs when a patient experiences either a depressed mood or anhedonia (loss of interest in pleasurable activity), nearly every day, over a period of at least 2 weeks.[2] In addition, in major depression, the depressed mood or anhedonia is accompanied by a number of cognitive or somatic symptoms. Cognitive changes may include poor concentration or indecision, as well as thoughts of worthlessness, hopelessness, guilt, or death. Somatic symptoms may include changes in appetite or weight, changes in sleep, decreased energy, or changes in psychomotor activity. As with all psychiatric illnesses, significant functional impairment—major problems in relationships, at work, or in self-care—needs to be present in order for the condition to be considered pathological.

Particularly in patients with serious illness and perhaps even more so in the acute care setting, differentiating normal states of sadness from major depression can be quite challenging, even for experienced clinicians. Patients with advanced illness will commonly experience episodes of intense sadness; many endure periods of anhedonia, low motivation, and even hopelessness; and it should be expected that seriously ill patients will also contemplate death. Taken individually, none of these phenomena should be assumed to indicate the presence of pathological depression. Similarly, the somatic dimensions of major depression (e.g., changes in sleep, low energy, changes in weight and appetite) frequently overlap with the physical symptoms seen in advanced medical illnesses, and so these alone are not reliable indicators of depression in this population. Instead, experts in palliative care psychiatry give greater weight to the emotional and cognitive symptoms of depression, as well

---

1 A major depressive episode may be seen in bipolar disorder as well, and screening for the absence of historical periods of mania or hypomania will distinguish major depression from bipolar disorder. This distinction is important therapeutically, as antidepressant therapy is likely to be ineffective, and may be harmful, in depressed patients with bipolar disease.

2 If neither depressed mood nor anhedonia is present, major depression should not be diagnosed; other conditions need to be considered.

Table 6.1 Distinguishing among Major Depressive Disorder and Its Look-Alikes

Condition	Characteristics	General Approach to Treatment
Major depressive disorder (MDD) [10]	A. Five or more of the following present, over at least 2 weeks, and at least one of the symptoms is either depressed mood or anhedonia: 　1. Depressed mood (or, in children/adolescents, irritable mood) 　2. Anhedonia: markedly reduced interest/pleasure in most activities 　3. Changes in weight or appetite 　4. Insomnia or hypersomnia 　5. Psychomotor agitation or retardation 　6. Fatigue or diminished energy 　7. Feelings of worthlessness or excessive guilt 　8. Poor concentration or indecisiveness 　9. Recurrent thoughts of death, suicidal ideation, or suicidal behavior B. Symptoms cause clinically significant distress or functional impairment C. Symptoms are not the result of substances or a medical condition D. Symptoms are not better explained by one of the psychotic disorders E. The patient has never experienced mania or hypomania	Drug therapy + Psychotherapy
Persistent depressive disorder [10]	Formerly called dysthymia; conceptualized as a chronic depressive illness (whereas MDD is episodic), of mild to moderate severity, *with no history of a major depressive episode* Expanded in DSM-5 to include more serious/persistent forms in which full criteria for a major depressive episode are continuously met over a period of at least 2 years	Drug therapy + Psychotherapy Frequently challenging to treat, may warrant lower threshold to consult with specialist
Unspecified depressive disorder [10]	Clinically significant distress from depression, accompanied by functional impairment, but which does not meet criteria for any of the more specific depressive illnesses NOTE: this should not be used for patients experiencing normal sadness without clear functional consequences	Continued assessment/ clarification of diagnosis + Psychotherapy

(Continued)

Table 6.1 (*Continued*)

Condition	Characteristics	General Approach to Treatment
Adjustment disorder with depressed mood [10]	Emotional/behavioral symptoms that develop within 3 months of an identifiable stressor Symptoms are disproportionate to the severity or intensity of the stressor May occur with features of depression, anxiety, behavior, or any combination NOTE: if criteria are met for MDD, MDD should be diagnosed and not adjustment disorder	Supportive counseling aimed at bolstering coping skills Problem solving aimed at resolving/removing stressor
Grief [10]	In grief, the predominant emotional state is characterized by emptiness and loss; in MDD, it is depressed mood and/or inability to experience pleasure In grief, dysphoria often occurs in waves, generally triggered by thoughts/memories of the deceased; in MDD, dysphoria is unrelenting, and cognitions center on worthlessness/hopelessness In grief, the mood state is reactive (i.e., individuals can have periods of happiness, laughter, etc. in relation to pleasant or humorous experiences); in MDD, the mood state can be pervasive or intractable In grief, self-esteem may be preserved, and if feelings of guilt are present, they are usually constrained to the relationship with the deceased In grief, thoughts of death often concern "joining" the deceased; in MDD, they are aimed at ending one's own life and rooted in feelings of hopelessness and worthlessness NOTE: bereavement is no longer an exclusion criteria for MDD. Even in the setting of bereavement, if criteria are met for MDD, MDD should be diagnosed and appropriate treatment initiated	Supportive counseling/ psychotherapy
Demoralization [11]	Marked by subjective incompetence (sense of failure), hopelessness, and despair Often, reactivity of mood is preserved Insufficient evidence for demoralization as a separate diagnostic category	

as changes in mood from baseline, and the intensity and time course of symptoms [12]. Thus, feelings of worthlessness, hopelessness, guilt, or thoughts of suicide are likely to indicate major depression, whereas changes in appetite or level of energy may represent symptoms of the underlying medical illness. Similarly, true anhedonia, in which the patient is *disinterested* in the things that once gave pleasure (and not simply unable to engage in those activities due to physical limitations), helps to identify major depression.

While major depression is the illness most clinicians have in mind when they refer to a patient as being "clinically depressed," several other important conditions may overlap with, or may be mistaken for, MDD. *Adjustment disorder* occurs in the context of an identifiable stressor, in which the patient experiences marked distress (in the form of depression, anxiety, or behavioral disturbances) to a degree in excess of the intensity of the stressor. In theory, the approach to "treatment" in adjustment disorder is nonpharmacologic, aimed at bolstering coping strategies or resolving/removing the stressor. *Grief*, the emotional experience associated with a significant loss, is also a distinct experience from major depression, though the two conditions have in common the experience of a depressed mood [13]. Of note, in the most recent iteration of the Diagnostic and Statistic Manual of Mental Disorders (DSM), the "bereavement exception" was removed from the diagnosis of MDD, so that even in the setting of bereavement, MDD should be diagnosed (and treatment considered) if criteria are met [10]. This distinction is important because the general approach to addressing grief, in the absence of major depression, should be with supportive therapeutic interventions and not drug therapy, though medication for specific symptoms, such as insomnia, can be helpful for brief periods. *Demoralization syndrome* captures a suite of psychological phenomena commonly seen in patients with advanced, serious illnesses, which may overlap with major depression [11]. At the core of demoralization syndrome is a sense of subjective incompetence, arising from the loss of purpose and meaning that may result from a serious medical illness. As distinct from depression, in which anhedonia robs patients of the ability to experience pleasure, demoralization syndrome is marked by profound hopelessness, robbing patients of the ability to imagine a fulfilling future. Also, the demoralized patient retains the reactivity of mood (i.e., they can experience happiness in relation to positive events), which is frequently lost in depression. There is considerable debate, beyond the scope of this chapter, as to whether or not demoralization syndrome can be reliably distinguished from major depression.

Finally, two common neurocognitive disorders, *delirium* and *dementia*, may also sometimes be mistaken for depression, particularly when marked by social withdrawal, psychomotor retardation, and abulia (diminished motivation). In both conditions, however, the predominant symptom is a significant cognitive disturbance, with an onset that is generally insidious (in the case of dementia), or acute/subacute (in the case of delirium). While cognitive deficits are seen in major depression, these tend to arise only after the emergence of changes in mood or the development of anhedonia.

6.3.2 Differential Diagnosis: Anxiety Disorders and Anxiety Symptoms

Anxiety symptoms may be the hallmark of a mental illness, the consequence of a physiologic problem, or the reaction to psychosocial stressors. In terms of psychiatric conditions, anxiety disorders encountered most often in palliative care settings include adjustment disorder with anxiety, generalized anxiety disorder, panic disorder, and posttraumatic stress disorder. The features that distinguish these conditions are described in Table 6.2. Other psychiatric conditions may mimic or exacerbate

Table 6.2 Anxiety Disorders Commonly Encountered in the Palliative Care Setting

Condition	Characteristics	General Approach to Treatment
Adjustment disorder with anxiety [10]	Emotional/behavioral symptoms that develop within 3 months of an identifiable stressor	Supportive counseling aimed at bolstering coping skills
	Symptoms are disproportionate to the severity or intensity of the stressor	Problem solving aimed at resolving/removing stressor
	May occur with features of depression, anxiety, behavior, or any combination	
	Symptoms do not meet criteria for any particular anxiety disorder	Symptom-focused, time-limited drug treatments
Generalized anxiety disorder [10]	A state of excessive and uncontrollable anxiety or worry, lasting at least 6 months and impacting day-to-day activities	Drug therapy + Psychotherapy
	People suffering with generalized anxiety are often described as worriers by their friends and families	
Panic attack/ panic disorder [10]	Sudden onset of intense discomfort apprehension, fearfulness, terror, or a feeling of impending doom, usually occurring with symptoms such as shortness of breath, palpitations, chest discomfort, a sense of choking, and fear of "going crazy" or losing control, often in unexpected situations	Psychotherapy (cognitive behavioral) + Drug therapy
	Panic attacks are discrete, usually lasting 15–20 min	
	Panic disorder is marked by recurrent panic attacks occur, accompanied by worry about future attacks, with significant impairment in psychosocial functioning	
Posttraumatic stress disorder [10]	Reexperiencing of a traumatic event, with symptoms of increased arousal, nightmares, intrusive memories, hypervigilance, and avoidance of reminders of the event	Drug therapy + Psychotherapy

anxiety, and these should be distinguished from a primary anxiety disorder. In particular, depression, dementia, and delirium may each present with strong anxiety components. In the palliative care population, and perhaps even more so in the acute hospital setting, symptoms of anxiety may commonly result from physiologic derangements due to an underlying medical illness, such as advanced COPD or hyperthyroidism. What's more, among seriously ill patients, particularly those approaching death, the social, spiritual, and existential dimensions of distress often manifest as anxiety. Table 6.3 enumerates some of these nonpsychiatric causes of anxiety.

Characterizing the source and nature of a patient's anxiety will enable hospitalist clinicians to more effectively intervene to alleviate suffering associated with anxiety. In general, anxiety disorders are addressed through a combination of psychotherapy and long-term antidepressant therapy, while symptoms of anxiety that result from physiologic disturbances and psychosocial stressors are best approached by seeking to address the underlying cause of anxiety, and medication therapies are typically symptom driven and used on an as-needed basis.

Table 6.3   Common Nonpsychiatric Causes of Anxiety in the Palliative Care Setting

Physical Conditions
　　Respiratory failure (dyspnea, hypoxia, increased respiratory effort)
　　Fatigue/weakness
　　Uncontrolled pain or other physical symptoms
　　Insomnia
　　Hypoglycemia, sepsis, fever, hypertension
　　CNS malignancy
　　Drugs (steroids, opioids, withdrawal states, adverse drug reactions such as akathisia)
　　Delirium
Practical Issues
　　Concerns about finances
　　Fear of unknown/hospital/treatment
　　Uncertainty about future/lack of information/inadequate information
Social Issues
　　Isolation/inadequate support
　　Concerns about family/caregivers
　　Disrupted family/peer relationships
Existential and Spiritual Concerns
　　Religious doubt/loss of faith
　　Loss of role
　　Sense of purposelessness
　　Hopelessness
　　Fear of mental impairment
　　Fear of loss of independence
　　Fear of dying
　　Feelings of guilt/regret

Source: Adapted from Irwin [14].

6.4 MANAGEMENT OF DEPRESSION AND ANXIETY IN PALLIATIVE CARE

Effective treatments exist for depression and anxiety, even in seriously ill patients. What's more, there is substantial overlap in the management strategies for these two conditions. Many nonpharmacologic approaches to depression are also useful in the management of anxiety, and even the standard drug treatments are often effective as long-term therapy for both conditions. There is a substantial body of high-quality evidence that supports combined treatment with medication and therapy for patients with MDD or anxiety disorders. The role for drug treatments is less clear in patients with symptoms of depression and anxiety that do not fit the clear diagnostic pattern of a psychiatric illness. However, most (though not all) drug therapies for depression and anxiety are relatively well tolerated and have few serious potential side effects and few drug–drug interactions. In this setting (where there is uncertain effectiveness but low expected harm), many experts in psychiatric palliative care encourage a low threshold to consider carefully supervised, time-limited therapeutic trials of medication—with consideration of a specialist referral if these initial strategies are ineffective.

6.4.1 Management of Depression in Palliative Care

The "gold standard" treatment for MDD includes a combination of patient and family education, psychotherapy, and antidepressant medication. Each of these approaches is employed in addressing depression in the palliative care setting [15], and they can be provided in the acute care environment.[3]

Psychotherapy. Even the busy hospitalist can provide valuable psychosocial support at the bedside. Some of the most basic elements of establishing rapport—use of active listening skills, seeking to clarify patients' concerns, engaging loved ones, and mobilizing support systems—will go a long way toward reducing distress. Chochinov [16] captures this succinctly: "comfort is often conveyed by a committed presence, various forms of affirmation, compassion and innumerable acts of kindnesses." Beyond this, formal psychotherapy interventions may be available through consultation with mental health specialists in the acute care setting, and these should be considered for any patient with high levels of psychological distress, irrespective of the etiology. Though the quality of evidence varies widely, a number of different psychotherapies have been shown to improve symptoms of depression in seriously ill patients, including cognitive-behavioral therapies [17], supportive–expressive group therapy [18], dignity therapy [19], and meaning-centered psychotherapy [20]. Awareness of these modalities and knowledge about local access to psychotherapy providers will enhance the hospitalist's ability to pair patients with appropriate interventions.

3 Electroconvulsive therapy (ECT) is also a highly effective treatment for depression, particularly suited for those with treatment-resistant depression and a prognosis of several months or more. Some hospitalist clinicians may have access to ECT, particularly those practicing in tertiary-care centers. Consideration of ECT should always involve consultation with a psychiatrist.

Pharmacotherapy. For hospitalist clinicians, drug treatments are the mainstay of depression management. In general, the antidepressant agents typically used in healthy patients are also recommended in palliative care, but other drug treatments may be warranted in this setting as well.

STANDARD ANTIDEPRESSANTS. Antidepressant drugs commonly used in the palliative care setting are described in detail in Table 6.4. Since these agents are essentially indistinguishable on the basis of efficacy in alleviating depression, familiarity with other distinguishing features (Table 6.5) will enable the hospital clinician to select from among different drugs. Among the standard antidepressant drugs, *selective serotonin reuptake inhibitors* (SSRIs), such as fluoxetine, sertraline, and citalopram, are perhaps the most familiar and widely used. Relative to the tricyclic antidepressants (TCAs),[4] which used to be considered first-line agents, SSRIs tend to have fewer autonomic and anticholinergic side effects. Side effects common to SSRIs include transient nausea, GI upset, and headache, and most of these agents can cause significant sexual side effects. Some of these drugs, particularly citalopram, may carry a dose-dependent propensity to prolong the QTc interval. Relative to the SSRIs, the *serotonin/norepinephrine reuptake inhibitors* (SNRIs), such as venlafaxine and duloxetine, have similar efficacy in treating MDD, may be more effective in certain anxiety disorders, and have strong data for efficacy in reducing neuropathic pain. As a class, SNRIs share a similar side effect profile with the SSRIs. Finally, several other agents with unique mechanisms of action—notably bupropion and mirtazapine—are also considered first-line antidepressants. Bupropion has mild stimulant properties and is frequently used in patients with significant fatigue or anergia, while mirtazapine can improve anorexia and insomnia at the low end of its dose range.

PSYCHOSTIMULANTS. Standard antidepressant therapies frequently fall short near the end of life, because the time course to effectiveness can be protracted: while some patients will experience improvement early in the course of therapy, those who fail to respond quickly need to remain on the drug for roughly 8 weeks at the target dose in order to adequately gauge response. By contrast, psychostimulants have been shown to produce rapid antidepressant effects, and a therapeutic trial can often be completed in a small number of days. For this reason, in situations where the expected prognosis is short, psychostimulants may be considered first-line agents for treating depression [23]. Typically, treatment is initiated at a low dose and titrated daily until either the clinical target is reached, or unwanted side effects emerge, such as anxiety, restlessness, or insomnia. Patients with existing anxiety or with cardiac tachyarrhythmias should be monitored closely for adverse effects.

---

4 Tricyclic Antidepressants (TCAs) are rarely used for the management of depression in palliative care, due in particular to their anticholinergic effects and the risks of delirium in medically ill patients. However, in patients who are refractory to first-line antidepressants, or who have had success in the past with TCAs, these may warrant consideration. TCAs do have strong evidence of efficacy in reducing neuropathic pain, but even for this indication the SNRIs are often preferred due to their favorable side effect profile.

Table 6.4 Drug Treatments for Major Depression and Anxiety Disorders in the Palliative Care Setting

Drug	Condition		Dosing/Titration	Notes
	Depression	Anxiety		
Selective Serotonin Reuptake Inhibitors (SSRIs)				
Citalopram	✓	✓ (chronic)	Depression: 20 mg PO qDAY, increasing after >1 week, to 40 mg PO qDAY	Less sedation and dry mouth than TCAs
				Often have sexual side effects
				Adequate trial requires ~6–8 weeks at therapeutic dose
			Anxiety: 10 mg PO qDAY, increasing by 10 mg every 1–2 weeks, to 40 mg PO qDAY	Well-tolerated
				Few drug–drug interactions
				Taper to DC, when possible
				Significant risk of QTc prolongation at doses >40 mg qDAY
				Available routes: PO (tabs, liq)
Escitalopram	✓	✓ (chronic)	Depression: 10 mg PO qDAY, increasing after >1 week, to 20 mg PO qDAY	Well tolerated
			Anxiety: 5 mg PO qDAY, increasing by 5–10 mg every 1–2 weeks, to 20 mg PO qDAY	Few drug–drug interactions
				Taper to DC, when possible
				Available routes: PO (tabs, liq)
Fluoxetine	✓	✓ (chronic)	Depression: 20 mg PO qDAY, increasing after >1 week, to 40 mg PO qDAY	Many drug–drug interactions
			Anxiety: 10 mg PO qDAY, increasing by 10 mg every 1–2 weeks, to 60 mg PO qDAY	Wide dose range: 5–80 mg qDAY
				Do not need to taper to DC (very long $t_{\frac{1}{2}}$)
				May be activating in some patients
				Available routes: PO (tabs, caps, liq)
Paroxetine	✓	✓ (chronic)	Depression: 20 mg PO qDAY, increasing after >1 week, to 40 mg PO qDAY	Many drug–drug interactions
			Anxiety: 10 mg PO qDAY, increasing by 10 mg every 1–2 weeks, to 60 mg PO qDAY	Significant discontinuation syndrome (very short $t_{\frac{1}{2}}$); taper to DC; use caution when oral route is unreliable
				Available routes: PO (tabs, liq)

Sertraline	✓	✓ (chronic)	Depression: 50 mg PO qDAY, increasing by 50 mg every > 1 week, to 200 mg PO qDAY Anxiety: 25 mg PO qAM, increasing by 25–50 mg every 1–2 weeks, to 200 mg PO qDAY	Well tolerated Few drug–drug interactions Taper to DC, when possible Available routes: PO (tabs, liq)
Serotonin/Norepinephrine Reuptake Inhibitors (SNRIs)				Effective adjuncts for neuropathic pain Sometimes have a mild stimulant effect Often have sexual side effects Adequate trial requires ~6–8 weeks at therapeutic dose
Venlafaxine	✓	✓ (chronic)	Depression: (extended release) 75 mg PO qDAY, increasing by 75 mg every 4 days, up to 225 mg PO qDAY Anxiety: (extended release) 37.5 mg PO qDAY, increasing by 37.5–75 mg every 1 week, up to 225 mg PO qDAY	Many common adverse effects (e.g., insomnia, headache, hypertension) Effective in neuropathic pain (higher doses) Significant discontinuation syndrome (very short $t_{1/2}$); taper to DC; use caution when oral route is unreliable Extended-release formulation permits qDAY dosing Available routes: PO (tabs, caps)
Duloxetine	✓	✓ (chronic)	Depression: 30 mg PO qDAY, increasing by 30 mg every 1 week, up to 120 mg PO qDAY Anxiety: 30 mg PO qDAY, increasing by 30 mg every 1 week, up to 120 mg PO qDAY	Effective in neuropathic pain Doses > 120 mg qDAY rarely more effective Significant discontinuation syndrome; taper to DC; use caution when oral route is unreliable Available routes: PO (caps)

(*Continued*)

Table 6.4 (*Continued*)

| Drug | Condition | | Dosing/Titration | Notes |
	Depression	Anxiety		
Miscellaneous Antidepressants				
Bupropion	✓	×	Depression SR formulation: 150 mg PO qAM, increasing after 3 days to 150 mg PO BID XL formulation: 150 mg PO qAM, increasing after 3 days to 300 mg PO qAM and then increasing after 2 weeks to 450 mg PO qAM	Effective as single agents, also used to augment effectiveness of SSRI/SNRI Weak norepinephrine and dopamine reuptake inhibitor Contraindicated with seizures or eating disorders Mild stimulant effect: useful in patients with low energy but may cause insomnia (with BID dosing, PM dose should not be given after 1400h) May improve concentration May augment antidepressant effect and reduce sexual side effect of SSRIs Multiple formulations available (IR, SR, XL); XL formulation permits qDAY dosing Available routes: PO (tabs)
Mirtazapine	✓	✓ (chronic)	Depression: 15 mg PO qHS, increasing by 15 mg every 1–2 weeks, up to 45 mg PO qHS Anxiety: 7.5 mg PO qHS, increasing by 7.5–15 mg every 1–2 weeks, up to 45 mg PO qHS	Exact mechanism of action is unknown (increases central serotonergic and noradrenergic activity) At lower doses, causes sedation and stimulates appetite; useful in patients with insomnia and anorexia Causes orthostatic hypotension Available routes: PO (tabs, ODT)
Psychostimulants				
Methylphenidate	✓	×	Depression: 2.5 mg PO BID, increasing by 5 mg/day (divided) every 5 days, up to ~15 mg PO BID	Rapid antidepressant effect Consider first line when prognosis <2 months May worsen/cause anxiety May worsen/cause insomnia (BID dosing should be scheduled at 0800 + 1400 h) Doses >30 mg/day usually not necessary Available routes: PO (tabs, caps, liq)

Medication	Chronic	Acute	Dosing	Notes
Experimental "Antidepressants"				
Ketamine	✓	?		Moderate-strength data in healthy populations using IV route Very limited data in palliative care/hospice setting: single open-label trial of daily oral administration suggests reductions in depression and anxiety Reserved for experimental use until better data available
Benzodiazepines				Effective anxiolytics but should be used with great caution in palliative care setting Cause sedation, confusion/delirium, falls, disinhibition Avoid short half-life agents (e.g., alprazolam)
Lorazepam	×	✓ (acute)	Anxiety: 0.25–2 mg PO q 1 h PRN anxiety	Wide dose range; adjust to desired effect or side effect, and then consider scheduled dose based on demand $t_{1/2}$ = 12 – 14 h Safer in liver failure than clonazepam Available routes: PO (tabs, liq)/SL/SC/IM/IV
Clonazepam	×	✓ (acute)	Anxiety: 0.125–1 mg q 1 h PO PRN anxiety	Wide dose range; adjust to desired effect or side effect, and then consider scheduled dose based on demand $t_{1/2}$ = 30–40 h Despite long $t_{1/2}$, many patients require BID–TID dosing Clonazepam 0.25 mg ≈ lorazepam 1 mg Available routes: PO (tabs, ODT)
Off-Label "Anxiolytics"				
Gabapentin	×	? (acute)	Anxiety: 50–300 mg PO q 1 h PRN for anxiety (NTE 3 doses or 600 mg/24 h)	Consider for off-label PRN use in anxiety Effective in neuropathic pain Requires dose adjustment in renal failure Available routes: PO (tabs, caps, liq)

(Continued)

Table 6.4 (*Continued*)

Drug	Condition Depression	Condition Anxiety	Dosing/Titration	Notes
Trazodone	✓	? (acute)	Depression: rarely used for this indication Anxiety: 25–50 mg PO q 1 h PRN anxiety (may titrate to 200 mg/dose, NTE 400 mg/24 h)	Antidepressant, potentiates CNS serotonergic activity Off-label treatment of insomnia is the most common use Adverse effects: sedation, restlessness, dry mouth, priapism (rare) Wide dose range; adjust to desired effect or side effect, and then consider scheduled dose based on demand Available routes: PO (tabs)
Valproic acid	✗	? (acute)	Anxiety: 250 mg PO BID	Antiepileptic and mood stabilizer with unknown mechanism of action (involving increased CNS GABA) Avoid or use with caution in hepatic impairment Available routes: PO (caps, liq)/IV

Notes:

- Dosing guidelines reflect a general, initial strategy, based on current references [21] and clinical experience of the authors. Consult with local experts/resources for specific concerns (e.g., dosing strategies in incomplete responders or dose adjustments in hepatic/renal insufficiency).
- All first-line antidepressants (SSRIs, SNRIs, bupropion, mirtazapine) have an FDA indication for major depressive disorder. FDA indications for anxiety disorders vary by drug and by the specific disorder, but in general, the first-line antidepressants (except bupropion) are also effective in anxiety disorders, though their use may be off-label. Use of other agents on this table is off-label.

Table 6.5   Factors to Consider in Choosing an Antidepressant in the Palliative Care Setting

Factor	Consideration
Prognosis	If prognosis is <2 months, consider psychostimulants as first line
Personal history	If the patient has previously had a good response with an agent, consider a rechallenge with the same agent
Family history	If a family member (especially first-degree relative) has had a favorable response with an agent, consider using the same agent
Common side effects	When possible, seek to match common side effects with patient's symptoms or goals of care
	Example: consider mirtazapine in patients with anorexia and insomnia
	Example: consider bupropion in patients with anergia/fatigue
Presence of neuropathy	Consider SNRIs or TCAs. May permit reduced use of opioids and help to limit polypharmacy
Discontinuation syndromes	If loss of the oral route is anticipated, consider avoiding agents with significant discontinuation syndromes (e.g., paroxetine, venlafaxine)
Drug–drug interactions [22]	Most first-line antidepressants are P450 substrates, and many also exhibit P450 inhibition. Many have P-glycoprotein activity, though these effects tend to be less well characterized. Check drug–drug interactions with a pharmacist or online resource

FUTURE AGENTS. Finally, several agents have recently emerged with promise for the rapid treatment of depression. Of these, ketamine currently has the strongest evidence: in a series of well-designed randomized trials, subanesthetic intravenous administration of ketamine in medically healthy subjects with depression has consistently produced rapid antidepressant effects [24]. Building on this data, a recent open-label pilot study has suggested a potential role for daily oral ketamine in the treatment of depression in hospice patients [25]. Further investigation will be necessary to clarify the role for this promising treatment for depression in palliative care.

6.4.2   Management of Anxiety in Palliative Care

Treatment of anxiety may include a combination of supportive care, psychotherapy, complementary or alternative therapies, and pharmacotherapy. As with depression, a combination of approaches is generally more effective than any one modality alone. Strong data supports the use of medication therapies for anxiety disorders, but the effectiveness of off-label, symptom-driven drug treatment is less clear. Because of the close links among anxiety, physiologic disturbances, and psychosocial stressors, it is vitally important to identify and address any physiologic or psychosocial conditions that may cause or amplify symptoms of anxiety; doing so will sometimes result in alleviation of anxiety without the need for pharmacologic interventions.

Nonpharmacological Interventions. As in the management of depression, hospital-ist clinicians can provide valuable supportive contact through careful listening, exploration of concerns, and mobilizing systems of support. Concerns about medical interventions, finances, family conflicts, future disability, dependency, existential questions, and dying do not resolve with medication. Patients and families are usu-ally receptive to exploration of the specific issues that are causing or exacerbating anxiety. Providing education about the expected course of serious illness and what to expect at each stage may further decrease patients' levels of anxiety and worry. Reinforcing that distressing symptoms will be managed aggressively will help reduce anticipatory worry over future suffering. In addition, as with depression, several formal psychotherapies have been shown to have strong efficacy in treating specific anxiety disorders, though for the most part these treatments have not been investi-gated in the acute care setting with palliative care populations.

Several complementary nonpharmacologic approaches have shown promise in reducing anxiety in palliative care settings. Relaxation training, for example, can be provided at relatively low cost and has long-term effects when practiced consistently [26]. Other nonpharmacologic interventions that target anxiety include music therapy, hypnotherapy, acupuncture, mindfulness meditation, aromatherapy, massage, and art therapy [27]. In general, it is recommended that clinicians have a low threshold to recommend treatment with these modalities, if they are locally available.

Pharmacotherapy. A recent Cochrane review found insufficient evidence to guide pharmacologic management of anxiety in adult palliative care populations [28]. In this context, drug treatments are guided by data from nonpalliative care populations or clinical expertise, and—as with other therapies in palliative care—interventions should be rooted in clear knowledge of goals of care and structured in time-limited therapeutic trials. Drug treatments for anxiety, detailed in Table 6.4, can generally be grouped on the basis of the duration of time required for a therapeutic trial.

ANTIDEPRESSANTS. Among the agents requiring a protracted therapeutic trial, a number of antidepressants have been shown to have efficacy in treating a variety of anxiety disorders, including both SSRIs and SNRIs. These agents are the drugs of choice for managing chronic anxiety disorders in patients with prognosis greater than 2 months. As with the treatment of depression, in the treatment of anxiety, individual antidepressants are difficult to distinguish on the basis of effectiveness—though some carry particular FDA-approved indications for specific anxiety conditions. Hence, the same strategies are used to select these agents when treating anxiety: knowledge of side effects, available routes of administration, cost, efficacy in family members, drug–drug interactions, etc. An impor-tant difference with respect to how these drugs are used in anxiety, however, concerns the dosing and titration: in general, it is recommended that therapy involve a lower initial dose, a slower rate of titration, and a higher target dose, relative to treatment in depression.

BENZODIAZEPINES. Just as in the management of depression, the slow titration of antide-pressants and the need for an extended therapeutic trial may not be practical for palliative care patients with a short prognosis. Benzodiazepines are often chosen for short-term, symptomatic management of anxiety, that is, when immediate relief is desired. Though these agents can be highly effective, they often cause serious adverse events in patients with advanced medical illnesses, such as confusion or delirium and gait instability or falls. Benzodiazepines should be used cautiously, if at all, in palliative care patients. Many experts advise against their use unless other, less harmful options have been unsuccessful and patients and family are thoroughly informed of the potential adverse effects. In general, very short half-life agents (e.g., alprazolam) are avoided altogether, because of likely problems with withdrawal and/or rebound anxiety. Instead, longer-acting formulations such as lorazepam and clonazepam are considered the agents of choice when benzodiazepines are used. Lorazepam is frequently chosen because it is available in several different routes, and its conjugative metabolism permits safer use in liver disease.

OTHER AGENTS. In light of the concerns around the use of benzodiazepines in seriously ill patients, coupled with the need for rapid relief of clinically significant anxiety when prognosis is short, some experts recommend off-label, time-limited therapeutic trials with other agents. Gabapentin, trazodone, and valproic acid, for example, are sometimes effective alternatives, and some experts recommend brief trials with these, based on clinical experience. Low-dose antipsychotic agents are sometimes used in a similar role, though there may be concerns about potential side effects (extrapyramidal symptoms, akathisia, sedation) and expense. Unfortunately, solid evidence for these therapies, beyond clinical experience, is lacking. For this reason, off-label use of psychotropic medication is often left to subspecialist clinicians.

6.5 CONSULTATION WITH OTHER SPECIALISTS

Knowing when to refer is perhaps the final competency in the care of hospitalized patients with symptoms of depression and anxiety. In complicated cases, or those where a second confirming opinion might be helpful, consultation can often benefit patients and families. Triggers for consultation can include preexisting psychopathology, refractory physical symptoms, ineffective initial treatments, diagnostic uncertainty, complicated family or interpersonal dynamics, concerns about polypharmacy or off-label use of psychiatric drugs, suicidal thoughts, or a desire for hastened death. Particularly in cases like these, relief of suffering often requires comprehensive, interspecialty care. Ideally, a psychiatrist with advanced palliative care psychiatry skills would be available for consultation. Alternatively, psychiatrists with subspecialty training in psychosomatic medicine (i.e., consult-liaison psychiatrists) can frequently facilitate more effective management in seriously ill patients. If the primary illness is oncologic, psycho-oncology specialists, where available, can fill the same role. In general, if psychiatric symptoms complicate management of the primary illness, or are a major source of suffering, or cannot be effectively addressed in the outpatient setting, then consultation from the acute care setting should not be delayed. The aim of consultation is to bring the right resources at the right time to the right patient, to ensure clinical excellence, produce favorable outcomes, and provide patient-centered care focused on symptom management and quality of life.

6.6 CONCLUSION

Patients with advancing, life-threatening illnesses frequently experience symptoms of depression and anxiety. If not identified and effectively addressed, these symptoms can seriously impair quality of life, increase morbidity and mortality, and may amplify distress in family, caregivers, and clinicians. As they may be the first to identify these symptoms, hospital clinicians can play a pivotal role in beginning to address psychological distress in seriously ill patients by early identification of symptoms of depression and anxiety, differentiating symptoms from disorders, initiating multi-modal treatments, and marshaling assistance from expert consultants when necessary. An interdisciplinary approach, rooted to the basic tenets of palliative care, can provide vital relief from depression and anxiety, even in the acute care setting.

REFERENCES

1. Satin JR, Linden W, Phillips MJ, Depression as a predictor of disease progression and mortality in cancer patients: a meta-analysis, *Cancer* 2009 Nov 15;**115**(22):5349–5361.
2. Hirdes JP, Freeman S, Smith TF, Stolee P, Predictors of caregiver distress among palliative home care clients in Ontario: evidence based on the InterRAI Palliative Care, *Palliat Support Care* 2012 Sep;**10**(3):155–163.
3. Zhang B, Nilsson ME, Prigerson HG, Factors important to patients' quality of life at the end of life, *Arch Intern Med* 2012 Aug 13;**172**(15):1133–1142.
4. Breitbart W, Chochinov HM, Passik S, Psychiatric symptoms in palliative medicine. In: Doyle D, Hanks GWC, Cherny NI, Calman K, editors. *Oxford Textbook of Palliative Medicine*, 4th ed. New York: Oxford University Press, 2011.
5. Wilson KG, Chochinov HM, de Faye BJ, Breitbart W, Diagnosis and management of depression in palliative care. In: Chochinov HM, Breitbart W, editors. *Handbook of Psychiatry in Palliative Medicine*. New York: Oxford University Press, 2000.
6. Wilson KG, Chochinov HM, Skirko MG, et al., Depression and anxiety disorders in palliative cancer care, *J Pain Symptom Manage* 2007 Feb;**33**(2):118–129.
7. Anderson WG, Alexander SC, Rodriguez KL, et al., "What concerns me is…" expression of emotion by advanced cancer patients during outpatient visits, *Support Care Cancer* 2008 Jul;**16**(7):803–811.
8. Wasteson E, Brenne E, Higginson IJ, et al., Depression assessment and classification in palliative care cancer patients: a systematic literature review, *Palliat Med7.* 2009 Dec;**23**(8):739–753.
9. Chochinov HM, Wilson KG, Enns M, Lander S, "Are you depressed?" Screening for depression in the terminally ill, *Am J Psychiatry* 1997 May;**154**(5);674–676.
10. American Psychiatric Association. *Diagnostic and Statistical Manual of Mental Disorders*, 5th ed. Arlington, VA: American Psychiatric Association, 2013.
11. Kissane DW, Clarke DM, Street AF. Demoralization syndrome—a relevant psychiatric diagnosis for palliative care. *J Palliat Care* 2001 Spring;**17**(1):12–21.
12. Block S, Perspectives on care at the end of life. Psychological considerations, growth, and transcendence at the end of life: the art of the possible, *JAMA* 2001 Jun 13;**285**(22):2898–2905.
13. Jacobsen JC, Zhang B, Block SD, Maciejewski PK, Prigerson HG. Distinguishing symptoms of grief and depression in a cohort of advanced cancer patients. *Death Stud* 2010 Mar;**34**(3):257–273.
14. Irwin SA, Fairman N, Montross L, UNIPAC 2: alleviating psychological and spiritual pain. In: Storey CP, editor. *UNIPAC*, 4th ed. Glenville, IL: American Academy of Hospice and Palliative Medicine, 2012.
15. Block SD, Assessing and managing depression in the terminally ill patient. ACP-ASIM E-of-Life Care Consensus Panel. American College of Physicians—American Society of Internal Medicine, *Ann Intern Med* 2000 Feb 1;**132**(3):209–218.

16. Chochinov HM, Dying, dignity, and new horizons in palliative end-of-life care, *CA Cancer J Clin* 2006 Mar–Apr;**56**(2):84–103.
17. Akechi T, Okuyama T, Onishi J, Morita T, Furukawa TA, Psychotherapy for depression among incurable cancer patients, *Cochrane Database Syst Rev* 2008 Apr 16;**2**:CD00537.
18. Kissane DW, Grabsch B, Clarke DM, et al., Supportive-expressive group therapy for women with metastatic breast cancer: survival and psychosocial outcome from a randomized controlled trial, *Psychooncology* 2007 Apr;**16**(4):277–286.
19. Chochinov HM, Kristjanson LJ, Breitbart W, et al., Effect of dignity therapy on distress and end-of-life experience in terminally ill patients: a randomized controlled trial, *Lancet Oncol* 2011 Aug;**12**(8):753–762.
20. Breitbart W. Poppito S, Rosenfeld B, et al., Pilot randomized controlled trial of individual meaning-centered psychotherapy for patients with advanced cancer, *J Clin Oncol* 2012 Apr 20;**30**(12):1304–1309.
21. Micromedex Drugdex [database on the Internet]. Ann Arbor, MI: Truven Health Analytics; 2014. Available at www.micromedexsolutions.com. Accessed on August 5, 2014.
22. Sandson NB, Armstrong SC, Kozza KL, An overview of psychotropic drug-drug interactions, *Psychosomatics* 2005 Sep-Oct;**46**(5):464–494.
23. Candy M, Jones L, Williams R, Tookman A, King M, Psychostimulants for depression, Cochrane *Database Syst Rev* 2008 Apr 16;**2**:CD006722.
24. Aan Hset Rot M, Zarate CA Jr, Charney DS, Mathew SJ, Ketamine for depression: where do we go from here? *Biol Psychiatry* 2012 Oct 1;**72**(7):537–547.
25. Irwin SA, Iglewicz A, Nelesen RA, et al., Daily oral ketamine for the treatment of depression and anxiety in patients receiving hospice care: a 28-day open-label proof-of-concept trial, *J Palliat Med* 2013 Aug;**16**(8):958–965.
26. Ayers CR, Sorrell JT, Thorp SR, Wetherell JL, Evidence-based psychological treatments for late-life anxiety, *Psychol Aging* 2007 Mar;**22**(1):8–17.
27. Johnson EL, O'Brien D, Integrative therapies in hospice and home health: introduction and adoption, *Home Healthc Nurse* 2009 Feb;**27**(2):75–82.
28. Candy B, Jackson KC, Jones L, Tookman A, King M, Drug therapy for symptoms associated with anxiety in adult palliative care patients, *Cochrane Database Syst Rev* 2012 Oct 17;**10**:CD004596.

ADDITIONAL RESOURCES

American Psychiatric Association. DSM-5 Diagnostic Criteria Mobile App. Available for Mac OS at https://itunes.apple.com/us/app/dsm-5-diagnostic-criteria/id662938847?mt=8. Accessed on July 28, 2014. Available for Android at https://play.google.com/store/apps/details?id=com.apa.dsm.v&hl=en. Accessed on July 28, 2014.
Block, SD, Psychological issues in end-of-life care, *J Palliat Med* 2006;**9**:751–772.
Chochinov HM, Breitbart W, editors. *Handbook of Psychiatry in Palliative Medicine*. 2nd ed. Oxford: Oxford University Press, 2009.
Gibson CA, Lichtenthal W, Berg A, Breitbart W. Psychologic issues in palliative care. *Anethesiol Clin N Am* 2006;**24**:61–80.
Irwin SA, Fairman N, Montross L. *UNIPAC*. 4th ed. *UNIPAC 2: Alleviating Psychological and Spiritual Pain*. CP Storey, editor. Glenville: American Academy of Hospice and Palliative Medicine, 2012. Available at http://www.aahpm.org/resources/default/unipac-4th-edition.html. Accessed on July 28, 2014.
Medical College of Wisconsin. End-of-Life/Palliative Education Resource Center: Fast Facts. Available at http://www.eperc.mcw.edu/EPERC/FastFactsandConcepts. Accessed on July 28, 2014.

Section 2

Communication and Decision Making

Chapter 7

Effective Communication with Seriously Ill Patients in the Hospital: General Principles and Core Skills

Kristen A. Chasteen and Wendy G. Anderson

7.1 INTRODUCTION

7.1.1 Why Hospitalists' Communication with Seriously Ill Patients Matters

Hospital communication is crucial to ensuring that seriously ill patients and their families receive adequate information about their illness and prognosis, receive adequate emotional support, and are able to make treatment decisions that are consistent with their goals of care. Seriously ill patients are often hospitalized at turning points in patients' illness trajectories: a new acute illness, exacerbation of chronic illness, or progression of terminal illness [1]. Many patients die in hospitals and even more are hospitalized in the months preceding death [2]. Because of the severity of illness and rapid pace of diagnostic testing in the hospital, patients often need to assimilate large amounts of information and participate in rapid decision making. Hospitalization is often a time of significant anxiety and emotional distress [3]. Communication of bad news and discussion of preferences for end-of-life care frequently occur in the hospital [4]. Effective communication with hospitalized patients is becoming an increasingly important quality measure. Good communication reduces patients' psychological distress, lessens physical symptoms, increases adherence to treatments, and results in higher satisfaction with care [5]. Additionally, better communication skills are associated with reduced clinician burnout and fewer malpractice claims [6, 7].

Hospital-Based Palliative Medicine: A Practical, Evidence-Based Approach, First Edition.
Edited by Steven Pantilat, Wendy Anderson, Matthew Gonzales, and Eric Widera.
© 2015 John Wiley & Sons, Inc. Published 2015 by John Wiley & Sons, Inc.

7.1.2   Hospitalists Need Skills to Address Their Unique Needs in Discussing Serious Illness

Hospitalists are in many ways well positioned to discuss care preferences with seriously ill patients. They work in teams and coordinate with multiple services and disciplines. They are not constrained to a clinic schedule, so may be able to build trust by visiting patients in multiple short segments throughout the day, or in longer segments of time if needed. After a discussion, they can follow up in a short time frame, compared to waiting for a clinic visit weeks later.

Hospitalists also face unique challenges in meeting patients' communication needs. They often meet patients for the first time in the hospital, and may only follow them for a few days. Hospitalists often have daily schedules that are less predictable than a routine clinic day. They have to quickly establish rapport and build trust, since they are often discussing serious information even during the first encounter [1, 3]. The communication section of this book offers skills and strategies to meet the specific communication needs of hospitalists.

7.1.3   What Patients and Families Want in Hospital Communication about Serious Illness

Empirical research illustrates that patients want clear, honest information about their disease process and treatment options [8]. However, they do not want to discuss more information than they are ready to hear [9]. Most patients want to know realistic information about prognosis; yet, a significant minority do not want this information [8, 10]. Patients want clinicians to convey empathy and support hope [10]. They want to establish relationships with clinicians who see them as individuals [9] and want to trust clinicians with whom they discuss end-of-life concerns and prognosis [11]. Though hospitalists may worry that their limited relationships are a barrier, research indicates that seriously ill patients want and may even prefer to discuss end-of-life care preferences with hospitalists [12].

Based on this evidence, we suggest three goals for communicating with seriously ill hospitalized patients: (1) conveying desired information clearly, (2) supporting patients and families emotionally, and (3) helping patients and families make decisions that are consistent with their goals. The communication section of this book provides practical evidence-based advice to meet these goals. In this chapter, we detail the general principles and core skills involved in four main domains of hospital communication: opening the encounter, responding to informational concerns, responding to emotional cues, and handling the special situations of discussing bad news, responding to families who say "don't tell," and balancing truth telling with hope.

7.1.4 How to Use this Chapter

Effective communication can be learned, but achieving competence requires more than just reading a book. Practice, feedback, and reflection are essential. We recommend implementing skills described in this book one at a time in practice, and reflecting alone or with a colleague to evaluate what happened when the skill was used and how the patient reacted. Communicating with seriously ill hospitalized patients will continue to be challenging; however, effective communication skills can improve the experience and outcomes for hospitalized patients and help clinicians feel more engaged with their work. We organized the chapter by phases of the encounter: opening, during, and closing; we address special situations at the end of the chapter.

7.2 KEY STEPS WHEN OPENING THE ENCOUNTER

7.2.1 Sit-Down

The simple act of sitting rather than standing during hospital encounters has a large impact on the patient–clinician interaction. When physicians sit down, patients perceive that encounters last longer and are more satisfied with interactions [13]. The importance of sitting during discussions of serious illness cannot be overemphasized.

7.2.2 Effective Introductions

A warm greeting, good eye contact, and a careful introduction help hospitalists quickly establish rapport. Some patients do not understand the hospitalist model and may feel worried that their primary care physician is not involved. Their concerns may by lessened by a good introduction. Developing an introductory script to use with all new patient encounters may help [14]. Specifics may vary by practice setting. Key components should include name, role (particularly when practicing with trainees), and how hospitalists work in partnership with the primary care physician. For example, "Hello. I'm Dr. Jones. Your doctor, Dr. Fitzpatrick, has asked me to see any patients of hers who need to come to the hospital because I specialize in hospital care. I will send her a full report [or call her after we talk] so she'll know exactly what's going on [14]."

7.2.3 Ask about the Patient as a Person

Asking something about the patient's life outside of the hospital can help to quickly establish rapport and show patients that clinicians see them as individuals: "I know that we are meeting for the first time. Can you tell me something about yourself so I can get to know you a little better?" [15].

7.2.4   Eliciting Concerns and Setting the Agenda

Eliciting concerns is an important beginning to any interaction [16] and can be especially important in discussions of serious illness. Most patients have concerns at hospital admission, yet many are not addressed in encounters with hospitalists [17]. It is especially important to begin discussions of serious illness, such as goals of care discussions or family meetings, by eliciting patient concerns.

Concerns are most effectively elicited with open-ended questions and active listening. Questions like "How are you coping with all of this?" let the patient know that the clinician is interested in the patient's concerns [18]. The phrase "tell me more," for example, "Tell me more about what information you need at this point?" or "Tell me more about what you mean by that," can be helpful to elicit concerns, particularly if the clinician feels that there is misunderstanding [15].

Once concerns have been elicited, the clinician and patient can set a collaborative agenda for the discussion. For example, "I would like to ask you some questions about the treatment you've had so far, and then we can discuss your concern about your chemotherapy treatment delay. Does that sound okay?"

7.3   KEY SKILLS TO USE THROUGHOUT THE ENCOUNTER

7.3.1   Responding to Concerns and Cues

Patient concerns often have both informational and emotional components [18]. Concerns can be elicited by the clinician as described earlier; patients also may spontaneously give cues about their concerns. To respond effectively, clinicians must first recognize concerns and cues, and determine whether they are primarily informational, emotional, or both. Patients indicate need for information in either statements or questions, for example, "I don't understand the test results," or "What is the prognosis doctor?"

In emotional cues, patients indicate their experience of distress. Emotional cues can be verbal, for example, "I'm scared to face the next steps," or nonverbal, for example, fidgeting, crying, or looking down. Emotional cues are sometimes masked by what appears on the surface to be a request for biomedical information. For example, a patient may say, "I just don't understand why the antibiotics aren't working. There must be something stronger." It is tempting to only see this statement as a request for information; however, it may also be an expression of negative emotion, such as worry or frustration.

Responding to Informational Concerns: "Ask–Tell–Ask" Technique. Hospitalized patients want information about their illness and how it will affect them yet often struggle to understand the huge amount of information conveyed to them by different clinicians. Hospitalized patients often lack an accurate understanding of even basic information about diagnoses and treatments [19]. Also, clinicians need to ensure that patients get the information they want and need, but do not give more detail than patients are ready to hear [8]. The "ask–tell–ask" technique (Table 7.1) allows

Table 7.1 Responding to Informational Cues: "Ask–Tell–Ask" [15]

Encounter Dialogue	Analysis
Patient: "How long do you think I have?"	
Clinician: "First, to make sure I give you the most helpful answer, do you find numbers or percentages helpful or just a general estimate?"	**1st Ask** to find out exactly what information the patient wants
Patient: "I guess I'm more just wondering what to expect"	
Clinician: "Let's first focus on how this illness is likely to impact your life over the next months. The main thing I'm worried about is that you will start to feel weaker"	**Tells** only the information the patient wants. Uses plain language
Clinician: "Is that the kind of information you were hoping for?"	**2nd Ask** to check if the patient's informational needs were met

clinicians to give only the amount of detail that the patient wants and to make sure that the information provided is understood [15].

"ASK." The first step is to ask the patient what they already know and what they want to know, for example, "Can you tell me what you understand of your disease?" and "Can you tell me what information would be most helpful?" This first "ask" allows the clinician to tailor the type of information that is provided to what the patient actually needs. This step is particularly important in the hospital, where patients are often receiving information from multiple different members of the clinical team.

"TELL." The next step is to tell the information to the patient in plain language, in a short statement conveying no more than three pieces of information at a time [15]. It is also helpful to start by conveying a big-picture message before disclosing more detailed biomedical information.

"ASK." The second "ask" checks patient understanding or perspective, for example, "What questions do you have so far?" or "What do you think of what I've said?" The clinician can also ask the patient to restate what was said in his/her own words. For example, "To make sure I did a good job explaining this, can you tell me what main points you are taking away?" or "How will you explain this to your husband?" The "ask–tell–ask" cycle usually needs to be repeated several times throughout the encounter so that information is always conveyed in small segments.

Responding to Emotional Cues: Expressing Empathy. Clinicians often focus on the informational aspect of cues and frequently miss emotional cues, yet responding to emotional cues is an essential aspect of both relationship and trust building and discussions of serious illness [18].

Hospitalization can be a time of significant negative emotion, including anxiety, sadness, and shock. Hospitalized patients frequently express negative emotion to clinicians [3]. Clinicians often cannot "fix" the causes of these emotions, but they can show emotional support by listening and expressing empathy. Expressing empathy is simply acknowledging the presence of a patient's emotion without judgment and without trying to alter it [18]. Clinician expression of empathy is associated with decreased patient anxiety, increased satisfaction, and improved medical outcomes [20–22]. Clinician expression of empathy encourages the patient to share his/her perspective and concerns, which helps the clinician clarify goals of care and tailor treatment plans to match the patient's goals [3].

Clinicians can express empathy both nonverbally and verbally. Nonverbal techniques can be summarized by the acronym S-O-L-E-R (Table 7.2) [18]. Allowing for silence and simply bearing witness to patient emotion can also be powerful ways to express empathy. The N-U-R-S-E acronym [15] and "I wish" statements [23] are useful tools to verbally express empathy (Table 7.3).

Expressing Verbal Empathy: N-U-R-S-E [15]

NAME. Naming the emotion is a useful way for clinicians to show that they are attuned to the patient's experience, for example, "I sense that you're feeling anxious about the MRI." It is safer to be suggestive rather than declarative, for example, "Some people in this situation would be angry" rather than "I can see that you're angry about this." Understating the emotion may also be less threatening, for example, "It sounds like this experience has been frustrating" rather than "This experience has clearly made you mad."

Table 7.2   Nonverbal Expressions of Empathy: S-O-L-E-R [18]

S	Face the patient *squarely*
O	Adopt an *open* body posture
L	*Lean* toward the patient
E	Maintain *eye* contact
R	Maintain a *relaxed* body posture

Table 7.3   Responding Verbally to Emotional Cues [15, 23]
Statement from a patient admitted with a severe COPD exacerbation: "I still can't even get out of bed without struggling to breathe? I'm so sick of this"
Empathic Responses

NURSE	
Name	"It sounds like you're worried that your trouble breathing has not improved"
Understand	"It must be hard to feel so short of breath"
Respect	"I'm impressed that you have been so committed to doing all the treatments to help your breathing"
Support	"I'm committed to doing everything possible to help you feel better"
Explore	"Can you tell me more about how this trouble breathing is affecting you?"
I wish...	"I wish we had been able to help you feel better more quickly"

UNDERSTAND. Expressing appreciation of the patient's situation or emotions is a useful way to express empathy and build rapport, for example, "It sounds like it is very difficult for you to be spending so much time in the hospital" or "It must be hard to experience this much pain."

RESPECT. Showing respect is a good way to express empathy, that is, "It sounds like you've done a lot of research on your illness." Praising coping skills or caregiving skills are ways to show respect, for example, "I'm impressed by how much support you've provided to your children during your illness" or "You've taken excellent care of your mom."

SUPPORT. Even though hospitalists may only have short-term relationships with patients, it is possible to offer statements of support, for example, "This is a lot of news to take in. I will be here all day if you have questions" or "I will work with you to determine the next steps."

EXPLORE. Patients often offer either verbal or nonverbal clues about their emotions initially. Asking a question may allow them to elaborate and state their emotions and concerns more explicitly, for example, "What are you most worried about?" "Tell me more" can be a helpful tool in this context, for example, "Can you tell me more about how you feel about this?"

Expressing Verbal Empathy: "I Wish" Statements

Clinicians often find it difficult to respond empathically to patient expressions of hopelessness or disappointment in the limitations of medicine. Clinicians may be struggling with their own guilt, disappointment, and feelings of failure when they have not been able to cure a patient's illness. In these situations, the temptation may be to say "I'm sorry this happened to you." Quill and colleagues suggest that using an "I wish" statement is a better way to acknowledge emotion without risking interpretation as pity [23]. For example, a daughter of a patient with advanced dementia and recurrent aspiration pneumonias asks, "Can't you do anything to stop these infections?" A clinician response of "I wish we had better treatments to prevent these complications of dementia. It sounds like it's very hard to see your mom so sick" conveys empathy and aligns the clinician and daughter. "I wish" statements can also be used in response to patients who express unrealistic hopes. A patient dying of advanced cancer says "I want to stay alive until my daughter gets married next year." A response of "I wish I could promise you that. It sounds like it is hard to think about leaving your family" conveys empathy without providing false hope [23].

7.4   CLOSING THE ENCOUNTER

Effective communication at the end of an encounter helps ensure patient understanding and provides a final opportunity to build rapport. Given the large amount of information conveyed in a hospital encounter, it is helpful to close the encounter by summarizing what was discussed. The end of the encounter is a good place to use the second "ask," from the "ask–tell–ask" technique, for example, "What are the main points that you're taking away from our discussion?" Providing a concrete plan for what will happen next and the expected time frame is also essential. Plans may include diagnostic tests, treatments, discharge plans, and when the clinician will see the patient next. Lastly, thanking the patient for their time helps build rapport and foster a respectful relationship.

7.5 SPECIAL SITUATIONS

7.5.1 Discussing Bad News

Hospitalists are often discussing bad news with patients, including new diagnoses, worsening of chronic illness, and disease progression to terminal illness and death. Prior research has shown that patients prefer to hear bad news in a quiet place and have clear communication about diagnosis, prognosis, treatment options, and how it will affect their lives; full attention of the physician; time to ask questions; and emotional support [18]. Discussing bad news is stressful for clinicians. Hospitalists have the added challenge of discussing bad news with patients who they have only known for a short time. Baille and colleagues have outlined a road map to help clinicians discuss bad news, which is summarized by the acronym SPIKES [24] (Table 7.4).

S: Setting Up and Preparing for the Conversation. Reviewing the medical facts and speaking with relevant consulting services prepares clinicians to convey accurate information. Emotional preparation is also helpful. Some clinicians use mindfulness techniques like pausing to notice their breathing to help prepare. The clinician should ask the patient who they want to be present when discussing serious information. Arranging to have chairs for everyone and a private, relatively quiet space, is essential. Setting phones and pagers to silent or asking a colleague to respond to pages helps minimize interruptions.

P: Assess the Patient's Perception. Discussing bad news is another important time to use the "ask–tell–ask" technique. Clinicians should first find out what the patient already knows so that the discussion can be tailored to the current degree of understanding, for example, "I want to make sure that we are on the same page. Can you tell me what you understand of your illness at this time?" The clinician may realize that the patient has significant misunderstanding about the disease, for example, "The chemotherapy is working and my cancer is getting better," or that he/she already has full understanding of the bad news, for example, "I know that I'm dying."

I: Ask for an Invitation to Discuss the Bad News. It is helpful to ask the patient's permission prior to discussing bad news and to assess how they like to hear information. For example, asking "How would you like me to talk to you about the test results? Would you like me to discuss all of the details or just the big-picture and then focus on treatment options?" Obtaining permission from the patient can also serve as a warning statement, that is, "I have some serious news to discuss about the test results, is now an okay time to talk?" If a patient declines the invitation, the clinician can offer to follow up at a different time or can request to speak to a surrogate who may be willing to discuss the information.

K: Impart Knowledge by Disclosing the News in Plain Language. After gaining permission to share, the next step is to convey the bad news in plain language.

Table 7.4   Discussing Bad News [24]

Patient admitted with pneumonia but now with worsening respiratory status. Likely needs transfer to a higher level of care

SPIKES Protocol	Encounter Dialogue	Analysis
Setup	Clinician: "Is it okay if I sit down so we can talk?"	Establishes appropriate setting. Asks patient's permission to initiate discussion
	Patient: "Sure"	
Perception	Clinician: "I want to make sure we have been clear in our communication. What is your understanding of what is going on with your lung infection?"	Assesses the patient's perception
	Patient: "I know it's a bad infection. I thought it was being treated with the antibiotics, but I don't feel better"	
Invitation	Clinician: "Is it okay if I discuss what I see is happening with your lung infection?"	Asks for the patient's permission before proceeding
	Patient: "Of course. I want to know"	
Knowledge	Clinician: "I'm worried about your breathing"	Offers a warning statement
	"I see that you are working harder to breathe and you need more oxygen"	Shares the information in plain language
	"The infection in your lungs seems to be getting worse instead of better"	Conveys the big picture
	Patient: "Oh my gosh"	Expresses emotion
	Clinician: Remains silent, continues eye contact and attention	Silence allows time for additional patient response
	Patient: "I thought that this infection was easy to treat. I can't believe this is happening"	Expresses emotion
Empathize	Clinician: "It sounds like you're worried"	Names the emotion
	Patient: "I'm very worried. I came to the hospital as soon as I started to get sick. I thought I caught it in time"	Expresses more emotion
	Clinician: "You did everything right"	Conveys empathy by offering respect
	"I wish the treatments had helped you get better quickly"	"I wish" statement
	Patient: "I do too"	
	Clinician: "Is it okay if I move forward and talk about the next steps in your care?"	Makes sure the patient is ready to move on
	Patient: "Yes, please do"	

(Continued)

Table 7.4   (*Continued*)

SPIKES Protocol	Encounter Dialogue	Analysis
Summarize and strategize	Clinician: "We know that your breathing is getting worse. There are several things that I think will help your breathing and make sure that we can monitor you closely. I'll talk about each of them"	Begins to summarize and discuss next steps

Consider using a warning statement if not already done, for example, "I'm sorry the news isn't what we were hoping for." It is important to discuss only small chunks of information at a time and to convey a "big-picture" message. After the main news is conveyed, the clinician should pause and allow time for the patient to process the news and express emotion.

E—Respond to Emotion. After hearing bad news, patients often experience strong emotion, including sadness, anger, or shock. It is important to respond empathically to patient emotion, prior to giving more information. Patients are unlikely to retain complex information while they are experiencing strong emotion. The clinician should continue to express empathy, using nonverbal (silence, SOLER) and verbal (NURSE, "I wish") methods, until the patient is ready to continue. If the clinician is not sure if the patient is ready to hear more information, it is helpful to ask, for example, "Are you ready to talk about the next steps in your care?"

S—Summarize the Plan. At the end of the discussion, it is helpful to summarize the information and concretely describe the next steps. Consider asking the patient to summarize in his/her own words to check for understanding.

7.5.2   Responding to Families Who Say "Don't Tell"

Clinicians often struggle with how to respond when a family member asks them to refrain from sharing bad news with the patient. It is helpful to start by trying to gain better understanding of the family's perspective [10]. "Tell me about your concerns" is a more helpful response than "we need to discuss this news with her." It is the cultural norm in many countries to withhold negative medical information from the patient and instead have family members make decisions [25]. Families often feel that hearing bad news will cause increased suffering or have a negative impact on the patient's health. This is again a place to respond empathically to emotion, that is, "I can see you're worried about how this news will affect your mom." Empathic responses help to build trust and help reassure family that the clinician will talk to their family member in a sensitive way. The clinician can then say something like "I'm fine with discussing this news with only you (the family member), if that is what your mom wants. I would like to first ask your mom what she prefers." The clinician can then make a careful plan with the family about the next steps, including discussing what language will be used, for example, "Some patients want to know all of the information about their illness, and others prefer for their doctor to discuss that information with their family. What would you prefer?"

7.5.3   Balancing Truth Telling with Hope

Most patients want detailed information about their illness and what to expect; however, they also want truth telling to be balanced with hope [8]. It is helpful to realize that an entire spectrum of hope can exist and evolve over time, including hope for cure, hope for living longer, hope for having time with loved ones, and hope for having a peaceful death [18]. The core communication principles outlined in this chapter help clinicians achieve the balance between truth telling and hope that is appropriate for each patient. Asking patient permission ensures that patients are only told bad news and prognostic information that they are ready to hear. Responding empathically to patient emotion with NURSE and "I wish" statements helps to convey hope and support even when prognosis is poor. In patients with incurable disease, open-ended questions like "What else are you hoping for?" and "Can you tell me more?" allow clinicians to reframe hope and help patients identify goals that are possible. Table 7.5 provides suggestions for phrases to avoid as well as preferred alternatives to help clinicians respond empathically and maintain patient hope.

Table 7.5   Better Words to Say [26]

Avoid	Use Instead	Rationale
"I understand what you're going through"	"It sounds like this has been a difficult situation"	Every person experiences illness differently. Express empathy, but do not assume that you completely understand the patient's experience
"It could be worse" "It's not that bad"	"It sounds like this has been a tough time for you"	Do not minimize a patient's experience or emotion. Express empathy
"There is nothing more we can do"	"I wish we had a treatment that would cure your illness. We do have a lot we can do to help you feel better"	Express empathy. Focus on what CAN be done
"Withdrawal of care"	"To respect his wishes, we will stop the breathing machine and use medications to help with his comfort"	Reframe stopping life-sustaining treatments as honoring the patient's wishes. Emphasize the care that will be provided
"Would you like us to do everything?"	"How were you hoping we could help?"	"Everything" can mean many different things. Start with open-ended questions to explore the patient's goals

Table 7.6   Additional Resources

Resource	Description
Oncotalk® http://depts.washington.edu/oncotalk/	Developed for oncology fellows. Useful for all clinicians. Learning modules, videos, and links to additional communication resources. "Tough talk" section focuses on how to teach communication skills
VitalTalk iPhone app http://vitaltalk.blogspot.com/ (accompanying blog)	Five-step concise guide to discussing bad news with videos. Directs clinicians to prepare to use the communication skills in a clinical encounter and debrief afterward. App format is convenient for busy clinicians
Back A, Arnold R, Tulsky J. *Mastering Communication with Seriously Ill Patients.* New York, NY: Cambridge University Press, 2009.	Practical, concise, book describing essential tools to improve communication skills. Helpful examples and analysis of patient encounters
http://endoflife.stanford.edu/	End-of-life online curriculum. Communication section has helpful tips, cases, videos, and pre-/posttests

REFERENCES

1. Anderson WG, Kools S, Lyndon A, Dancing around death: hospitalist-patient communication about serious illness, *Qual Health Res* 2013;**23**(1):3–13.
2. Teno JM, Gozalo PL, Bynum JP, et al., Change in end-of-life care for medicare beneficiaries: site of death, place of care, and health care transitions in 2000, 2005, and 2009, *JAMA* 2013;**309**(5):470–477.
3. Adams K, Cimino JE, Arnold RM, Anderson WG, Why should I talk about emotion? Communication patterns associated with physician discussion of patient expressions of negative emotion in hospital admission encounters, *Patient Educ Couns* 2012;**89**(1):44–50.
4. Auerbach AD, Pantilat SZ, End-of-life care in a voluntary hospitalist model: effects on communication, processes of care, and patient symptoms, *Am J Med* 2004;**116**(10):669–675.
5. Griffin SJ, Kinmonth AL, Veltman MW, Gillard S, Grant J, Stewart M, Effect on health-related outcomes of interventions to alter the interaction between patients and practitioners: a systematic review of trials, *Ann Fam Med* 2004;**2**(6):595–608.
6. Levinson W, Roter DL, Mullooly JP, Dull VT, Frankel RM, Physician-patient communication. The relationship with malpractice claims among primary care physicians and surgeons, *JAMA* 1997;**277**(7):553–559.
7. Ramirez AJ, Graham J, Richards MA, et al., Burnout and psychiatric disorder among cancer clinicians, *Br J Cancer* 1995;**71**(6):1263–1269.
8. Parker SM, Clayton JM, Hancock K, et al., A systematic review of prognostic/end-of-life communication with adults in the advanced stages of a life-limiting illness: patient/caregiver preferences for the content, style, and timing of information, *J Pain Symptom Manage* 2007;**34**(1):81–93.
9. Wright EB, Holcombe C, Salmon P, Doctors' communication of trust, care, and respect in breast cancer: qualitative study, *BMJ* 2004;**328**(7444):864.
10. Clayton JM, Hancock KM, Butow PN, et al., Clinical practice guidelines for communicating prognosis and end-of-life issues with adults in the advanced stages of a life-limiting illness, and their caregivers, *Med J Aust* 2007;**186**(Suppl 12):S77, S79, S83–108.

11. Walczak A, Butow PN, Davidson PM, et al., Patient perspectives regarding communication about prognosis and end-of-life issues: how can it be optimised? *Patient Educ Couns* 2013;**90**(3):307–314.

12. Dow LA, Matsuyama RK, Ramakrishnan V, et al., Paradoxes in advance care planning: the complex relationship of oncology patients, their physicians, and advance medical directives, *J Clin Oncol* 2010;**28**(2):299–304.

13. Swayden KJ, Anderson KK, Connelly LM, Moran JS, McMahon JK, Arnold PM, Effect of sitting vs. standing on perception of provider time at bedside: a pilot study, *Patient Educ Couns* 2012;**86**(2):166–171.

14. Darves B, What should you say after "hello"? *Today's Hospitalist* April 2008.

15. Back AL, Arnold RM, Baile WF, Tulsky JA, Fryer-Edwards K, Approaching difficult communication tasks in oncology, *CA Cancer J Clin* 2005;**55**(3):164–177.

16. Marvel MK, Epstein RM, Flowers K, Beckman HB, Soliciting the patient's agenda: have we improved? *JAMA* 1999;**281**(3):283–287.

17. Anderson WG, Winters K, Auerbach AD, Patient concerns at hospital admission, *Arch Intern Med* 2011;**171**(15):1399–1400.

18. Back AL, Anderson WG, Bunch L, et al., Communication about cancer near the end of life, *Cancer* 2008;**113**(Suppl 7):1897–1910.

19. Makaryus AN, Friedman EA, Patients' understanding of their treatment plans and diagnosis at discharge, *Mayo Clin Proc* 2005;**80**(8):991–994.

20. Epstein RM, Hadee T, Carroll J, Meldrum SC, Lardner J, Shields CG, "Could this be something serious?" Reassurance, uncertainty, and empathy in response to patients' expressions of worry, *J Gen Intern Med* 2007;**22**(12):1731–1739.

21. Fogarty LA, Curbow BA, Wingard JR, McDonnell K, Somerfield MR, Can 40 seconds of compassion reduce patient anxiety?. *J Clin Oncol* 1999;**17**(1):371–379.

22. Hojat M, Louis DZ, Markham FW, Wender R, Rabinowitz C, Gonnella JS, Physicians' empathy and clinical outcomes for diabetic patients. *Acad Med* 2011;**86**(3):359–364.

23. Quill TE, Arnold RM, Platt F, "I wish things were different": expressing wishes in response to loss, futility, and unrealistic hopes, *Ann Intern Med* 2001;**135**(7):551–555.

24. Baile WF, Buckman R, Lenzi R, Glober G, Beale EA, Kudelka AP, SPIKES-A six-step protocol for delivering bad news: application to the patient with cancer, *Oncologist* 2000;**5**(4):302–311.

25. Kagawa-Singer M, Blackhall LJ, Negotiating cross-cultural issues at the end of life: "You got to go where he lives", *JAMA* 2001;**286**(23):2993–3001.

26. Pantilat SZ, Communicating with seriously ill patients: better words to say, *JAMA* 2009;**301**(12):1279–1281.

Chapter 8

Family Meetings and Caring for Family Members

Sara K. Johnson

8.1 WHY CARE FOR FAMILIES OF PALLIATIVE CARE PATIENTS?

By definition, palliative medicine aims to provide care both to patients and their families; this premise of inclusion of family is also considered a standard for end-of-life care. It is important to recognize that the term "family" is broadly used in palliative medicine and applies to a myriad of relationships—relative, legal, financial, emotional—that the patient has within his or her support system.

Evidence reveals improved patient, family, and medical system outcomes when using a holistic approach to care of seriously ill patients that includes care of their families. For patients, maintaining strong communication with family members, including their involvement in decision-making, defines quality end-of-life care [1]. Patients also express preferences to have family members involved in medical decision-making, and some even defer decision-making completely to their families. Notably, supportive family members are associated with improved patient quality of life and less symptom burden [2]. Ensuring their families are not burdened, both emotionally and otherwise, is also important to patients at the end of life [1].

Family members of seriously ill patients also benefit from attention to their needs. Many seriously ill patients require significant assistance from family caregivers; this demanding role frequently results in anxiety and depression and is associated with increased risk of mortality [3]. Not surprisingly, family satisfaction with end-of-life care in the hospital is higher, and the likelihood of complicated bereavement is lower with better communication and emotional support from clinicians [3].

From a logistical standpoint, it is often necessary to include families intimately in patients' medical care, as a large proportion of hospitalized patients are unable to make medical decisions. Unfortunately, in hospital settings, communication with families needs improvement: as many as half of family members of seriously ill

Hospital-Based Palliative Medicine: A Practical, Evidence-Based Approach, First Edition.
Edited by Steven Pantilat, Wendy Anderson, Matthew Gonzales, and Eric Widera.
© 2015 John Wiley & Sons, Inc. Published 2015 by John Wiley & Sons, Inc.

patients do not understand their loved one's diagnosis, prognosis, or treatment [4]. Surrogate decision-makers who perceived better communication from physicians had family members with a shorter lengths of life-sustaining treatments [5]. This is consistent with studies on communication interventions for families of hospitalized patients at high risk of death, which have shown decreased hospital and ICU length of stays and less resource utilization [6, 7].

As outlined, focusing care on not only the patient during hospitalization, but also on family members, has positive effects on patients, families, and medical systems.

8.2 EFFECTIVE COMMUNICATION WITH FAMILY MEMBERS

There are various approaches to improve communication with seriously ill patients' families in the hospital: family meetings (see Tables 8.1 and 8.2), involving interprofessional team members (e.g., nursing, social work, and spiritual care), and education in a variety of media, perhaps even brochures [8]. Communicating well with families involves noting and responding to statements made by family members, which can be missed during family meetings [9]; an important aspect of good communication is empathic responses to the emotions of families, as outlined in Chapter 7.

8.2.1 Assistance with Surrogate Decision-Making

Many seriously ill patients are unable to make medical decisions, in which case we turn to surrogate decision-makers to assist with guiding medical care. The designated surrogate decision-maker is either a patient-appointed healthcare power of attorney or, if that is lacking, typically the next of kin. The standard approach to surrogate decision-making is substituted judgment: the surrogate decision-maker decides on the treatment course the patient would choose for him- or herself if he or she were able. However, the process is often not straightforward. Surrogate decision-makers are frequently inaccurate in their assessment of patients' preferences for treatment and, perhaps not surprisingly, err on the side of providing more interventions than patients would want, rather than less [10]. There is often conflict perceived with staff and significant emotional distress associated with this role [11].

The role of surrogates in medical decision-making varies, with a spectrum of involvement, from the surrogate making the choice without input from the physician, to

Table 8.1   General Principles for Family Meetings

- The patient or family should do most of the talking
- Communication style should be open, honest, and clear
- Specific types of physician statements during conferences are associated with increased family satisfaction: nonabandonment statements, reassurance of priority of patient's comfort, and support for decision made by family
- Note and respond to emotions of family members using empathic statements

Table 8.2 Framework for a Family Meeting

BEFORE the Family Meeting

WHY Are You Meeting? The Goal Should Be Clear in Your Mind

"To help the patient and family [decide on whether or not to continue life-supportive therapies, etc.]"

WHO Should Be at the Meeting? The Participants

Yours: Important medical providers and interdisciplinary team members

Decide Who is LEADING the Meeting

Patient's: The primary decision-maker is essential. Ask who else desired by patient or family to be present

WHERE? The Setting

In patient's room or not? Ideal is an area that is private, quiet, with seating for all participants if possible

WHAT Is Going On Medically? WHAT Are the Options? Discuss at PREMEETING

Meet ahead of time with medical and interprofessional team members to get everyone updated: What is the likely diagnosis or prognosis? What are the treatment options and likely benefits and burdens? What are the disposition options? What are subspecialists' recommendations?

DURING the Family Meeting

Start with Introductions

Set the Agenda

State your agenda AND elicit patient/family's

"We want to update you on your father's health and discuss options for next steps for his medical care. Is there anything else you were hoping to talk about during this [x] minute meeting?"

Sharing of Knowledge

Elicit Perception of Patient and/or Family: Use an Open-Ended Question

"What have you been told about what is going on with your father's health right now?"

"I know we have had a lot of discussions about your father's medical situation, but to make sure I have been explaining well, I would like to hear your understanding of what is going on with his health right now?"

Give Medical Information: Be Direct, Concise, Honest, and Avoid Medical Jargon

If you are giving bad news, consider using a "warning shot"

"Unfortunately, I have bad news; your father's lung and kidney failure are getting worse and he is likely going to die in the hospital"

Give the News and Then Stop Talking

Respond to Emotion: Use Empathic "NURSE" Statements and Give the Family the Time They Need

Name emotion: "I cannot imagine how difficult it is to hear that the infection is worse"

Understand: Legitimize emotion—"I can imagine this news would make anyone upset"

Respect statement: "You have taken incredible care of your mother throughout her illness"

Supportive statement: "No matter what happens, we will deal with it together"

Explore emotion: "Tell me more about how you are feeling right now."

Eliciting Values and Goals: Open-Ended Questions to Assess What Patient Would Want

"If your father were able to be here and discuss his health with us, what do you think he would want given how sick he is?"

Decision-Making

Integrate the medical information with patient's values

Make a RECOMMENDATION

Summarize and Wrap Up

Discuss plan and how family can contact you, and assure nonabandonment

AFTER the Family Meeting

Debrief with Other Providers and Carry Out Plan

Table 8.3   Best Practice Approach to Assist Surrogate Decision-Makers

1. Educate them on role of surrogate decision-maker
2. Consider assessing their preferred role in decision-making
3. Offer your recommendation
4. Navigate family conflict and help them arrive at a consensus
5. Pace of decision-making should be on timeline of the family
6. Guilt alleviation with MD support for decision made about end-of-life care
7. Honest communication throughout and keep them involved in treatment plan

shared decision-making, to the physician deciding alone (paternalistic). Shared decision-making has been highlighted as the ideal model; however, surrogate decision-makers vary in their preferences for what role in decision-making they desire to have [12]. Notably, many surrogate decision-makers prefer to have the consensus and involvement of their family when deciding on medical treatment for a loved one [13] and are more confident in their roles when physician communication is better [5]. Surrogates cite that having enough time to process information and make decisions is important [13, 14] and that having the physician help to facilitate family consensus is helpful [15].

It is clear that to assist surrogate decision-makers in these serious choices, it is crucial to have thorough, clear, and open communication with them that includes the aspects listed in Table 8.3 [12, 13, 16, 17].

8.2.2   The Family Meeting: A Framework for Family Decision-Making

Family conferences are a tool that can meet the needs of family members, including assistance with decision-making and improved communication. Family members of seriously ill patients have been found to have less psychological distress and more consensus between family members with scheduled "proactive" family meetings in the ICU [7, 8].

What follows is a framework on how to approach leading a family meeting (see Table 8.2). The evidence base on how to approach family meetings is growing, and though there is no definitive consensus on structure, many observed and recommended meeting components in the literature are similar to this framework [3, 18–20]. Further, though we often think of a family meeting as one occurrence, most families will need multiple meetings over the course of a patient's hospital stay, so it is important to not try to accomplish too much over one meeting. For example, a first meeting might establish concerns that the outcome might be poor, another confirms that the patient is not doing well, another describes the process of withdrawing life support, and a final meeting prepares to transition to comfort care.

BEFORE the Family Meeting. Preparation is key and the most important aspect of a successful family meeting. Premeeting planning should include the following.

WHY ARE YOU MEETING? THE GOAL. One should have a clear discussion goal for a family meeting and keep in mind that the reason for the meeting should not be only the medical team's agenda but also the patient's and family's agenda. A useful way to frame this is, "Our goal is to help the family/patient [fill in the blank]." For example, it could be "...to help the family understand how critically ill a loved one is" or "to help the family/patient make a decision about continuation versus withdrawal of life-sustaining therapies." It is also important to speak with the patient and family before the meeting about what you want to talk about: to prepare them, as well as to assess what they wish to discuss. Though it is important to set a goal before a meeting, it is also important to adjust this goal based on feedback from the family. For example, if you hoped to address code status, but the family does not feel ready to, this topic may need to be deferred to a later meeting.

WHO SHOULD BE AT THE MEETING? THE PARTICIPANTS. A successful family meeting is dependent on ensuring that the appropriate people are at the meeting. Consider which medical providers and interprofessional team members should attend, and who is important to be there from the patient and family's perspective. If the agenda includes discussing cancer prognosis and treatment options, it will be helpful to have an oncologist present; if you will be discussing a hemodialysis decision, a nephrologist. Ideally, providers who have an established relationship with the patient should attend, such as a primary care provider or primary oncologist; however, in reality this if often not feasible. At the very least, having discussed the situation with subspecialists or primary providers will provide you with important information and credibility.

Involvement of multiple disciplines in family meetings increases the likelihood that families' needs for information and emotional support will be met. For example, in family meetings nurses and social workers are often able to clarify medical terminology, ensure families understand information and are emotionally supported. During meetings, nurses can provide important insights into patient's status and symptom control. Spiritual care providers help families with emotional support and decision-making in the context of their faith. These interprofessional providers can also follow up with families to clarify and reiterate key information and answer questions.

When considering the participants from the patient's perspective who need to be present, several factors need to be considered, particularly assessment of the patient's decision-making capacity. If the patient has capacity, ask who he or she wishes to be involved in the family meeting and decision-making process. Keep in mind that sometimes patients do not want to be involved in either the meeting or decision-making, which can be influenced by cultural factors or just personal preference. If the patient does not have decision-making capacity, you should ensure the appropriate designated decision-maker(s) participate(s) in the meeting, and determine who they wish to have present. If a key person is unable to attend the meeting, consider a phone conference.

From the medical team perspective, it is helpful to identify ahead of time the individual who will lead the meeting. This person should be available for the duration of the meeting, and if needed should arrange for colleagues to cover for acute issues during that time. It is not this person's job to know all the answers, but rather to guide the discussion and move it forward, and defer specialty questions to the consultants in the room, or other individuals who may be best poised to answer. This is an excellent learning opportunity for trainees, who can lead the meeting to either a predetermined juncture or to whenever assistance is needed from a more experienced team member.

WHERE? THE SETTING. Ideally, meetings should be held in an area that is private, quiet, and with seating for all participants. This may be difficult if meeting in a patient's room, and the next best option is ensuring that the facilitator and key decision-makers are seated. It is also recommended that tissue and water be on hand. When patients are unable to participate in the discussion, for example, in the ICU, families may feel uncomfortable asking key questions about prognosis in the presence of the patient, for fear the patient may overhear [21].

WHAT IS GOING ON MEDICALLY? WHAT ARE THE OPTIONS? THE MEDICAL PREMEETING. A 5- to 10-min premeeting between medical providers and interprofessional staff is one of the most important aspects of a successful family meeting. This allows all the healthcare providers to be up to date on medical facts and gives time to review with colleagues the important issues in the patient's care, including prognosis and treatment options. If subspecialists, or other providers, have recommendations, this is the time to discuss them. It is important to acknowledge and attempt to work through disagreements in the medical information at this time to avoid any surprises during the meeting due to differing opinions or new medical information. If important subspecialists cannot attend, get the information you need before the meeting to help the patient and family make a decision.

DURING the Family Meeting: General Approach. As outlined in Table 8.1, there are general points to keep in mind during family meetings:

- The patient or family should do most of the talking. In end-of-life conferences, families allowed to speak more than providers during the meeting have increased satisfaction with clinician communication and report less conflict with providers [22]. This means providers must be able to tolerate periods of silence, particularly when emotional news has been given, to allow family members time to process and speak their minds.
- Communication style should be open, honest, and clear [14]. Providers should limit details and medical jargon. Euphemisms for death and dying should be avoided; if you believe a patient is going to die from his or her illness, say it but with compassion: "Unfortunately, I'm concerned your father is going to die in the hospital from his pneumonia and kidney failure." You can ask for permission to discuss difficult things they may not wish to know: "Do you want to talk about how much time he may have left?"
- Specific types of physician statements during conferences have been associated with increased family satisfaction: nonabandonment statements, reassurance of priority of patient's comfort, and support for the decision made by family [23]. Nonabandonment statements include those that assure you will ensure the patient does not suffer, you will allow the family to be with the patient if they wish, and you are available if needed [24].
- In family meetings, the opportunities to support family members by acknowledging and addressing their emotions are often missed [9], which can keep meetings from being productive. Emotional responses should be noted and

responded to with empathic statements, which can be remembered with the acronym "NURSE" (see Chapter 7 for details). Examples of these statements are in Table 8.2 [25].

DURING the Family Meeting: Logistics

INTRODUCTIONS. An easy and important way to start is go around the room for all persons to introduce themselves and their role.

AGENDA SETTING. This should be a very brief dialogue of what everyone is hoping to discuss at the meeting. State your agenda, for example, "We want to update you on your father's health and discuss options for next steps for his medical care." This is an excellent time to highlight if a decision needs to be made in a particular time period, as decisions often do not need to be made during the meeting. This is also the time to elicit the patient and family's agenda. For example, "We want to make sure that this meeting best addresses your needs—what do you feel are the things that are most important for us to discuss?" If there is a time frame for your meeting, it is appropriate to state the time frame at the beginning and work with families to prioritize topics for discussion, deferring other topics until a later time.

SHARING OF KNOWLEDGE

Elicit Perception of Patient and/or Family: Open-Ended Question. This should be an open-ended question of what the patient's or family's current understanding is of the medical situation. For example, the facilitator can ask, "What have you been told about what is going on with your father's health right now?" If you have been the provider telling them what is going on and you know what they have been told, this is still an important step, especially with new family members who can be around for meetings, though the phrasing could be different. For example, "I know we have had a lot of discussions about your father's medical situation, but to make sure I have been explaining things well, I would like to hear your understanding of what is going on with his health right now." This open-ended question serves two purposes. The first is to understand how the patient and family perceive the current medical situation. This helps in identifying the information needs of the patients as well as what aspects of care need to be clarified. At times the open-ended question about the patient's current health can reveal how profound the family's understanding is of a dire situation, even if you haven't explicitly discussed that with them. For instance, a response of "We know he's dying and want to take him home with hospice. How would we do that?" would change the course of the discussion quickly. Conversely, you may find out that the perception of the patient/family is not as up to date as you thought, even though information you relayed previously seemed clear. A response from a family member of a patient with terminal cancer in the ICU with multiorgan failure who states that "She is getting better, she's breathing on her own with the machine; we just need to get her stronger to get more chemotherapy to beat her cancer" is going to alert you that you will need to spend more time discussing certain medical information or the underlying emotional needs of the family.

The second purpose of starting with open-ended questions is that it allows a period for family members, or patients, to express any pent-up emotions, particularly frustration and anger, that would otherwise obstruct any productive conversations. Once their emotion has been discussed and acknowledged, most people will be able to move beyond it to the cognitive parts of the discussion.

Give Medical Information: Just Say It. As in the aforementioned, it is crucial to be clear, concise, and honest when relaying medical information. One should have in mind prior to the meeting what the important medical information is, such as the biopsy result, a worsening prognosis, or that the organ failure is worsening despite significant ICU support. It is important to avoid medical jargon or ambiguous words or euphemisms. If you think the patient is dying or is likely to die, use those words, so there are not misperceptions about what you are saying. Focusing on the details of every medical issue is not necessary, nor particularly helpful, though how much medical detail you discuss will depend on the family's health literacy and questions. Start with where their perception is; this is the time to correct any misconceptions and to give any new news. If you are giving bad news, it is helpful to use a modifier, often called a "warning shot." This brief alert to the impending bad news allows for some preparation that the information you have is not good. Examples of a warning shot with a quick, clear delivery of the bad news are: "We have some bad news; the biopsy showed cancer," or "Unfortunately, your father's lung and kidney failure are getting worse, and he is likely going to die in the hospital." Once you have given the bad news, stop talking and give the family time to take this in.

RESPOND TO EMOTION   After you have given medical information, allow time for the normal emotional reactions that many family members will have in the setting of bad news. Silence after giving bad news is important, as it shows you are acknowledging the difficulty of the situation, and most people will not hear what is being said after difficult news if the conversation starts before they are done with emotional processing. Using empathic statements, as outlined in Chapter 7, are useful to acknowledge and support the emotions the family is feeling. For example, "I cannot imagine how difficult this is for your family to go through." Most people will be able to move on from the emotional place after a few minutes; however, if the emotion is too great, you need to recognize that and consider stopping the meeting here with plans for follow-up discussions. Keep in mind that not all people will have an emotional reaction at this time, but pausing allows time if needed.

ELICITING VALUES AND GOALS: OPEN-ENDED QUESTIONS   This is the point at which you want to determine what is important to this patient/family, so that you can help them in making a decision for medical care consistent with their values and goals. There are many open-ended questions you can use to assess this, even as simple as "We are only seeing your father while he is sick, tell us about him." Other examples are, "Knowing this information, what are you worried about as you look ahead?" and, to highlight the surrogate decision-maker role, "If your husband were able to be here and discuss his health with us, what do you think he would want?" This is a key

Table 8.4   Responding to Difficult Family Statements

Example of Family Statements	Response Approach and Examples
"She's a fighter"	Acknowledge this truth they are relaying:
	"I can see she has been fighting this illness, and now, the situation is different and the treatment is not working. It may be time to focus her fight on other issues"
"She wants to live"	Again, acknowledge this truth while reflecting that you would wish this for her as well:
	"Clearly, she has a lot to live for; I wish we had treatments that would cure her illness"
"Don't tell her she is dying"	If the patient has decision-making capacity, let the family know that you will, without going into specifics, ask the patient what she wishes to know. It can be helpful for the family members to hear how you are going to phrase the question ahead of time:
	"Some patients wish to discuss all their medical information with their doctor themselves, while others want instead to have their family members discuss it with their doctor. Which would you prefer?"
	Another example:
	"How much do you want to know about what is going on with your health?"

time to allow the family to do the majority of the talking. There can be statements made by family members that can be challenging to respond to; some common examples and possible responses are shown in Table 8.4.

DECISION-MAKING Now that everyone has the same information about the medical situation, and the patient's goals, you can start to make decisions about how to best proceed with integrating that information. The treatment options should be discussed with avoiding medical jargon and being clear, with allowing time for the family to have all questions answered. When discussing treatment options, be mindful of how you describe an option of focusing on comfort and foregoing life-prolonging therapies. Specifically, describing the option of focusing on comfort as "…or, we can do nothing" or "…we can stop everything" does not accurately describe this treatment route, nor would family members want medical providers to "do nothing" for their loved one. Keep the conversation focused on what we would be doing in a more palliative-focused treatment plan, "We can remove the breathing tube and aggressively treat any pain or shortness of breath he may have."

It is rare that a decision needs to be made right in the meeting, so there is no need to force one. It often helps if you directly say that "You do not need to make a decision right now, we can allow you to talk as a family and discuss a decision tomorrow" or even say "in 15 minutes" if the decision is an urgent one.

MAKE A RECOMMENDATION This can be an important step, with some data to support that many people want physicians to give input on which treatment option to choose [12]. The majority of families in an ICU study did want a medical provider's recommendation on limitations of life-supporting therapies, though others did not [17]. If you are not sure if a recommendation is desired by the patient and the family, ask: "Would it be helpful to hear our recommendation?" Recommendations should be based on the values and goals previously elicited during a family meeting. There are many ways to give a recommendation, but one approach that integrates information already obtained during the meeting would be: "I'm hearing that your grandmother has always been a very active and independent person who never wanted to live in a nursing home. Since she had this severe stroke and will not be able to eat on her own again or be independent, I would recommend that we focus her medical care on her comfort and quality of life and not put in a feeding tube. Does that sound consistent with her wishes?"

SUMMARIZE AND WRAP UP Not all meetings end with a decision, but all meetings must come to an end: either outline the decision and what the next steps will be, or close the meeting with plans for follow-up for more discussions (e.g., "There is still a lot to discuss, and we are out of time. We should plan another meeting"). The decision may even be a time-limited trial, such as 3 more days of ventilatory support to see if the patient improves or not, though there should be discussion about how improvement, or the lack thereof, will be assessed (see Chapter 12). Physician statements that are particularly helpful to families are validation statements about the decision and assurances of ensuring patient comfort and that the patient will not be abandoned, regardless of the decision made [23]. For example, "Your grandmother is fortunate to have such a supportive family who is able to carry out her wishes. We will make sure she is comfortable no matter what happens." It is also helpful to make clear the plans for follow-up and how the family can get in contact with members of the team if they have any questions or needs that arise.

AFTER the Family Meeting. For all medical providers involved, it can be helpful to spend a few minutes both to discuss the logistics of how to carry out the plan discussed and to debrief on the meeting, as they can be filled with difficult emotions for all involved. Also, discussing what went well, what did not, and what could have been done differently can provide learning opportunities for all involved on how to improve communication with patients and families.

8.3 ADDITIONAL INTERPROFESSIONAL SUPPORT FOR FAMILIES

Palliative medicine is an interprofessional field for good reason, as there are many domains of patients' and families' lives affected by serious illness. The key is to be attuned to and ask about the common areas of needs, and get families in touch with the right interprofessional provider to get them the appropriate assistance.

8.3.1   Opportunities to Ask Questions and Clarify Information

Most families are unable to understand detailed and emotionally laden information such as a bad news or a poor prognosis after one meeting. Further, large meetings with physicians and multiple clinicians can be intimidating for families. It is important to identify clinicians with whom families feel comfortable and who have time to discuss what occurred in the family meeting in a more relaxed setting. These clinicians may be physicians with whom families have a preexisting relationship, nurses, social workers, or palliative care clinicians.

8.3.2   Spiritual and Religious Care

Religious and spiritual beliefs are important to many patients and families during end of life [11]; therefore, it is important to ask about these needs for patients and family members in a sensitive way. If patients and family members desire spiritual or religious support, you should make a referral to chaplaincy or spiritual care services. Also, be aware of signs of negative religious coping (i.e., punishment, abandonment by God) that would particularly benefit from spiritual care involvement.

8.3.3   Psychosocial Support

During critical illness, there are many practical concerns that patients and family members will have, in addition to the emotional burdens that arise as well, and these areas are within the expertise of social workers. Many families lose income during loved one's illness, whether due to the patient's or caregiver's inability to work, so financial concerns are common [26]. As mentioned previously, many family members will deal with anxiety, depression, and PTSD symptoms during and after a loved one's hospitalization or death. Encouragement should be made to appropriate family members to make contact with a mental health provider or their primary care provider, or if possible social work can get them local mental health resource information. Referrals for bereavement support can often be made to local hospice agencies, or social work can get them material on local grief support groups.

8.3.4   Support for Families with Children

For families with children, special attention to the children's needs is valuable. Often family members are unsure how to, or how much to, tell children about a family member's illness or death and dying. Another component is the complexity of children's grief, as there are age-specific grief responses that can be seen. If your hospital has child-life services, consultation with a child-life specialist and the family (with or without the children) is an excellent option. If you do not have child-life resources available, Table 8.5 lists online resources for interested families.

Table 8.5   Additional Resources on Family Meetings and Caring for Families

Medical College of Wisconsin Fast Facts #016, #149, #223, #224, #225, and #227
http://www.eperc.mcw.edu/EPERC/FastFactsandConcepts
ONCOTALK
http://depts.washington.edu/oncotalk/
MD Anderson Cancer Center, I*CARE Videos, *Managing Difficult Communication*
http://www.mdanderson.org/education-and-research/resources-for-professionals/
  professional-educational-resources/i-care/complete-library-of-communication-videos/
  managing-difficult-communication.html
Specific Resources for Families with Children
The Dougy Center, Child Grief Resources
http://www.dougy.org/grief-resources/
The American Academy of Child and Adolescent Psychiatry, Child Grief Resources
http://www.aacap.org/AACAP/Families_and_Youth/Facts_for_Families/Facts_for_
  Families_Pages/Children_And_Grief_08.aspx

REFERENCES

1. Singer PA, Martin DK, Kelner M, Quality end-of-life care—patients' perspectives, *JAMA* 1999 Jan 13;**281**(2):163–168. PubMed PMID: WOS:000077966800037. English.
2. Manning-Walsh J, Social support as a mediator between symptom distress and quality of life in women with breast cancer, *J Obstet Gynecol Neonatal Nurs* 2005 Jul–Aug;**34**(4):482–493. PubMed PMID: 16020416.
3. Rabow MW, Hauser JM, Adams J, Supporting family caregivers at the end of life: "they don't know what they don't know," *JAMA* 2004 Jan 28;**291**(4):483–491. PubMed PMID: 14747506.
4. Azoulay E, Chevret S, Leleu G, et al., Half the families of intensive care unit patients experience inadequate communication with physicians, *Crit Care Med* 2000 Aug;**28**(8):3044–3049. PubMed PMID: 10966293.
5. Majesko A, Hong SY, Weissfeld L, White DB, Identifying family members who may struggle in the role of surrogate decision maker, *Crit Care Med* 2012 Aug;**40**(8):2281–2286. PubMed PMID: 22809903. Pubmed Central PMCID: 3530841.
6. Ahrens T, Yancey V, Kollef M, Improving family communications at the end of life: implications for length of stay in the intensive care unit and resource use, *Am J Crit Care* 2003 Jul;**12**(4):317–323; discussion 24. PubMed PMID: 12882061.
7. Lilly CM, De Meo DL, Sonna LA, et al., An intensive communication intervention for the critically ill, *Am J Med* 2000 Oct 15;**109**(6):469–475. PubMed PMID: 11042236.
8. Lautrette A, Darmon M, Megarbane B, et al., A communication strategy and brochure for relatives of patients dying in the ICU, *N Engl J Med* 2007 Feb 1;**356**(5):469–478. PubMed PMID: 17267907.
9. Curtis JR, Engelberg RA, Wenrich MD, Shannon SE, Treece PD, Rubenfeld GD, Missed opportunities during family conferences about end-of-life care in the intensive care unit, *Am J Respir Crit Care Med.* 2005 Apr 15;**171**(8):844–849. PubMed PMID: 15640361.
10. Shalowitz DI, Garrett-Mayer E, Wendler D, The accuracy of surrogate decision makers: a systematic review, *Arch Intern Med.* 2006 Mar 13;**166**(5):493–497. PubMed PMID: 16534034.
11. Abbott KH, Sago JG, Breen CM, Abernethy AP, Tulsky JA, Families looking back: one year after discussion of withdrawal or withholding of life-sustaining support, *Crit Care Med.* 2001 Jan;**29**(1):197–201. PubMed PMID: 11176185.
12. Johnson SK, Bautista CA, Hong SY, Weissfeld L, White DB, An empirical study of surrogates' preferred level of control over value-laden life support decisions in intensive care units, *Am J Resp Crit Care* 2011 Apr 1;**183**(7):915–921. PubMed PMID: WOS:000289318800018. English.

13. Schenker Y, Crowley-Matoka M, Dohan D, Tiver GA, Arnold RM, White DB, I don't want to be the one saying "we should just let him die": intrapersonal tensions experienced by surrogate decision makers in the ICU, *J Gen Intern Med* 2012 Dec;**27**(12):1657–1665. PubMed PMID: WOS:000312072200015. English.

14. Apatira L, Boyd EA, Malvar G, et al., Hope, truth, and preparing for death: perspectives of surrogate decision makers. *Ann Intern Med* 2008 Dec 16;**149**(12):861–868. PubMed PMID: 19075205. Pubmed Central PMCID: 2622736.

15. Tilden VP, Tolle SW, Garland MJ, Nelson CA, Decisions about life-sustaining treatment. Impact of physicians' behaviors on the family, *Arch Intern Med* 1995 Mar 27;**155**(6):633–638. PubMed PMID: 7887760.

16. Vig EK, Starks H, Taylor JS, Hopley EK, Fryer-Edwards K, Surviving surrogate decision-making: what helps and hampers the experience of making medical decisions for others, *J Gen Intern Med* 2007 Sep;**22**(9):1274–1279. PubMed PMID: 17619223. Pubmed Central PMCID: 2219771.

17. White DB, Evans LR, Bautista CA, Luce JM, Lo B, Are physicians' recommendations to limit life support beneficial or burdensome? Bringing empirical data to the debate, *Am J Respir Crit Care Med* 2009 Aug 15;**180**(4):320–325. PubMed PMID: 19498057. Pubmed Central PMCID: 2731809.

18. Fineberg IC, Kawashima M, Asch SM, Communication with families facing life-threatening illness: a research-based model for family conferences, *J Palliat Med* 2011 Apr;**14**(4):421–427. PubMed PMID: 21385083.

19. Lautrette A, Ciroldi M, Ksibi H, Azoulay E, End-of-life family conferences: rooted in the evidence. *Crit Care Med* 2006 Nov;**34**(11 Suppl):S364–S3672. PubMed PMID: 17057600.

20. Curtis JR, Patrick DL, Shannon SE, Treece PD, Engelberg RA, Rubenfeld GD, The family conference as a focus to improve communication about end-of-life care in the intensive care unit: Opportunities for improvement, *Crit Care Med* 2001 Feb;**29**(2):N26–N33. PubMed PMID: WOS:000167333000006. English.

21. Anderson W, Cimino J, Ungar A, et al., Keys to communicating about prognosis in the ICU: a multicenter study of family, provider, and expert perspectives, *J Pain Symptom Manage* 2013 Feb;**45**(2):382. PubMed PMID: WOS:000315684600119. English.

22. McDonagh JR, Elliott TB, Engelberg RA, et al., Family satisfaction with family conferences about end-of-life care in the intensive care unit: increased proportion of family speech is associated with increased satisfaction, *Crit Care Med* 2004 Jul;**32**(7):1484–1488. PubMed PMID: 15241092.

23. Stapleton RD, Engelberg RA, Wenrich MD, Goss CH, Curtis JR, Clinician statements and family satisfaction with family conferences in the intensive care unit, *Crit Care Med* 2006 Jun;**34**(6):1679–1685. PubMed PMID: 16625131.

24. West HF, Engelberg RA, Wenrich MD, Curtis JR, Expressions of nonabandonment during the intensive care unit family conference, *J Palliat Med* 2005 Aug;**8**(4):797–807. PubMed PMID: 16128654.

25. Pollak KI, Arnold RM, Jeffreys AS, et al., Oncologist communication about emotion during visits with patients with advanced cancer, *J Clin Oncol* 2007 Dec 20;**25**(36):5748–5752. PubMed PMID: 18089870.

26. Covinsky KE, Goldman L, Cook EF, et al., The impact of serious illness on patients' families. SUPPORT investigators. Study to understand prognoses and preferences for outcomes and risks of treatment, *JAMA* 1994 Dec 21;**272**(23):1839–1844. PubMed PMID: 7990218.

Chapter 9

Assessing Goals of Care: A Case-Based Discussion

Elizabeth Lindenberger and Amy S. Kelley

Whether healthy or facing serious illness, people go through life with a sense of identity, what gives meaning to their lives, and what hopes they hold for the future. "Goals of care" (GOC) refer to those things that are most important to patients as they journey through illness. GOC are likely to change over time as an illness progresses, as prognosis changes, or as patients adjust to disease. Potential GOC may include hope for cure or life prolongation, relief of suffering, maintaining functional independence, or location of death [1, 2]. Patients may have multiple GOC at once, for example, achieving disease cure and relief of pain and other symptoms. Simultaneous goals may be supported by encouraging patients to both "hope for the best, and prepare for the worst [3]."

Eliciting and negotiating GOC require skilled communication on the part of the medical provider. These skills include assessing a patient's understanding of the disease, providing information about disease and prognosis, responding to emotion, and exploring concerns, hopes, and spirituality. Providers must also be prepared to explore the cultural, religious, or spiritual background of a patient and family, as these factors may influence personal GOC. Through skilled discussions, physicians can help guide patients and families toward care plans that best match their goals [4]. Of further benefit, studies demonstrate that GOC discussions for seriously ill patients are associated with less aggressive medical interventions, lower costs, and increased hospice referrals at the end of life [5, 6].

In this chapter, we will use a patient vignette to illustrate the process of discussing GOC. Each segment offers a step-by-step list of "tasks" as well as specific language. Several key topics (e.g., religion and spirituality) and possible challenges (e.g., using an interpreter) are also addressed.

Hospital-Based Palliative Medicine: A Practical, Evidence-Based Approach, First Edition.
Edited by Steven Pantilat, Wendy Anderson, Matthew Gonzales, and Eric Widera.
© 2015 John Wiley & Sons, Inc. Published 2015 by John Wiley & Sons, Inc.

The Case of Ms Lopez

One morning on a hospitalist shift, you are called to admit Ms Lopez, a 64-year-old woman with idiopathic pulmonary fibrosis (IPF) presenting with shortness of breath (SOB) and hypoxia. Ms Lopez was in her usual state of health until 2 days prior, when she began experiencing worsening cough and dyspnea. She reports requiring more of her home oxygen in order to ambulate a few feet to the bathroom and subjective fevers. In the emergency department, she was found to be hypoxic both by oxygen saturation and ABG, tachypneic to the 30s, but was otherwise stable and not currently requiring intubation. Her chest X-ray showed some bilateral infiltrates that could be consistent with infection. A computed tomography (CT) is recommended for further evaluation. She is being admitted for a probable acute exacerbation of her pulmonary fibrosis, possibly triggered by pneumonia.

Ms Lopez has been hospitalized 4 times this year for acute exacerbations of her IPF. She generally improves with supportive care including oxygen, antibiotics, and steroids. Over the past 2 years, she has been intubated twice for hypoxic respiratory failure. The pulmonologist's note from her last admission states that this is a progressive and incurable condition. Due to her illness and recurrent hospitalizations, she has become increasingly weak and fatigued and is losing weight. Functionally, she can only walk a few steps before having SOB and needing to rest, even with 2l of oxygen by nasal canula. She requires help with daily tasks like preparing meals and getting dressed. She has a large and supportive family who help to care for her, and her younger sister, Josephine, recently moved in with her. Because of her poor functional status, she is not a transplant candidate.

You plan to admit her, start antibiotics and steroids, and closely monitor her respiratory status. Given her history, you assume that she would want to be intubated if her condition declined, but you are not sure when or if GOC were discussed with her. You cannot find evidence of a prior discussion in her chart.

9.1   ROAD MAP FOR DISCUSSING GOALS OF CARE

The discussion of GOC is a process. The first conversation may lead to a fuller understanding of the medical circumstances by the patient or family (Part I); may develop a deeper understanding of the patient's identity, values, and concerns by the medical team (Part II); and even may result in mutual agreement about the GOC at that point in time (Part III). Providers must remember, however, that goals and preferences may shift over time and the discussion of GOC should continue over the course of an illness. Here, we lay out steps for discussing GOC. These steps may not all be completed in one encounter, and the discussion need not be strictly linear. We will illustrate each step with phrases and questions that may be useful in your own clinical practice.

9.1.1   Part I: Lay the Groundwork for Discussing GOC

The first and most fundamental task in identifying GOC is ensuring the patient and/ or family's accurate understanding of the medical circumstances (Table 9.1). The level of detail of this understanding will vary widely across individuals based upon their personal desire for information. Rarely do patients desire to know medical details, such as the specific results of laboratory test, nor is this level of detail necessary for full understanding and informed decision-making. In fact, some details may distract from or muddle the big-picture message. For example, a patient may understand that he has lung cancer that has spread and that it is not possible to cure his disease. Therefore, it is best to begin by finding out what the patient already knows about her condition. Corrections or clarifications can then be addressed as needed. After providing information, confirming understanding is essential before moving on. Following these steps will save time later by avoiding misunderstandings.

Table 9.1   Ensuring Accurate Understanding of the Medical Circumstances

Task	Suggested Language
Prepare for the discussion: • Set a time and minimize interruptions • Who does the patient want to be present • Ensure a private setting where the patient, family, and providers can sit comfortably	"I'd like to find a time to talk more about your medical condition and the treatment plans. Who would you like to have there when we talk?"
Assess the patient's understanding of her condition and the current medical situation	"Just so we're on the same page, could you tell me what you have heard about your medical condition?"
Explore how much information the patient wants to know	"I wondered if you could tell me what the other doctors have told you so far" "Are you the type of person who wants information in detail?"
Ask permission before giving new information	"Is it okay if I explain what the test showed?" "Would now be a good time to discuss your test results?"
Provide information: • Give small pieces, starting with the big picture • Avoid medical jargon • Pause before providing additional pieces of information	"The CT scan shows that your condition has gotten worse" "Unfortunately, we do not have any treatment that can fix the underlying problem"
Check for the patient's emotional response and respond explicitly to emotional data	"This must come as a shock" "I can't imagine how painful it is to hear this news" "I wish things were different" "It must be so hard facing this uncertainty"
Confirm patient's understanding before moving on	"How will you describe what I told you to your sister?"

Case—Ms Lopez: Ensuring Accurate Understanding

You ask Ms Lopez about setting up a meeting to discuss her condition and her medical plan. She says that while her family is wonderful and extremely supportive, she worries about burdening them with this sad information. Therefore, she would like to have only her sister Josephine present during the meeting. You come back later that afternoon when Josephine is visiting. In the meantime, you have received the CT chest report. It reveals bilateral ground-glass abnormalities and honeycombing, increased since the study 6 weeks prior and consistent with progression of IPF, and a new left lower lobe consolidation, suggestive of acute lobar pneumonia.

The patient is in a private room, so you bring in a few extra chairs and ask her nurse to also join you for the meeting. Ms Lopez understands her lung disease is bad, and she says she has been told that it will only get worse. She tells you, though, that she has always been very independent and tough. She worked as a high school math teacher for 28 years, until she had to start oxygen therapy 3 years ago. While she has been told that there is no cure for the disease, she keeps hoping that something new may be discovered that will help her.

She is not surprised by the current CT scan because this has happened before. She hopes she will get better this time without having to go on the ventilator machine. You tell her, "Unfortunately, we do not have any treatment that can fix the underlying problem." The patient is silent and her sister reaches out to hold her hand. After several seconds, you add, "I wish things were different." She looks you in the eyes and says, "Me too. I know we can't fix my lungs completely, but there must be some things we can do to help me breathe."

9.1.2   Part II: Assess Goals and Values

Assessing goals and values involves four components (Table 9.2). The first step is to explore communication preferences. Patients' personal and cultural backgrounds may impact how they prefer to receive information. Some patients, for example, may prefer to have their families make medical decisions for them.

The second step is to explore what gives life meaning to the patient, that is, what people and activities are most important and what he or she most enjoys. The third step is to identify your patient's concerns about the future. What does your patient most fear, and what has been most difficult about being ill.

The fourth step to assessing goals and values is a cultural and spiritual assessment. Providers should address any unique cultural values that may affect decision-making [7]. Spiritual and religious beliefs may also impact patients' health in a variety of ways, including illness beliefs, coping strategies, and community supports. Exploring spirituality helps providers incorporate beliefs and traditions into individualized treatment plans and also encourages patients and families to draw support from their spiritual traditions. Spiritual support by inpatient medical teams may also improve health outcomes at the end of life. In one study of terminally ill patients well supported by religious communities, receiving spiritual support from the medical team was associated with fewer aggressive interventions and higher rates of hospice use [8].

Table 9.2   Assessing Goals and Values

Task	Suggested Language
Identify communication preferences	"Some people want to know everything about their medical condition, and others do not. How much would you like to know?"
	If a patient prefers to have family be primary decision-makers, then:
	"Would you like me to speak with them alone, or would you like to be present?"
Explore what gives life meaning	"Before we talk about next steps, I wondered if you could tell me more about what your life is like when you are not in the hospital"
	"What is important to you?"
	"What do you enjoy?"
	"What is most important to you if your time is limited?"
Identify concerns	"What concerns do you have about the future?"
	"What else?"
	"What's the hardest part of this for you and your family?"
Assess unique cultural values	Is there anything that would be helpful for me to know about how you and your family view serious illness? Are there any cultural beliefs, practices, or preferences that affect you during illness?
Assess spirituality	"Do you consider yourself spiritual or religious?"
• F—Faith and belief	If yes, continue below
• I—Importance	"Have your beliefs influenced how you take care of yourself in your illness?"
• C—Community	"Are you part of a spiritual or religious community?"
• A—Address in care	"Is this of support to you? How?"
	"How would you like me to address these issues in your health care?"

A spiritual assessment involves exploring how patients' beliefs and faith traditions affect their relationship with illness. The FICA tool, outlined in the following, is one widely used method of spiritual assessment [9]. A spiritual assessment may begin with an invitation such as "Is it ok if I ask you about your spiritual beliefs?"

9.1.3   Part III: Confirm Goals and Develop Treatment Plan

The hardest part is done! Through skillful questions and empathetic responses, you have elicited a fuller understanding of the patient and her goals and values. This is the critical information that cannot be gleaned from a radiology study or lab report, and yet is fundamental to developing a patient-centered treatment plan.

Case—Ms Lopez: Assessing Goals and Values

You ask Ms Lopez how her life has been outside of the hospital and what things are most important to her. She shares she lived alone for many years, worked hard, was independent. Her health decline has made her more dependent on others, and this has been difficult for her. At the same time, she is close with her family and has great support from friends, particularly several former teachers with whom she used to work. When asked about concerns, she is most worried about her mother's well-being and how she will be able to cope when she dies. She also worries about being a burden on her family, particularly Josephine when she becomes increasingly ill and dependent. She notes that she trusts Josephine immensely and feels she is the one who best understands what she is going through and how hard these changes have been. When asked about spirituality, she states she is Catholic and that her religion is extremely important for her. She both draws strength from her spirituality and also meaning about her disease. She believes her illness is part of God's plan, even though she does not fully understand.

She only remembers pieces of her past ICU admissions, but she remembers being in pain and so frustrated she could not communicate. She also recalls how distressing it was for her mother. Her mother is 86 and thinks of nothing but her children. She doesn't speak English and is fearful of the hospital and doesn't understand how ill her daughter is. When Ms Lopez is in the hospital, her mother prays constantly, and Ms Lopez worries that one of these times it will be too much for her.

Ms Lopez says that she hopes to recover and return home but that she wants to avoid going to the ICU. She knows she is going to die from her disease and would rather be comfortable and surrounded by her family when that happens. She wants Josephine to make her medical decisions if she becomes too sick to talk. She knows she needs to tell her mother about her condition, but she can never find the words. She wants to protect her.

The next tasks, outlined here, are to confirm the central or primary goal and then translate that into a recommended medical plan (Table 9.3). First, restating or confirming the primary goal may require the provider to "translate" a value to a clinical goal. For example, the patient may have described being happiest when at home and hopes for maximizing her time with her grandchildren. The provider may translate this to the primary goal of being at home, having care delivered in the home setting, and efforts made to avoid hospitalization. This translation or restating allows the patient the opportunity to confirm or correct the primary goal so that everyone understands and agrees about what the treatment plan is aiming to achieve.

Once the primary goal is confirmed, the provider can recommend a congruent treatment plan. While the patient is the expert in her own values and goals, she has likely not had the years of medical training and experience that are required to determine whether a specific medical intervention or diagnostic procedure will support her reaching those goals or work against that effort. Depending upon the patient's goal, these suggestions may include a recommendation to not attempt resuscitation and, rather, to ensure comfort at the time of death.

Table 9.3 Confirm Goal and Develop Treatment Plan

Task	Suggested Language
Restate primary goal(s) and confirm shared understanding	"Thank you for sharing that with me. It sounds like the most important thing is to maximize your time with your family" "Given what you have told me, it sounds like as long as you are comfortable, you want to continue treatments that may extend your life. Even if that means being in the hospital" "I am glad to know your faith gives you peace amidst this uncertainty. I understand that you would want to try medicines to see if your condition can improve, but because you know you are dying from this disease, you would not want to have machines keep you alive artificially"
Ask permission to give recommendation, once the primary goal of care is clear	"Now that I understand what is most important to work toward, could I make some recommendations?" "Given what you have told me, may I recommend some next steps?"
Provide recommendations for plan of care to meet goals: what will be done and what will not be done	"In order to maximize your time with your family, I recommend that we plan for you to go home with services from a hospice team, who can manage your pain and help support you and your family. In the meantime, we will add a medication to try to control your nausea. I also recommend that if you were to die in the hospital, that we focus on making you comfortable and do not attempt CPR or put you on a breathing machine" "We will continue treatments and medicines focused on trying to get you through this episode and back home. We will also add medicine to help make your breathing more comfortable. Knowing that we can't change the underlying disease, if your condition gets worse, we will work to keep you comfortable and allow you to die peacefully"
Confirm understanding and agreement: • Reaffirm nonabandonment regardless of the goals of care • Answer questions • Make arrangements for follow-up	"What questions do you have?" "We have to talk about a lot of difficult things; what else concerns you?" "We will continue to check on you to be sure we are making progress on your pain" "I will see you in the morning and we can talk more then"

Case—Ms Lopez: Confirming Goals and Developing Treatment Plan

You repeat back to Ms Lopez the primary goals she has identified: she hopes to recover enough from this current episode to return home to spend more quality time with her family; she wants medicines and treatments that will help achieve that goal, but does not want to have machines used to prolong her life; she wants Josephine to be her health-care agent when/if she is too ill to make decisions; and she is very concerned about how her mother will cope with her declining health. She confirms what you said is correct and would like to hear your recommendations. You recommend the following plan: continue antibiotics, steroids, and nebulizers; add low-dose morphine to further relieve SOB as needed; record a DNR/DNI order so that she would not be intubated in an emergency; and organize a time to talk together with her mother and include the hospital chaplain, Father Ritchie, in the conversation.

She is surprised and grateful when you offer to help talk to her mother and explain what is happening. She agrees that the rest of the plan sounds good, and is glad to know that hospital team will be working hard to get her better enough to go home, but that she will not have to put her family or herself through another period on the ventilator. You agree that Josephine will help to arrange a time to bring her mother in to visit. You promise to follow up tomorrow morning.

9.1.4   After the Discussion

After any full or partial discussion of goal of care, it is critical to document the conversation. The following chapter deals with this topic in detail including the completion of HCP, MOLST, DNR, etc. as appropriate.

It is also important to spend a few minutes after the discussion to debrief with your team or review the conversation by yourself. What was said? What questions or phrase did you use that worked well? Did you feel stuck at any point? Are there alternative questions or phrases you would try in a similar situation? Aim to take away a learning point from every communication encounter. By doing so, you will build a large repertoire of skills for future use.

9.2   USE OF INTERPRETERS

A large and growing number of seriously ill patients in the United States are non-English-speaking immigrants. Accurate and sensitive language interpretation is critical when discussing complex GOC issues with non-English-speaking patients and families. Appropriate use of language interpreters not only increases comprehension but also associated with decreased health disparities and improved clinical outcomes. Use of professional interpreters, whether in-person or by telephone, is the standard of care for language interpretation in the medical setting. Ad hoc interpreters, in contrast, refer to family members or hospital staff (e.g., nurses) who have second language skills but are not trained as professional interpreters. Use of professional interpreters improves comprehension, especially when complex treatment decisions are being addressed, and decreases cultural misunderstandings. Avoiding the use of family interpreters also decreases the potential for serious emotional burdens that can occur when they are playing the dual role of family member and interpreter. It is recommended that even physicians who are native speakers in the patient's language consider using a professional interpreter for complex family meetings, especially when there are clinicians or family members present who do not speak the language. It is difficult and risky to lead a family meeting while simultaneously serving as interpreter.

When using an interpreter, it is important to speak directly to the patient and family rather than to the interpreter. Patients and families should be assured that all professional interpreters are trained to protect patient confidentiality and privacy. Direct communication and eye contact improve both verbal and nonverbal communication and also emphasize the primary therapeutic alliance, which is between the clinician and the patient and family. The clinician should also take extra efforts to keep phrases short and simple, avoid medical jargon, ask patients and families for understanding after information is given, and encourage questions.

When serious and complex medical issues are discussed, for example, communicating bad news or withholding or withdrawing treatments, professional interpreters may feel emotionally burdened by the process. Preparing interpreters before and debriefing them after a family meeting may decrease the burden on interpreter and also improve communication between provider and patient/family. Strategies for preparation and debrief with interpreters are outlined in Table 9.4 [10].

Table 9.4 Communicating with Interpreters

Recommendation	Things to Say
Prepare the interpreter before the meeting	"Before we go into the room, I want to tell you about our goals for this meeting and some topics we will be discussing"
	"I would like you to translate everything that is said, word for word. I will try and pause frequently to give you a chance to translate exactly"
	"Please let me know if there are any words I am using that are not easy to translate and that may lead to understanding. One example of a specific, technical term I may use is hospice"
	"Are there any cultural concerns I should know about?"
Debrief with the interpreter after the meeting	"Tell me about how the meeting went for you?"
	"Do you have any concerns about the family's understanding or the impact the discussion may have had on the family?"
	"Is there anything the family said that you did not have a chance to interpret?"

Case—Ms Lopez: Discussion with Patient and Her Mother Using Interpreter

A meeting is arranged with Ms Lopez and her mother to help her communicate her diagnosis and the progression disease. The patient's sister Josephine is also present. Josephine offers to translate, but you explain that you have invited a hospital interpreter to assist so that she can focus on participating in the discussion rather than on interpreting. You meet with the interpreter outside of the room before starting the meeting to explain the goals and content of the discussion. You also instruct her to translate everything that is said, word for word, exactly. You then introduce the interpreter to the family and explain to the family that all hospital interpreters are trained to protect patient privacy and confidentiality and that the service is free of charge.

You begin the family meeting, speaking directly to the family and using the interpreter to translate. Following reintroductions and greetings, you ask the patient's mother what she has been told so far about what is going on with her daughter's health. She becomes tearful and says, "I know she is very sick." You ask if it is ok with her for you to share information. You explain that you have already spoken with her daughters and that it is important to them that she also understands all that is going on. Ms Lopez and Josephine nod. You affirm that she is correct, that her daughter's disease is serious, and that what is most important to her daughter is to focus on comfort, spending time with her family, and being at home. The patient's mother becomes very tearful but expresses relief at understanding the situation. She explains that she had already assumed the worst. She expresses that she wants to support her daughter in going home and that she and her whole family will be committed to caring for her. You hold her hand as she cries, and you tell her, "I know this is very difficult. I am so impressed by how much love and support there is in this family." After a short silence, you explain that you are recommending hospice services to help provide maximum support to the patient and family at home after hospital discharge.

Following the meeting, you debrief with the interpreter privately outside of the room. She states she feels that the patient's mother understood the conversation well. When asked if there was any other information that you should know, she states that she thinks the mother's faith is important to her because she said quietly to herself several times, "God will take care of her."

9.2.1 When Surrogates Are Making Decisions

When patients are critically ill or have lost decisional capacity for other reasons, surrogate decision-makers become responsible for treatment decisions. The surrogate's role is to exercise substituted judgment, that is, to make decisions as the patient would have made them using what is known from the patient's previously expressed goals and values. This role can be extremely difficult for many surrogates, as the desire to honor the patient's goals and values may conflict with other emotions such as fear of responsibility for patient's death, desire to avoid family conflict, and hope for their loved one to recover [11]. Effective communication with surrogates may alleviate decision-making burdens and promote effecting honoring of patients' goals and values (see Chapter 10).

Table 9.5   Helpful Language When Speaking with Surrogates [12, 13]

The Approach	Things to Say
Bring the patient's "voice" into the decision-making process	"What gave his life meaning? What things were most important to him as a person?" "If your husband were sitting here with us, what would he say?"
Respond to emotion For example, the surrogate says: "He's a fighter"	"Yes, I can see that is a very strong person. He has fought very hard through this disease."
"I want you to do everything!"	"I can only imagine how hard this is for you. Could you tell me more about what you mean by 'everything'?"
Recognize the importance of time and support for surrogates	"This is very difficult. Our team is here to support you and your whole family through this process"

Discussing GOC with surrogates involves all of the same steps as outlined earlier for patients. Additionally, effective communication includes discussion and processing of the surrogate's role. Table 9.5 outlines language that may be helpful in framing the role of the surrogate and decreasing the stress and burden of surrogate decision-making.

9.3   CONCLUSION

Discussing GOC with seriously ill patients is a critical skill that should occur in an ongoing manner over time. Understanding patients' goals helps ensure that treatment decisions match patients' values and preferences. It is not uncommon for patients' goals to change over time and to include simultaneously the hope for life prolongation as well as relief of suffering. Eliciting and negotiating GOC requires several key skills, including assessing a patient's understanding of the disease, providing information about prognosis and treatment options, responding to emotion, and exploring concerns, hopes, and spirituality. Discussing GOC with surrogates becomes necessary when patients lack decisional capacity and requires a similar approach. In these situations, clinicians must additionally use strategies for bringing the patient's "voice" into the decision-making process. Lastly, when caring for patients and families who are non-English speaking, clinicians should use professional interpreters to ensure effective communication.

REFERENCES

1. Steinhauser KE, Christakis NA, Clipp EC, McNeilly M, McIntyre L, Tulsky JA, Factors considered important at the end of life by patients, family, physicians, and other care providers, *JAMA* 2000;**284**(19):2476–2482.
2. Quill T, Norton S, Shah M, Lam Y, Fridd C, Buckley M, What is most important for you to achieve?: an analysis of patient responses when receiving palliative care consultation, *J Palliat Med* 2006;**9**(2):382–388.

3. Back AL, Arnold RM, Quill TE, Hope for the best, and prepare for the worst, *Ann Intern Med* 2003;**138**(5):439–443.

4. Mack JW, Weeks JC, Wright AA, Block SD, Prigerson HG, End-of-life discussions, goal attainment, and distress at the end of life: predictors and outcomes of receipt of care consistent with preferences, *J Clin Oncol* 2010;**28**(7):1203–1208.

5. Wright AA, Zhang B, Ray A, et al., Associations between end-of-life discussions, patient mental health, medical care near death, and caregiver bereavement adjustment, *JAMA* 2008;**300**(14):1665–1673.

6. Zhang B, Wright AA, Huskamp HA, et al., Health care costs in the last week of life: associations with end-of-life conversations, *Arch Intern Med* 2009;**169**(5):480.

7. Lum H, Arnold R, Asking about cultural beliefs in palliative care #216, *J Palliat Med* 2012 Jun;**15**(6):714–715.

8. Balboni TA, Balboni M, Enzinger AC, et al., Provision of spiritual support to patients with advanced cancer by religious communities and associations with medical care at the end of life, *JAMA Intern Med* 2013;**173**(12):1109–1117.

9. FICA Spiritual History Tool. Available at http://www.gwumc.edu/gwish/clinical/fica-spiritual/fica-spiritual-history/index.cfm. Accessed June 10, 2013.

10. Schenker Y, Smith AK, Arnold RM, Fernandez A, "Her husband doesn't speak much English": conducting a family meeting with an interpreter, *J Palliat Med* 2012;**15**(4):494–498.

11. Schenker Y, Crowley-Matoka M, Dohan D, Tiver GA, Arnold RM, White DB, I don't want to be the one saying 'we should just let him die': Intrapersonal tensions experienced by surrogate decision makers in the ICU, *J Gen Intern Med* 2012;**27**(12):1657–1665.

12. Weissman DE, Quill TE, Arnold RM, Helping surrogates make decisions# 226, *J Palliat Med* 2010;**13**(4):461–462.

13. Quill TE, Arnold R, Back AL, Discussing treatment preferences with patients who want "everything," *Ann Intern Med* 2009;**151**(5):345–349.

Chapter 10

Documenting Goals of Care and Treatment Preferences in the Hospital: A Case-Based Discussion

Lynn A. Flint, Rebecca L. Sudore, and Brook Calton

10.1 PRACTICAL IN-HOSPITAL DOCUMENTATION

Patient-centered care is essential for those facing life-limiting illness. However, care cannot be patient-centered without knowing the patient's goals. Studies [1–3] have found that discussing patient's wishes for end-of-life care results in improved quality of life for patients, less anxiety for caregivers, and care consistent with patient's goals which often translates to receipt of less resource-intensive care near the end of life. This impact can be multiplied if these discussions result in clear documentation that is easily and consistently accessible to all members of the care team.

We suggest a five-step process for advance care planning documentation, summarized in Figure 10.1. This figure emphasizes that both goals of care discussions and documentation are ongoing and complementary processes. In her research, Freid [4] has demonstrated that treatment preferences change over time. Given this fact, goals of care discussions should occur at every hospitalization, transition in care, and change in clinical status for a patient. Using prior documentation as a starting point can make these difficult conversations easier (step 1). The results of these discussions should inform iterative documentation, including updating advance directive forms (step 2) as well as hospital orders (step 3) and progress notes (step 4). Finally, the information obtained should be handed off to providers rotating onto the service or covering providers in such a way that patient safety is maintained and patients' wishes are honored (step 5).

Hospital-Based Palliative Medicine: A Practical, Evidence-Based Approach, First Edition.
Edited by Steven Pantilat, Wendy Anderson, Matthew Gonzales, and Eric Widera.
© 2015 John Wiley & Sons, Inc. Published 2015 by John Wiley & Sons, Inc.

Case—Ms Lopez: Documentation Needs

In Chapter 9, "Assessing Goals of Care in a Diverse Population: A Case-Based Discussion," we met Ms Lopez, a 64-year-old woman with worsening idiopathic pulmonary fibrosis (IPF). Ms Lopez' case continues here.

Ms Lopez has been admitted to the hospital for an exacerbation of IPF. Early in her hospital stay, during discussions of goals of care, she shares that her primary goal is to return home as soon as possible and to spend quality time with her family. You recommend that she continue antibiotics, steroids, and nebulizers but that she avoid cardiopulmonary resuscitation (CPR) and mechanical ventilation, because the chance of leaving the hospital after these interventions would be very low. You also add low-dose morphine as needed to further relieve shortness of breath.

To help ensure Ms Lopez' wishes are followed, you plan to document the details and decisions from the conversation in your hospital orders, progress note, and an advance care planning note.

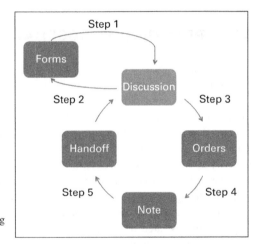

Figure 10.1   Iterative advance care planning documentation.

10.1.1   Step 1: Using Advance Care Planning Forms to Inform Goals of Care Discussions

The first task in documenting goals of care is to review patient's medical record for past goals of care discussions and documentation, and/or to ask patients if they have previously completed advance directive forms. *Advance health-care directives* are legal documents that list a patient's preferences for life-sustaining treatments and/or the person whom they would like to make decisions should they not be able to make them on their own (a surrogate or health-care proxy). Some hospital systems may include copies of a patient's advance directive in the medical record. You can also ask the patient or their family to supply a copy.

Documentation of whether the patient has an advance directive, its content, and the stability of preferences should be included in an admission note. If an advance directive can be obtained, note the date the document was signed, as it may have been executed in the distant past. Asking patients to describe previous discussions concerning advance directive completion could provide a good starting point for your current discussion. Confirm that the listed health-care proxy is correct, as is the alternate proxy, and that their contact information is accurate. Review any treatment preferences outlined in the document to ensure the patient still feels similarly. Potential questions include: "Your prior advance directive said X. Do you still feel the same way? Have you changed your mind about any of your preferences?"

If no prior documentation is available, education can be provided about the advance care planning process; this can often provide a smooth transition into discussion of goals of care or, at the very least, identification of a surrogate decision-maker should the patient lose capacity to make medical decisions.

10.1.2   Step 2: Completing Advance Care Planning Forms Based on Goals of Care Discussions

After the discussion, the next step is to document the outcomes of this discussion on a legal, advance care planning form (summarized in Table 10.1). Inpatient social workers can often help with this task once the wishes are known.

An *advance health-care directive*, which includes a *health-care proxy* document, an *instructional directive*, or both, can be critically helpful. In a recent study by Silveira [5] of adults who were over age 60 and died between 2000 and 2006, 42% required decision-making about treatment in the final days of life, and 70% of those patients lacked decision-making capacity. The *health-care proxy* helps medical providers know

Table 10.1   Advance Care Planning Forms

Name of Document	Description	Pros	Cons
Advance health-care directive	Includes health-care proxy and/or instructional directive	Allows patients to specify preferences for medical treatment	Language is sometimes vague and difficult to apply to specific situations
State-approved out-of-hospital orders for life sustaining treatment (i.e., POLST, MOLST)	Lists specific treatment preferences (i.e., no CPR, no feeding tube, etc.)	Actionable medical order that travels with patients across settings	Lists but does not legally appoint health-care agent Developed only for patients who have serious, progressive, chronic illness
Out-of-hospital DNR form	Lists specific preference not to have CPR	Recognized as medical order outside the hospital	Does not specify other treatment preferences Can only use if choosing DNR

whom the patient has chosen to make decisions on their behalf. The *instructional directive* may then give some guidance to clinicians and surrogate about the types of treatments a patient would want in given situations. Instructional directives often contain standardized language about various treatments in different clinical scenarios.

State-approved physician orders for life-sustaining treatment forms (a.k.a. POLST) translate a seriously ill patient's preferences for life-sustaining interventions into actionable medical orders. The POLST is a standardized form that provides instructions regarding CPR and medical orders that indicate the patient's desired level of medical intervention (i.e., intubation, artificial nutrition, antibiotics, rehospitalization). Once signed by the patient (or their legally designated surrogate decision-maker if the patient has lost decision-making capacity) and their medical provider (typically MD though varies by state), the form serves as a standing medical order. The POLST form can then travel with the patients as they move from one setting to another, thereby ensuring that their physician orders travel with them. The states participating in the POLST program are listed at http://www.polst.org/programs-in-your-state.

A POLST form is different from an advance directive. The POLST forms provide *specific* orders for *current* treatment; in contrast, advance directives specify patient preferences for *future* treatment. In addition, POLST forms are only intended for patients with serious, life-limiting illness or patients with advanced chronic illness (such as frail nursing home patients), whereas all patients may complete an Advance Directive. We recommend that, if available, a POLST form is used as a complement to the advance directive in patients with serious or life-limiting illness.

An older iteration of the POLST form is the *out-of-hospital do not resuscitate* form, which is also a physician's order. This form must be signed by a medical provider (check your state's laws for details) and refers only to a patient's desire to forgo CPR. This document is intended for use outside of the hospital.

Laws related to advance directives, POLST-type forms, and oral advance directives vary by state. Please refer to the "American Bar Association, Commission on Law and Aging" (website: www.abanet.org/aging) to review state-specific laws related to advance directives. A list of suggested advance directive resources is provided at the end of the chapter.

Case—Ms Lopez: Completing Advance Care Planning Forms

You decide to complete a traditional advance directive and a POLST form with Ms Lopez.

On her health-care proxy document, she lists her sister, Josephine, as her health-care agent. She lists her brother, who also lives locally, as an alternate agent, should Josephine not be able to make decisions. Ms Lopez plans to discuss her end-of-life wishes with her brother, since he was not present at the conversations in the hospital. Ms Lopez decides against listing her mother as her alternate agent as she worries she will have difficulty making decisions under stress. On her instructional directive, she specifies that she does not want to have CPR or intubation. In the instructional directive's space where additional wishes can be written, she notes her desire to continue other medical treatments, including antibiotics, as well as her desires to have effective symptom management and to spend as much time at home as possible. A POLST form specifying her code status and desire not to have artificial nutrition is also prepared.

10.1.3   Step 3: Writing Medical Orders

Hospital orders for treatment preferences are most often focused on code status orders, and should be addressed or acknowledged as a regular part of the admission process for patients with serious illness.

However, code status orders like do not resuscitate (DNR)/do not intubate (DNI) do not define all subsequent medical decisions. For instance, the order "DNR" only applies to the decision to withhold CPR in the event of cardiopulmonary arrest. Similarly, "DNI" order only applies to the decision to withhold mechanical ventilation. Of note, DNR and/or DNI orders do not imply other medical treatments should be withheld. Many patients who are on DNR/DNI status may still want antibiotics, blood transfusions, dialysis, and even IV vasopressors and ICU care. For this reason, if a patient expresses a desire not to have a particular treatment, such as dialysis or transfer to the ICU, this should be written as a separate order.

Case—Ms Lopez: Writing Treatment Preference Orders

After completing your progress note, you write the following orders:
"Do not resuscitate."

"Do not intubate."

"No bipap or noninvasive positive pressure ventilation."

"No ICU transfer."

10.1.4   Step 4: Writing a Progress Note

Once you have had an advance care planning discussion with a patient, no matter how brief, document the details in a designated section of your admission or progress note. Your institution may have their own advance care planning note titles. If not, consider titling your note, "Advance Care Planning Discussion Note."

The following pieces of information should always be included in your progress note:

- WHO: Who was present for the discussion.
- WHEN: Date and time of your discussion, including time spent (the latter for billing purposes).
- REVIEW: If an existing advance directive was reviewed, list which document, the date it was executed, preferences reviewed with the patient, and any changes.
- SURROGATE: Surrogate and an alternate health-care agent, and contact information.

Depending on the clinical situation, some or all of the following information may also be helpful to include:

- GOALS AND VALUES: General values such as a desire to focus on comfort or longevity or acceptable/unacceptable health states
- MEDICAL TREATMENT PREFERENCES: That is, code status, artificial nutrition, and why these choices were made and explanations of any time-limited treatment trials decided upon between the medical team and patient
- LEEWAY: Leeway allowed to surrogate in decision-making (i.e., should wishes on instructional directive be followed strictly or does health-care agent have flexibility to make end-of-life treatment decisions they feel are in line with the patient's goals and values)
- Any additional preferences for care at the end of life (place of death, spiritual/cultural traditions, particular family members or friends to be contacted, burial preferences, etc.)

Case—Ms Lopez: Writing Your Note

After you finish working with Ms Lopez, you open a new "Advance Care Planning Discussion Note" note in the electronic medical record and write the following note:

January 1, 2014, 11:20AM.

I met with Ms Lopez and her sister, Josephine Lopez (WHO), for approximately 40 min (WHEN) to discuss goals of care. We reviewed her current medical condition and treatments (REVIEW).

She acknowledged how difficult it has been to live with a chronic lung condition and how hard it is to be in the hospital. She understands her lungs are unlikely to improve dramatically. Based on this understanding, she stated her main goal is to spend quality time with her family at home (GOALS). She does not want machines to prolong her life (VALUES). I confirmed with her that she does not want attempts at CPR or intubation should she suffer cardiac or respiratory arrest (treatment preferences). She has had bipap in the past, felt it to be uncomfortable, and does not want this intervention again. Additionally, while she does want treatments to maximize her comfort, she wants to be alert for as long as possible, even if that means she is slightly less comfortable (GOALS).

Ms Lopez confirmed that if she were to lose the capacity to make medical decisions, she would want her sister to make health-care decisions for her (SURROGATE). If her sister cannot make decisions, her brother would be the alternate. Ms Lopez decided not to choose her mother as her health-care agent as she worries she would be unable to make difficult health-care decisions under stress. Ms Lopez stated she would like her end-of-life wishes regarding CPR and intubation to be strictly followed by her health-care agent (LEEWAY).

A new advance directive and POLST forms dated January 1, 2014 have been completed and copies have been provided to the patient; I will update her orders to reflect her wishes.

10.1.5   Step 5: Conveying Treatment Preference Information to Other Providers

The goal of sign-out is to transfer key information about advance care planning discussions and documentation to the next provider so that they can honor patients' preferences and start from where the prior provider left off in future discussions. Most goals of care conversations do not need to start from scratch and a prior conversation can serve as a very useful starting point.

Principles of effective sign-out for specific medical treatment apply for sign-out of advance care plans. When a patient is unstable and changes in condition are anticipated, the patient should be discussed verbally between the two providers, and the following details should be provided in a written sign-out:

- Surrogate decision-maker name and best contact number
- Alternate surrogate decision-maker name and best contact number
- Any specific preferences around resuscitation, mechanical ventilation, intensive care, and other procedures including conditions under which a procedure might be acceptable
- Reference to specific notes or advance care planning documents in the medical record where more information can be found

---

Case—Ms Lopez: Updating Sign-Out

At the end of your shift, you update your sign-out. For Ms Lopez, you write, "goals of care discussed today and documented in today's note. DNR/DNI, no BIPAP. Please contact her sister (phone number) if she has a change in condition. May increase opioids for comfort but she would like maximize her level of alertness for as long as possible."

10.2   TROUBLESHOOTING

The stress of serious illness can present challenges for patients, families and care teams. A variety of problems can arise. Strategies for approaching some common problems concerning advance care planning documentation are described here.

10.2.1   Patient's Stated Preferences Differ from Advance Directive

As previously discussed, patient's goals of care often change over time as their medical illness evolves. Thus, as Freid suggests [4], the goals of care and treatment preferences a patient expresses when faced with a real-life medical situation may differ from what they, or their physician, have documented previously.

As long as the patient has decision-making capacity at the time when goals of care are discussed, verbally expressed goals and preferences (e.g., preferences for CPR, rehospitalization, etc.) supersede any prior written documentation, including advance care planning documents such as advance health-care directives, information from progress notes, and medical orders. The same principle holds for appointing a health-care agent. An oral designation of surrogate supersedes a previous written directive. Please note that in some states, this appointment is only effective for the duration of their stay in the healthcare institution where the appointment was made, or 60 days, whichever comes first. For this reason, it is extremely important that all documentation, including advance health-care directives, be updated to reflect a patient's new preferences. If a change is made, it should be documented in your progress note or a specially designated advance directive note.

10.2.2   Patient Has Multiple Advance Health-Care Directives

In the event the patient has multiple advance care planning documents, the completed document with the most recent date is considered valid. After identifying the most recently dated document, the provider should confirm with the patient or surrogate decision-maker that the document is accurate. All other documentation should be updated to reflect the preferences specified in the advance care planning form, and, if possible, the correct advance care planning form should be scanned into the electronic medical record. Outdated advance care planning documents should be marked "void" and disposed of securely in a HIPAA-compliant manner.

10.2.3   Surrogate Decision-Makers' Preferences Differ from Patient Documentation

Instructional directives are rarely specific enough to direct all the medical decisions that need to be made when a seriously ill patient has a health crisis and lacks capacity to make decisions. Thus, providers typically look to legally designated surrogate decision-makers for guidance. In some instances, the surrogate decision-maker may request treatments that seem to conflict with the patient's instructional directive. For example, if a patient with advanced dementia and an instructional directive that specifies no aggressive life-sustaining measures should he or she be unable to recognize his or her family members becomes septic and the surrogate requests ICU-level care, this request conflicts with the previously executed directive.

A five-question framework for systematically addressing this type of conflict was recently proposed by Smith [6]. This approach, which relies on conversations between the physician and surrogate to understand the patient's previously expressed goals and values, can help providers reach an ethically sound decision. The questions are summarized as follows:

- Is the clinical situation an emergency that allows no time for deliberation?
- In view of the patient's values and goals, how likely is it that the benefits of the intervention will outweigh the burdens?
- How well does the advance directive fit the situation at hand?
- How much leeway did the patient provide the surrogate for overriding the advance directive?
- How well does the surrogate represent the patient's best interests?

These types of questions can reveal that a surrogate is making decisions in his own best interest rather than those of the patient. Often, this occurs when surrogates become overwhelmed by their own emotional needs (i.e., "I can't let her go). When the situation allows for time for conversation, the provider must acknowledge and address these feelings first before successfully working with the surrogate to make decisions in line with the patient's expressed goals and values. Occasionally, a surrogate may have a strong conflict of interest (i.e., pension, housing, inheritance). Depending on the severity of the situation, an ethics consultation or contact with adult protective services may be necessary to help resolve this conflict.

Case—Ms Lopez: Follow-Up

Ms Lopez is discharged from the hospital a few days later with copies of her newly completed advance directive and POLST form. Her symptoms are well controlled with assistance from home nursing services and her primary care doctor.

A few months later, Ms Lopez's breathing gradually worsens and she calls 911. Although she meets medical criteria for intubation, the paramedics carried out her DNI order in the field after reviewing her POLST form. Ms Lopez is readmitted to the hospital on your service. You review Ms Lopez's POLST, advance directive, and hospital notes documenting prior goals of care conversations. Upon admission, Ms Lopez is somnolent and unable to make her own medical decisions; you therefore discuss the medical plan for Ms Lopez's care with Josephine, her health-care agent. You confirm with Josephine that her sister would not want to be intubated or transferred to the ICU, and together, you elect for a time-limited trial of antibiotics along with symptom management. You write medical orders and a progress note accurately reporting the decisions.

Unfortunately, by morning, Ms Lopez is actively dying. Sitting with Josephine, you decide together that it is time to transition Ms Lopez to comfort care. Ms Lopez dies a few hours later, surrounded by her family. Josephine and her family, though incredibly sad, are very grateful to you for your compassionate care and excellent communication.

10.3 SUGGESTED RESOURCES

Resource	Details	Website
American Bar Association, Commission on Law and Aging	State-specific advance directive laws, advance care planning patient toolkit	www.abanet.org/aging
Caring Connections	Information on advance care planning and links to download blank, state-specific advance directives	www.caringinfo.org
Five Wishes	User friendly, handbook-style advance directive legal in 40 states	www.agingwithdignity.org
Physician Orders for Life-Sustaining Treatment	Additional program information and resources	www.polst.org
PREPARE	Internet, advance care planning tool for seniors	https://www.prepareforyourcare.org

REFERENCES

1. Zhang B, Wright AA, Huskamp HA, et al., Health care costs in the last week of life: associations with end-of-life conversations, *Arch Intern Med* 2009;**169**(5):480–488.
2. Detering KM, Hancock AD, Reade MC, Silvester W, The impact of advance care planning on end of life care in elderly patients: randomised controlled trial [published online March 23, 2010].*BMJ* 2010;**340**:c1345.
3. Bischoff KE, Sudore R, Miao Y, Boscardin WJ, Smith AK, Advance care planning and the quality of end-of-life care in older adults, *J Am Geriatr Soc* 2013 Feb;**61**(2):209–214.
4. Fried TR, Van Ness PH, Byers AL, Towle VR, O'Leary JR, Dubin JA, Changes in preferences for life-sustaining treatment among older persons with advanced illness, *J Gen Intern Med* 2007 Apr;**22**(4):495–501.
5. Silveira MJ, Kim SY, Langa KM, Advance directives and outcomes of surrogate decision making before death, *N Engl J Med* 2010 Apr 1;**362**(13):1211–1218.
6. Smith AK, Lo B, Sudore R, When previously expressed wishes conflict with best interests, *JAMA Intern Med* 2013 Jul 8;**173**(13):1241–1245.

Chapter 11

Prognostication: Estimating and Communicating Prognosis for Hospitalized Patients

Joshua R. Lakin and Eric W. Widera

11.1 WHAT IS PROGNOSTICATION?

Prognostication involves two separate tasks. The first requires clinicians to *estimate* prognosis, which is the probability of an individual developing a particular outcome over a specific period of time. The second is to *communicate* this information to the patient and/or family. These two tasks are fundamental skills for hospitalists to master as nearly every diagnostic or therapeutic medical decision requires some knowledge of a patients' prognosis. Furthermore, prognosis adds a crucial timeframe required for determining realistic and achievable goals of care for patients, families, and health-care providers.

11.2 WHY IS PROGNOSTICATION IMPORTANT?

Prognosis impacts many decisions in the normal process of admission to discharge for patients who are hospitalized. Upon admission, prognosis drives triage to higher or lower levels of care based on the likelihood of decompensation. During the hospital stay, knowledge about prognosis influences most diagnostic and treatment decisions. For instance, when older adults were asked about their end-of-life preferences, 44% desired CPR [1]. After learning the probability of survival, the number desiring CPR dropped by half to 22%. Prognostic information can also aid in targeting interventions to those likely to live long enough to benefit, as seen with decisions around preventative cancer screening and tight glucose control in diabetes or artificial nutrition for a patient with advanced cancer. Upon discharge, prognostication affects location of discharge and which interventions are continued. For example, decisions

Hospital-Based Palliative Medicine: A Practical, Evidence-Based Approach, First Edition.
Edited by Steven Pantilat, Wendy Anderson, Matthew Gonzales, and Eric Widera.
© 2015 John Wiley & Sons, Inc. Published 2015 by John Wiley & Sons, Inc.

on whether someone needs a short-term skilled nursing facility stay or long-term care are based on the likelihood that an individual will improve with physical and occupational therapy. Estimating prognosis is also is explicitly required for eligibility.

Another reason to develop skill in prognostication is that patients and their families desire this information, even if the prognostic information is uncertain [2]. The reasons surrogates cite for this desire include preparing for loss, allowing families to hope for the best and prepare for the worst, fostering trust in their doctors, and aiding in decision-making [2]. However, despite this need, physicians remain distressed by prognosticating and studies have demonstrated that both patients and physicians tend to overestimate prognosis. Part of this is due to lack of training. In a large survey in 1998, 7% and 6% of internists reported inadequate training in diagnosis and therapy, respectively, but 57% reported inadequate training in prognostication despite needing this information frequently [3].

11.3 OVERVIEW OF METHODS TO ESTIMATE PROGNOSIS

The estimation of prognosis can be conceptually broken down into three main methods: (1) clinician prediction of survival (CPS), (2) population-based averages and prognostic indices, and (3) a combined approach using all of these methods.

11.3.1 Clinician Judgment and Experience

Clinicians use a variety of inputs into individual predictions of survival, including pathological and clinical findings, diagnosis, comorbidities, past and ongoing therapy, and psychosocial factors. The combined weight and analysis of each of these factors is what eventually drives a clinician's estimate but, unfortunately, this process remains poorly understood. Nonetheless, while the process is not clear, the accuracy of clinician judgment has been studied. A systematic review of physicians' estimates of survival in cancer patients demonstrated that while clinicians can separate those at high risk of death from those at low risk of death, their prognostic estimates are poorly calibrated as there is a systematic bias toward optimism [4]. Further studies have shown that CPS is confounded by the doctor–patient relationship and by experience level. For instance, clinicians provide more optimistic prognoses to patients they have known for a long time, although this may be less of an issue for hospitalists who typically are meeting patients for the first time.

11.3.2 Population-Based Averages and Prognostic Indices

The factors involved in population-based averages and prognostic indices vary extensively, from patient- or population-based characteristics such as age, gender, and race displayed in a life table to specific biomarkers analyzed in regression models and

Table 11.1 Categories of Population Averages and Prognostic Tools

Tool	Examples
Life tables	Centers for Disease Control—National Vital Statistics Reports
Generalizing data from studies and trials	Overall survival in previously treated stage IIIB or IV non-small cell lung cancer [5]
Prognostic indices	ePrognosis.org, Palliative Performance Scale, Acute Physiology and Chronic Health Evaluation (APACHE)

then incorporated into an online tool. As displayed in Table 11.1, there are several categories of tools, and we have provided some specific examples within each category.

The use of life tables require knowledge of only a few key characteristics but, as a result, give a broad population-based estimate of median survival. This presents problems in populations such as the elderly where there is significant variation in life expectancy among patients of similar ages. Another method to determine population-based averages is to use published studies whose participants closely mirror the patient's clinical details and then apply the results from these studies to generate a prognosis. This method provides a more individualized estimate than does a life table but requires an accurate match between a specific patient and a study population. Because studies often exclude individuals who are hospitalized or who have multiple comorbidities in order to strengthen association statistics, using these studies for ill hospitalized patients is often difficult.

The last method to refine population-based estimates is to use well-validated prognostic indices. Prognostic indices are tools that utilize systematically selected characteristics from a particular population, such as functional status or lab results, to calculate a prognostic estimate. The use of prognostic indices requires knowledge of the accuracy, validity, and generalizability of a specific index. For instance, if a prognostic index was developed in a community-based setting, it will likely overestimate prognosis in hospitalized adults.

11.3.3 Combined Approach

Each of the aforementioned methods has its own benefits and drawbacks. Clinician estimates of survival have consistently shown to overestimate survival. Population-based averages and prognostic indices may avoid this bias, but the prognostic estimates derived from them may not be generalizable or individualized to the individual patient under the care of the hospitalist. Given this, we recommend using either population-based data from recent research studies or a prognostic index that closely approximates the patient's condition to "recalibrate" an educated, self-aware clinical judgment. We will now detail a few of these tools that will be most useful to hospitalists.

11.4 TOOLS FOR ESTIMATING NON-DISEASE-SPECIFIC PROGNOSIS

Many patients for whom hospitalists care have multiple chronic conditions, functional impairment, advanced illness, and/or cognitive impairment. Focusing on one specific disease when estimating prognosis fails to take in the interactions of all these factors. In addition, older adults are typically underrepresented in the development of most disease-specific prognostic indices and in clinical trials. Non-disease-specific prognostic indices, which have been created in multiple different settings including hospitals, nursing homes, home, and hospice, are typically most useful for these patients. A repository of published non-disease-specific prognostic indices for older adults can be found at www.ePrognosis.org. One prognostic index that is of particular importance for hospitalists and is included in ePrognosis is the Walter index. This index was developed in tertiary care hospitals and validated in community hospitals, making it useful to estimate all the causes for 1-year mortality [6].

For the elderly and those with advanced illness, one of the strongest markers for mortality is the performance or functional status of a patient. A number of tools focusing on functional status have been developed. Two of the most commonly used tools in palliative care and hospice include the Karnofsky Performance Status Scale (KPS) and the Palliative Performance Scale (PPS).

The KPS (Table 11.2) was devised as part of one of the first studies to show an association between performance status and survival, and it has since been validated, albeit only in cancer populations. The obvious challenge in using the KPS, as well as the other performance status scales, is that patients are often admitted to the hospital with an acute decline that may or may not be reflective of their baseline functional status.

Table 11.2 Karnofsky Performance Status Scale

Able to carry on normal activity and to work; no special care needed	100	Normal, no complaints; no evidence of disease
	90	Able to carry on normal activity; minor signs or symptoms of disease
	80	Normal activity with effort; some signs or symptoms of disease
Unable to work; able to live at home and care for most personal needs; varying amount of assistance needed	70	Cares for self; unable to carry on normal activity or to do active work
	60	Requires occasional assistance but is able to care for most of his personal needs
	50	Requires considerable assistance and frequent medical care
Unable to care for self; requires equivalent of institutional or hospital care; disease may be progressing rapidly	40	Disabled; requires special care and assistance
	30	Severely disabled; hospital admission is indicated although death not imminent
	20	Very sick; hospital admission necessary; active supportive treatment necessary
	10	Moribund; fatal processes progressing rapidly
	0	Dead

Building upon this tool is the PPS (Table 11.3), and it has been validated in a broader population but is also subject to similar biases as the KPS. Importantly, the PPS has been studied more recently in both cancer and noncancer hospitalized patients receiving palliative care and used to build survival estimates by PPS level [7]. The PPS and survival periods resulting from this data are also displayed in Table 11.3. The validation in hospitalized patients makes the PPS a useful performance status tool in informing prognosis in hospitalized patients. However, it is important to remember that the PPS is biased by the fact that prognostic data was collected as part of care by palliative care teams, so selection of patients is not a random set of those admitted to the hospital.

11.5 TOOLS FOR ESTIMATING DISEASE-SPECIFIC PROGNOSIS

The categories below represent categories of commonly seen diseases and syndromes in hospital medicine. Each subject examines the prognostic considerations and highlights available tools if any.

11.5.1 Cancer

There is significant heterogeneity between disease courses in different types of cancer, even with narrowed definitions such as "within metastatic solid tumors" [9]. For instance, metastatic breast and prostate cancer are associated with much longer survival times as compared to metastatic lung cancer. With tissue diagnosis and staging established with the aid of consultants such as oncology, surgery, gastroenterology, and interventional radiology, there are several means of estimating an initial disease-based prognosis. One method is through the use of published studies related to a particular diagnosis, specifically from treatment trials. While this can often be challenging for physicians, there are a large number of possibly relevant treatment trials that can provide guidance on prognosis for treatment versus supportive care at any particular point in an oncologic disease course. Of note though, most of these trials do not include patients who are hospitalized or who have poor functional status, multimorbidity, or organ dysfunction.

Using one of the performance status-based tools as described in the previous section is a foundation for hospitalists in cancer prognostication as there is often a dearth of other evidence from clinical trials in hospitalized, ill advanced cancer patients. Furthermore, in this population, performance status is consistently demonstrated to show an association with survival, although length of survival may depend on the underlying illness. For example, for patients with metastatic cancers with relatively good prognosis and treatment options, such as prostate or breast cancer, a KPS less than 60 correlates with a median survival of less than 6 months [10]. This is in contrast to cancers with poor prognosis, such as pancreatic or biliary cancers, which result in a median survival of less than 6 months for those with a much higher KPS score (less than 90) [10].

In addition to functional status, a range of symptoms and laboratory values have been demonstrated to correlate with survival. For instance, out of a myriad

Table 11.3 Palliative Performance Scale (PPS)[a] Tool [7] and Survival Statistics [8]

PPS Level	Ambulation	Activity and Evidence of Disease	Self-Care	Total Care	Conscious Level	Mean Survival Time in Days (95% CI)[b]	Median Survival Time in Days (95% CI)[b]	Range of Survival in Days[b]
100%	Full	Normal activity and work; no evidence of disease	Full	Normal	Full	n/a	n/a	n/a
90%	Full	Normal activity and work; some evidence of disease	Full	Normal	Full	n/a	n/a	n/a
80%	Full	Normal activity with effort; some evidence of disease	Full	Normal	Full	151 (92, 210)	71 (0, 196)	33–424
70%	Reduced	Unable to do normal job/work; significant disease	Full	Normal or reduced	Full	168 (133, 203)	110 (77, 143)	3–607
60%	Reduced	Unable to do hobby/house work; significant disease	Occasional assistance necessary	Normal or reduced	Full or confusion	104 (61, 147)	50 (33, 67)	7–624
50%	Mainly sit/lie	Unable to do any activity; extensive disease	Considerable assistance required	Normal or reduced	Full or confusion	58 (43, 72)	35 (29, 41)	2–320
40%	Mainly in bed	Unable to do any activity; extensive disease	Mainly assistance	Normal or reduced	Full or drowsy ± confusion	65 (36, 95)	31 (15, 47)	1–493
30%	Totally bed bound	Unable to do any activity; extensive disease	Total care	Normal or reduced	Full or drowsy ± confusion	32 (23, 41)	12 (9, 15)	1–249

PPS%	Ambulation	Activity and evidence of disease	Self-care	Intake	Conscious level			
20%	Totally bed bound	Unable to do any activity; extensive disease	Total care	Minimal to sips	Full or drowsy ±confusion	14 (8, 21)	6 (4, 8)	<1–123
10%	Totally bed bound	Unable to do any activity; extensive disease	Total care	Mouth care only	Full or drowsy ±confusion	5 (1, 9)	2 (1, 3)	<1–22
0%	Death	—	—	—	—	—	—	—

[a]Instruction for use of PPS (see also definition of terms)

[b]Survival times were taken from the initial PPS done during the first assessment at home or in the hospital by a regional palliative care team.

1. PPS scores are determined by reading horizontally at each level to find a "best fit" for the patient which is then assigned as the PPS% score.

2. Begin at the left column and read downward until the appropriate ambulation level is reached, and then read across to the next column and downward again until the activity/evidence of disease is located. These steps are repeated until all five columns are covered before assigning the actual PPS for that patient. In this way, "leftward" columns (columns to the left of any specific column) are "stronger" determinants and generally take precedence over others.

of symptoms studied, anorexia, weight loss, xerostomia, dysphagia, dyspnea, confusion, and cognitive decline have shown clear association with prognosis [4, 9]. The Palliative Prognostic Score combines a group of patient level characteristics (CPS, KPS score, symptoms, white blood cell count, lymphocyte count) into one prognostic score, recently updated and validated to include delirium as well [11].

11.5.2   Heart Failure

Like other diseases that involve chronic, progressive organ dysfunction, short-term survival is challenging to prognosticate for people with heart failure. It is clear though that the need for hospitalization in this population is associated with high mortality rates despite recent advances in heart failure management. In a study of 2.5 million Medicare beneficiaries hospitalized with heart failure, there was a reduction in in-hospital mortality from 5% to 4% between 2001 and 2005, although mortality at 30 days, 180 days, and 1 year remained unchanged at 11%, 26%, and 37%, respectively [12]. The prognosis is worse after each subsequent hospitalization for heart failure. The median survival in one study of older patients admitted for heart failure declined from 2.4 years in those with one hospitalization to 0.6 years for those with four hospitalizations [13]. The prognosis only worsens for the oldest old who have a median survival of 1 year after just a single hospitalization and a median survival of 6 months after two hospitalizations [13].

In addition to hospitalizations, there are several other markers of poor prognosis. These include patient demographic factors, heart failure severity, comorbid diseases, physical examination findings, and laboratory values including cachexia, hyponatremia, anemia, and NYHA Class. Two important prognostic tools to help clinicians estimate prognosis in heart failure include the EFFECT model and the Seattle Heart Failure Model. The EFFECT model was developed from a cohort of 2624 patients who presented with heart failure between 1999 and 2001. The factors used to stratify risk of death include age, comorbidities, and physiologic variables (respiratory rate, systolic pressure) and laboratory findings (blood urea nitrogen, serum sodium concentration, and hemoglobin) at the time of hospital presentation. Thirty-day-mortality risks range from 0.4% in the lowest risk group to 59% in the highest risk group. An online calculator for the EFFECT model can be found at www.ccort.ca/CHFriskmodel.aspx. The Seattle Heart Failure Model is a freely available although lengthy online calculator (http://depts.washington.edu/shfm/) that was developed and validated among outpatients participating in clinical trials, observational studies, and clinical registries. Caution is warranted though when generalizing the results to hospitalized patients or those with other major comorbidities such as renal failure, dementia, or cancer.

11.5.3   Advanced Dementia and Cognitive Decline

Individuals with advanced dementia typically have a prolonged period of severe functional disability, and during this time they are at risk of acute events such as pneumonias and urinary tract infections that are markers of very poor short-term

Table 11.4   Summary of Functional Assessment Staging (FAST)

Stage 1	No subjective or objective impairments in cognition
Stage 2	Mainly subject complaints of forgetting names and misplacing objects
Stage 3	Objective evidence of memory impairment; impairment beginning to affect work performance
Stage 4	Moderate cognitive decline with impairments in instrumental activities of daily living
Stage 5	Difficulty in naming current aspects of their lives with some disorientation
Stage 6 (a–e)	Difficulty dressing, bathing, toileting without assistance. Experiences urinary and fecal incontinence in stage 6d and 6e
Stage 7 (a–f)	Speech declines from less than six intelligible words per day (7a) to one or less (7b). Progressive loss of ability to ambulate (7c), sit up (7d), smile (7e), and hold head up (7f)

survival. For instance, the 6-month mortality rates exceeded 50% in one study of individuals with advanced dementia who are admitted to the hospital with either pneumonia or a hip fracture.

Hospice eligibility criteria for dementia require that individuals need to meet or exceed stage 7a on the Functional Assessment Stage (FAST) scale (Table 11.4) and must have at least one complication from their dementia (aspiration, upper urinary tract infection, sepsis, multiple stage 3–4 ulcers, persistent fever, weight loss >10% within 6 months). However, studies have shown that these criteria fail to accurately predict 6-month survival in those with advanced disease. The Advanced Dementia Prognostic Tool (ADEPT), which can be found online at ePrognosis.org, can help identify nursing home residents with advanced dementia at high risk of death within 6 months. Compared to the hospice eligibility criteria, the ADEPT had greater predictive value of 6-month prognosis.

11.5.4   Chronic Liver Disease

Two of the most commonly used prognostic models used in chronic liver disease are the Child–Turcotte–Pugh (CTP) score and the Model for End-Stage Liver Disease (MELD). The CTP uses five variables (serum bilirubin, serum albumin, prothrombin time, ascites, and encephalopathy) to categorize patients into one of three classes (A, B, or C). The largest drawback to the CTP is the subjectivity in grading ascites and encephalopathy, and its limited ability to stage the severity along a broad continuum seen in liver disease as individuals are only placed into three categories. MELD is a prospectively developed and validated continuous scoring system that calculates the severity of chronic liver disease across a broader spectrum than the CTP. It uses a patient's laboratory values for serum bilirubin, serum creatinine, and the international normalized ratio (INR) to predict survival. Mortality for patients awaiting liver transplantation is noted in Table 11.5. Of note, there are some conditions, such as hepatocellular carcinoma (HCC) and hepatopulmonary syndrome, in which the

Table 11.5   3-Month Mortality for Patients Awaiting
Transplantation Based on MELD Score [14]

MELD Score	3-Month Mortality (%)
<9	2
10–19	6
20–29	20
30–39	53
≥40	71

Source: Wiesner R, Edwards E, Freeman R, et al. Model for
end-stage liver disease (MELD) and allocation of donor
livers. *Gastroenterology* 2003;**124**:91–96. © Elsevier.

calculated MELD score overestimates survival. An online MELD calculator can be
found at http://www.mayoclinic.org/meld/mayomodel6.html.

11.5.5   Chronic Obstructive Pulmonary Disease

The course of chronic obstructive pulmonary disease (COPD) is characterized by a
chronic, slowly progressive decline in pulmonary function punctuated with sudden
and potentially life-threatening exacerbations. Among Medicare decedents with a
COPD diagnosis in 2009, 80% had hospitalizations in the last 90 days of life, and
nearly 1 in 5 had 3 or more hospitalizations in the last 90 days of life. COPD exacerbations that require hospital admissions are associated with increased mortality after
hospital discharge. In one study of 260 patients admitted for a COPD exacerbation,
the 1-year mortality was 28% [15]. Age, male gender, prior hospitalization for COPD
in the last 2 years, $PaCO2 \geq 45\,mmHg$ (6 kPa), and urea$>8\,mmol/l$ were all
independent risk factors for mortality. In patients hospitalized for exacerbation of
COPD, the presence of comorbidity is associated with the need for a readmission or
mortality within 3 months after hospital discharge.

11.5.6   End-Stage Renal Disease

There have been significant improvements in survival in the last decade for individuals with end-stage renal disease (ESRD). However, mortality remains high as
median survival after initiation of dialysis is only 3 years. This may be in part due to
a progressive increase in the average age of individuals initiating dialysis. These
older individuals have a life expectancy significantly lower than that of younger
patients, as those who are 75 years of age and older have 1- and 5-year survival prob-
abilities of 59% and 13% compared with 75% and 34% for the general dialysis
population. However, there is significant heterogeneity among patients of similar
ages. For instance, as a whole, nursing home patients fair much worse than community
dwelling older adults after initiating dialysis. In a study of 3702 nursing home

residents, 58% had died and only 13% had maintained their predialysis functional status at 1 year after initiating dialysis [16]. The majority (69%) of these patients were hospitalized at the time of initiating dialysis.

In addition to age, multiple other prognostic factors have been associated with mortality in chronic dialysis patients. A validated prognostic model developed by Cohen and colleagues combines several of these factors along with a clinician's estimation of survival. Cohen's prognostic model calculates 6-month and 1-year estimates of the risk of dying by combining age, serum albumin, presence or absence of dementia, and peripheral vascular disease with the surprise question: "Would I be surprised if this patient died within the next year?" Prognosis after the withdrawal of dialysis is short, with most individuals dying within 7–14 days after discontinuing long-term dialysis. However, patients with some residual kidney function may live for longer periods of time after stopping dialysis.

11.6 HOW TO COMMUNICATE PROGNOSIS TO PATIENT OR SURROGATE?

Patients and their surrogates are looking for prognostic guidance from their physicians for a number of reasons, even when this information is uncertain. Yet, for a number of reasons, delivering prognostic information remains one of the most difficult tasks that hospitalists do as part of their work [9]. In this section, we will focus on delivering news about a poor prognosis, first by working to build understanding of some of the demonstrated barriers to effective prognostic communication followed by a discussion on ways to surmount those barriers.

11.7 CHALLENGES IN COMMUNICATING PROGNOSIS

Barriers on both the physician and the patient/surrogate side of a discussion of bad news make this conversation particularly challenging. From the physician standpoint, providers clearly experience emotional stress as the bearer of bad news. This is compounded by providers' concerns about a possible negative impact of their news upon patients and their support systems. For example, in a survey of 500 attendees of a national clinical oncology meeting, participants raised concerns about being honest without destroying hope, dealing with patient's emotions, and talking about ending active treatment [17]. These barriers drive significant variation in physicians' delivery of prognosis. In one U.S. study, physicians working in five hospices said that they would provide frank disclosure only around 37% of the time, favoring instead either no disclosure or a conscious overestimate [18]. Awareness of these barriers and biases is critical for physicians as they develop and use strategies for delivering prognoses to patients and their families.

Furthermore, the delivery of prognostic information is influenced by an understanding of barriers on the patient and surrogate side as well. As mentioned before, numerous studies have shown that individuals and their families want to be informed of the likely prognosis and the trajectory that an illness is likely to take, yet they often do not feel that they receive as much information as they want. In addition, it is important for hospitalists to remember that the vast majority of people are using other inputs into their decision-making process. Boyd et al. demonstrated that only 2% of surrogates stated that their own prognostic estimates were solely based on prognostication information delivered by physicians [19]. Other contributors to decision-making include perceptions of individual strength, will to live, unique history, individual observations of physical appearance, surrogate presence, optimism, intuition, and faith. Most importantly, for some, these additional inputs were of greater importance than the information provided by physicians. Compounding all of this, we know that after receiving especially poor prognostic information, surrogates significantly misinterpret the information with a bias toward optimism. This optimism in interpretation of prognostic information occurs regardless of whether information is given as numerical or qualitative values [20]. In summary, inherently imperfect communication of an often uncertain prognosis is clouded significantly by provider biases, numerous and varying patient and surrogate needs, and a complicated and dynamic decision environment.

The description of these barriers raises the concern of whether or not it is then worth the effort to disclose prognosis in the context of planning for medical care, especially at the end of life. However, effective communication around end-of-life issues has been shown to provide benefits to patients and families, without worsening of anxiety, hopelessness, or depression. These benefits include improvements in quality of life, peacefulness, goal concordant care, and mood, as well as an increased sense of control and facilitation of future planning. As such, when planning these discussions, hospitalists should have an understanding of the barriers as described earlier but also know that, when done well, this type of discussion leads to better outcomes for patients and their families.

11.8   WAYS TO COMMUNICATE PROGNOSIS

Given these barriers and decision environment, communicating prognosis requires careful attention and skill. Developing comfort with a structured format for these conversations helps to provide a foundation for ensuring delivery of the required information consistently. We will first describe an example of a structured approach for difficult conversations and then suggest some language around the most difficult piece of this process: that of delivering the prognostic information specifically.

As an example of one such tool, Baile et al. have proposed a stepwise protocol for conveying difficult prognosis that we present here as a useful tool [17]. In their article, they first lay out four key goals of prognostic disclosure. These are as follows: (1) assess knowledge, expectations, and readiness of the patient and surrogate, (2) provide information in an intelligible means in line with the needs and expectations of the patient and surrogate, (3) support the recipient of the prognostic information, and (4) develop a cooperative plan for moving forward. The authors then propose six specific and stepwise tasks to employ as a tool to meet these goals based on the SPIKES mnemonic, details of which can be found in Chapter 7. We also have listed specific tasks for clinicians based on SPIKES in Table 11.6 in order to provide a useful tool for planning and executing prognostic disclosure discussions.

Table 11.6   SPIKES Mnemonic for Delivery of Prognosis

Step	Specific Tasks for Each Step

*S*et up *i*nterview	• Review the communication plan—have the key prognostic information needed before the meeting
	• Prepare for emotional responses to difficult information and questions—rehearse to prepare for possible negative internal feelings and strong emotional reactions from patients
	• Control the setting
	  ∘ Set up a private room
	  ∘ Gather enough chairs for providers, patient, and key significant others
	  ∘ Make sure everyone is seated strategically (meeting leader next to the patient, not opposed)
	  ∘ Have tissues within patient reach
	  ∘ Make contact with the patient—strong eye contact or, if appropriate, touching the patient on the hand or arm
	  ∘ Explicitly manage time and any unavoidable interruptions. For example, "We have your surgery team here for the first 20 min of this conversation but they will need to excuse themselves after that time"

Assess *p*erception	• Begin with an open-ended question like: "What have your doctors told you about your medical situation so far?" • Refine with more specific questions, such as: "What specific concerns do you have about the reasons we repeated the CT scan?" • Based on this information, work to structure prognostic information in order to tailor to the patient's current level of understanding
Obtain *i*nvitation	• Begin with questions such as: "Many people have questions about prognosis; they wonder about how long do I have (does she have)? I'm wondering if you have those questions." • If needed, provide further guidance: "Some patients like all of the information. Would you like me to discuss it all or try to summarize for you?" • Use this time to both gain permission from the patient to share bad news and gather a better understanding of which form of information will be best for the particular patient

Impart *k*nowledge	• Begin with a warning statement such as: "I'm afraid that what I have to tell you is bad news"
	• Proceed with small pieces of information
	  ∘ Begin at the patient's level of understanding
	  ∘ Use nontechnical words, that is, "spread" instead of "metastasized"
	  ∘ Check intermittently for understanding

Address *e*motions	• Observe the patient's emotions • Internally identify the emotion being expressed • If unclear, ask clarifying open-ended questions to explore the patient's emotion, for example, "Could you tell me what you're worried about?" • Validate your understanding of the emotion by making an empathic statement and/or gesture. For example, "Many other patients feel very sad just as you do" or "this seems to come as a large surprise to you"

(Continued)

Table 11.6   *(Continued)*

Step	Specific Tasks for Each Step
Summarize and strategize	• Assess the patient's understanding of the discussion and address gaps in knowledge. For example, "We have discussed a difficult topic today and have talked about a lot of medical information. Before we move on, I want to make sure I have done a good enough job. What have you heard from me today? Do you have questions I have not addressed?" • Discuss next steps and specific treatment or diagnostic decisions that need to be made • Describe a specific timeline for when these decisions need to be made and to which providers they must be communicated. Be clear about who will communicate decisions and when

11.9   TIPS FOR DELIVERING PROGNOSTIC ESTIMATES

In thinking about the specific task of delivering prognostic estimates, we find the following key elements to be critical:

1. Acknowledge uncertainty by giving ranges in prognostic estimates: Use ranges whether describing prognosis in terms of the time left to live or the probability of surviving for, or dying within, some specified period of time.

   "I am going to give you my best estimate of the time you have left, please know that some people will do worse and some people will do better."
   "I cannot predict exact times and I will tell you the range of time that I expect to be most likely."
   "However, I would be surprised if you died in a few days and I would also be surprised if you lived 6 months or longer." (If delivered after prognostic time range)
   "For people such as yourself, with this disease, who are mostly in bed as you are, I would estimate the time you have left to be measured in weeks. Unlikely to be days but also unlikely to be months."
   "Someone with your condition lives, on average, for days to weeks."
   "Your mother is very sick and I am worried that she only has hours to live."

2. Include the primary factors that led to prognosis when delivering prognostic information: As mentioned previously, surrogate decision-makers use various sources of information to come up with their own prognostic estimates, with only a small minority relying solely on a physician's estimate. Therefore, it would be important for physicians to describe the various factors that may be influencing their prognostic estimates.

   "Half of people like you, who have been admitted to the hospital for heart failure, will die in a year."
   "For someone with cancer of your type that has spread at diagnosis, 1 out of 5 will be alive at 5 years."
   "Based on the system we use to evaluate severe liver failure like yours, 70% of patients with your level of disease will die in 3 months."

3. Whether qualitative or quantitative statements are used to convey prognostic estimates, use both positive and negative framing: There is little data to suggest qualitative statements are any better or worse at conveying prognostic information than numeric or quantitative statements. Furthermore, there is mixed data on whether frequencies or percentages are better understood when delivering risk information. However, when delivering prognostic estimates, it can be very helpful to frame it both in positive and negative ways to decrease framing bias.

> Qualitative: "*It's very unlikely that he will survive. Saying it another way, that means it's very likely he will die from this terrible illness.*"
> Quantitative: "*I would say he has about a 5% chance of surviving. Saying it another way, that means there's about a 95% chance that he's going to die.*"

4. Explore whether the patient/surrogate's expectations for the future have changed after hearing the prognosis from the physician.

Studies have shown that surrogates' personal estimates of prognosis are different, and generally more optimistic, than what they understood to be the physician's prognostic estimate. The reasons for this discordance between understanding and appreciation include surrogates need to express optimism, skepticism about physicians' abilities to predict the future, different belief systems about illness, or distrust.

> "*Given this information and what I have told you about how long I think he has to live, what do you think about your father's prognosis?*"

5. Use supportive statements to connect with the patient throughout delivery of prognosis: These statements are helpful both for the clinician, often in order to express something that feels helpful or beneficial, as well as for patient support.

> "*I wish the news was better for you.*"
> "*I too hope that you are on the higher end of that range.*"
> "*We are committed to helping you get the most out of the time that you have left.*"

11.10 CONCLUSION

In summary, prognosis informs, in some way, all decisions around patient care for hospitalized patients. Generating a patient's individual prognosis is a key step in the concept of shared decision-making around these decisions. Patients and families who understand that the prognosis is limited make different decisions about their care, with many opting for less invasive therapies and more comfort-focused approach. Deriving a prognosis should be generated by a combination of clinical prediction of survival based on experience and expert consultation. Knowledge of the evidence that these estimates tend to be optimistic and the biases clinicians carry in making these estimates is the first step to refining a prognosis. Disease-specific and generalized actuarial tools build upon a clinician's estimate to generate a prognostic window or probability of survival in the course of a complicated disease. Even using a combination of all of these tools, predictions are imperfect. Compounding this challenge is the fact that communication of prognosis is difficult for clinicians and also fraught with known receptive types of challenges for patients and families. Knowledge of these barriers is paramount for clinicians in their daily decision-making with patients and their families. This chapter outlined the importance of prognosis and the means of generating a prognosis and highlighted communication strategies and barriers to generate a systematic approach for hospital-based clinicians in using prognostication in their daily work.

REFERENCES

1. Murphy DJ, Burrows D, Santilli S, et al., The influence of the probability of survival on patients' preferences regarding cardiopulmonary resuscitation, *N Engl J Med* Feb 24 1994;**330**(8):545–549.
2. Evans LR, Boyd EA, Malvar G, et al., Surrogate decision-makers' perspectives on discussing prognosis in the face of uncertainty, *Am J Respir Crit Care Med* Jan 1 2009;**179**(1):48–53.
3. Christakis NA, Iwashyna TJ, Attitude and self-reported practice regarding prognostication in a national sample of internists, *Arch Intern Med* Nov 23 1998;**158**(21):2389–2395.
4. Glare P, Virik K, Jones M, et al., A systematic review of physicians' survival predictions in terminally ill cancer patients, *BMJ* Jul 26 2003;**327**(7408):195–198.
5. Shepherd FA, Rodrigues Pereira J, Ciuleanu T, et al., Erlotinib in previously treated non-small-cell lung cancer, *N Engl J Med* Jul 14 2005;**353**(2):123–132.
6. Walter LC, Brand RJ, Counsell SR, et al., Development and validation of a prognostic index for 1-year mortality in older adults after hospitalization, *JAMA* Jun 20 2001;**285**(23):2987–2994.
7. Lau F, Downing GM, Lesperance M, Shaw J, Kuziemsky C, Use of Palliative Performance Scale in end-of-life prognostication, *J Palliat Med* Oct 2006;**9**(5):1066–1075.
8. Lau F, Maida V, Downing M, Lesperance M, Karlson N, Kuziemsky C, Use of the Palliative Performance Scale (PPS) for end-of-life prognostication in a palliative medicine consultation service, *J Pain Symptom Manage* Jun 2009;**37**(6):965–972.
9. Lamont EB, Christakis NA, Complexities in prognostication in advanced cancer: "to help them live their lives the way they want to", Jul 2 2003;**290**(1):98–104.
10. Salpeter SR, Malter DS, Luo EJ, Lin AY, Stuart B, Systematic review of cancer presentations with a median survival of six months or less, *J Palliat Med* Feb 2012;**15**(2):175–185.
11. Maltoni M, Scarpi E, Pittureri C, et al., Prospective comparison of prognostic scores in palliative care cancer populations, *Oncologist* 2012;**17**(3):446–454.
12. Curtis LH, Greiner MA, Hammill BG, et al., Early and long-term outcomes of heart failure in elderly persons, 2001–2005. *Arch Intern Med* Dec 8 2008;**168**(22):2481–2488.
13. Setoguchi S, Stevenson LW, Schneeweiss S, Repeated hospitalizations predict mortality in the community population with heart failure, *Am Heart J* Aug 2007;**154**(2):260–266.
14. Wiesner R, Edwards E, Freeman R, et al., Model for end-stage liver disease (MELD) and allocation of donor livers, *Gastroenterology* Jan 2003;**124**(1):91–96.
15. Slenter RH, Sprooten RT, Kotz D, Wesseling G, Wouters EF, Rohde GG, Predictors of 1-year mortality at hospital admission for acute exacerbations of chronic obstructive pulmonary disease, *Respiration* 2013;**85**(1):15–26.
16. Kurella Tamura M, Covinsky KE, Chertow GM, Yaffe K, Landefeld CS, McCulloch CE, Functional status of elderly adults before and after initiation of dialysis, *N Engl J Med* Oct 15 2009; **361**(16):1539–1547.
17. Baile WF, Buckman R, Lenzi R, Glober G, Beale EA, Kudelka AP, SPIKES-A six-step protocol for delivering bad news: application to the patient with cancer, *Oncologist* 2000;**5**(4):302–311.
18. Lamont EB, Christakis NA, Prognostic disclosure to patients with cancer near the end of life, *Ann Intern Med* Jun 19 2001;**134**(12):1096–1105.

19. Boyd EA, Lo B, Evans LR, et al., "It's not just what the doctor tells me:" factors that influence surrogate decision-makers' perceptions of prognosis, *Crit Care Med* May 2010;**38**(5): 1270–1275.
20. Zier LS, Sottile PD, Hong SY, Weissfield LA, White DB, Surrogate decision makers' interpretation of prognostic information: a mixed-methods study, *Ann Intern Med*, Mar 6 2012;**156**(5): 360–366.

Chapter 12

Managing Conflict over Treatment Decisions

Robert M. Arnold and Eva Reitschuler-Cross

12.1 USING A NONJUDGMENTAL STARTING POINT TO FIND COMMON VALUES AND GOALS

One of the most challenging and uncomfortable situations clinicians face is how to handle requests for therapy from patients or surrogate decision-makers that the clinicians believe will not change the reality of life-threatening illnesses. In particular, clinicians struggle with situations in which they are asked to "do everything" or when patients and family members are hoping for a miracle and are not ready to limit medical interventions.

A common response by clinicians is to try to convince patients and families of their expertise, and, failing to achieve this, develop negative internal feelings and judgments regarding the patient and family. As a consequence of these conflicts, patients and family members may feel misunderstood, abandoned, or betrayed, while clinicians feel that their expertise is disrespected.

Finding a nonjudgmental starting point can help clinicians escape these nonproductive, maladaptive responses to conflict. From this viewpoint, clinicians can clearly hear patients' and families' perspectives and stories, promoting compromise and common goals that may help resolve the conflict.

12.2 MANAGING CONFLICT

A helpful, stepwise approach to navigate and solve conflict is to (1) recognize conflict early, (2) attempt to understand the other person's perspective, (3) find common ground, and (4) devise a strategy based on common ground [1, 2].

Hospital-Based Palliative Medicine: A Practical, Evidence-Based Approach, First Edition.
Edited by Steven Pantilat, Wendy Anderson, Matthew Gonzales, and Eric Widera.

12.2.1 Recognizing Conflict Early

It is often difficult to recognize conflict early. By the time a conflict reaches a boiling point, involved individuals may have acted or spoken in ways that they regret, poisoning the relationship. Signs suggestive of early conflict include "closed" body language, sarcasm, and the feeling that the conversation is going in circles. Another clue is when clinicians begin forming negative judgments about patients and families or a desire to withdraw from the situation. When a clinician begins to see these early signs of conflict, it is time to move toward a nonjudgmental starting point.

12.2.2 Attempting to Understand the Other Person's Perspective

Shifting to a more constructive, nonjudging approach can be achieved by asking oneself the humanizing question, "Why is this otherwise reasonable and well-meaning person acting in this challenging and difficult way?" Three aspects are typically involved: (1) disagreements about the facts of the situation, (2) one's emotional reactions to the situation, and (3) how one's viewpoint limits the possible acceptable solutions [3].

Aspect 1: The Facts. Disagreements around the perceived facts of a situation often consume the greatest amount of time and energy during a difficult conversation. Often these disagreements are based on assumptions of the fundamental correctness of one's perspective. In medical conflicts, clinicians often believe that they know the factual truth of the medical situation, and that, if the patient or family were reasonable, they would agree with them. This leads clinicians to neglect their patients' viewpoints (which are as "true to them" as the clinicians' medical facts). For example, the doctor may believe the patient is very unlikely to get better, while the family believes their dad has a very strong will and will beat the odds; both viewpoints are "true."

There are a number of reasons why clinicians, patients, and families may not have the same set of facts [4]. It may simply be that the patient and family have not been told the medical information. Clinicians often speak in a manner that is strongly rooted in the medical culture, which may include scientific terms and jargon. Further, the terms clinicians use may be vague, especially when talking about prognostic issues. These may include using hedging phrases such as "cannot rule out" or trying to soften bad news by using phrases such as "may not do well" rather than "dying." Additionally, various clinicians contributing to a patient's care may have differing interpretations of the medical situation and give conflicting information. Finally, even when clinicians communicate clearly, they may still find that patients' and families' physical and emotional exhaustion may impede their ability to understand the clinician's words.

Patients and family members who understand the medical details may nonetheless be in disagreement with health-care providers over the interpretation of this information. This may be caused by cultural and socioeconomic factors, as well as prior experiences with the medical system. For example, a family that has been told incorrectly in the past that a patient is not likely to survive an acute exacerbation of a chronic condition may refuse to accept the idea that he will not survive this episode. Families also receive information from other well-trusted sources, including friends and other family members, Internet sites, and television advertisements, and this external information may be in conflict with the information provided by clinicians. Finally, families may not believe the prognostic data is applicable to their loved one who they feel is stronger than most.

Clinicians often fail to hear and understand the patients' nonbiomedical stories. Clinicians who spend time to learn these stories can better understand patients' reasons for what may seem to be unrealistic decisions. Physicians may also underestimate the quality of life of chronically ill patients and therefore fail to accept descriptions of their level of functioning. Families who are given ample time to share their view of the facts of the situation report higher satisfaction with care and less conflict [5].

The key to resolving the "facts" aspect of conflict is to remember that these conversations are rarely about getting the facts right; the question at hand is about what each side believes is important. Each human being has a different background, a unique story, and, therefore, different perceptions of a situation informed by personal values. In order to find a solution, a clinician needs to be willing to learn more about the patient's story. This is simply done by being curious, asking open-ended questions, and listening. After inquiring about the patient's understanding of the medical information and filling in any relevant knowledge gaps, further questions to ask are, "What do you think is going to happen?" or "What do you hope that further chemotherapy will do?" or "I would like to understand; tell me more about your father's illness."

Aspect 2: The Emotions. Many conflicts have emotions lying at their roots. For example, a young woman whose spouse is dying in an intensive care unit may request medical interventions that are not likely to change her spouse's condition. The woman's sadness interferes with her ability to hear medical information, to consider what her husband might think about the situation, or to consider losing him. Trying to convince her that treatment is "futile" rather than addressing her intense grief is likely to result in heightened conflict. Attending to emotions and showing empathy helps patients feel supported and respected. This may then allow clinicians to build alliances with patients and move toward a mutual solution.

Clinicians, however, tend to avoid talking about emotions due to time constraints, personal discomfort with emotional crises, and a fear of releasing an uncontrollable flood of emotions. Physicians and other clinicians are also trained to maintain medical objectivity, and attending to emotions may feel insufficiently objective. A clinician's medical training may not have sufficiently addressed methods to navigate emotional conversations.

In order to assure that one is tracking and responding to emotions, clinicians can ask themselves, "Have I given feedback that shows that I am trying to understand the other person's experience?" Responding to emotions can be done nonverbally (such as through eye contact, changes in body position, or touch) or through explicit statements. The acronym NURSE summarizes ways to respond verbally to emotions, as described in more detail in Chapter 7 (Table 12.1).

Table 12.1   Responding to Emotions: NURSE Statements

Strategy	Example
Name	"It sounds like you are feeling…"
Understand	"I understand that this is very scary"
	"I'm hearing you say…"
Respect/praise	"I am impressed that…"
Support	"I will be available for you"
Explore	"It would help me to know more about…"

Common emotions that arise during conflicts include guilt, anger, and denial. Patients may feel guilt or shame about previous decisions and hope that they can make up for these decisions by "trying harder now." Surrogate decision-makers may feel guilty about limiting life-sustaining therapies, as it may appear to be equivalent to abandoning their loved ones. A way to unburden surrogates of this guilt is by asking, "If your father were able to tell us for himself, what would he say about all of this?"

Anger that things are not going the way that one wished is common. A natural tendency in response to anger is to cut visits short and to try to avoid further contacts. In order to help the patient cope with his or her anger, it is important to continue to engage with the patient without personalizing the anger. It can help to normalize the anger, affirming to the patients that anger is a common response to loss. An example of a normalizing statement is, "It is common in this situation to feel very frustrated and angry." Such a statement helps to keep patients from developing anger as a maladaptive coping strategy.

Denial is a very challenging reaction clinicians encounter, and it often triggers frustration in clinicians. Patients and families displaying denial may be perceived as being unwilling to accept a reality despite extensive and repeated explanation. Furthermore, individuals in denial may be regarded as uneducated and stubborn. Denial is a defensive mechanism that in its adaptive role allows patients to gradually integrate new, painful realities into their lives and to minimize painful, possibly overwhelming emotions such as hopelessness, depression, and fear. To support patients in their transition from denial to realism, it is helpful to provide small bits of information gradually over time, to show support, and to check in repeatedly to assess a patient's understanding of the illness, along with their hopes and worries.

Difficult conversations and conflicts about treatment decisions also evoke strong emotions in clinicians. Unrecognized feeling may leak into their interactions with patients, inhibiting clinicians' ability to listen attentively, and often coloring the content of the interactions with sarcasm and frustration. When necessary, clinicians benefit from deferring interacting with patients until the deluge of their emotions passes.

Aspect 3: How Our Viewpoint Limits Possibilities. A subtle aspect of conflict involves the way in which personal and professional identities and viewpoints limit our ability to think creatively about possible solutions. Identity here refers to the sense of one's ideal role that one plays in any given situation. These identities are powerful because they represent one's core, ideal self-image. Calling these identities into question can easily make people feel unbalanced and vulnerable, which can stoke strong emotions that exacerbate conflict.

For example, a clinician who considers himself a good communicator may feel that he has failed if a patient's family insists on a medically unadvisable full-resuscitation order. Alternatively, a family member who considers it his duty to ensure that his loved one receives every possible treatment may feel that he has failed if he accepts the withholding of possible interventions.

In these situations, it is important to remember that the identities, which run far more deeply than the medical issue at hand, are playing powerful roles in how we perceive the conflict. Clinicians may easily fall into the trap of seeing themselves as good or bad, or competent or incompetent, which can lead them to feel unbalanced and vulnerable. In truth, the roles each individual plays are far more complex and nuanced. Recognizing the emotional of depth of these identities, and having a willingness to discard one's own good/bad dichotomy, can prevent struggles to maintain one's ideal identity and favor a successful resolution.

12.2.3 Finding Common Ground

After listening to and acknowledging a patient's or family's story, taking into account the contributors to conflict as detailed previously, it is helpful for clinicians to reply by summarizing what has been said, identifying what the conflict is about, and then checking in to ensure accuracy. An example would be to say, "It sounds like you are frustrated because you are getting mixed messages from the doctors. Some are saying that your mom might die and yet your doctors from home say that things may turn around. Is that accurate?"

The next step is to identify shared goals, such as providing for the patient's comfort, honoring the patient's wishes, and ensuring that the family is at peace with the medical decisions. A clinician's language should focus on shared interests rather than personalizing the conflict. For example, rather than saying, "You are wrong to think that the treatment you read about on the Internet would help you," one can shift to a shared interest by beginning, "I would like to make sure that you have access to the best treatments."

One strategy that can indicate to patients and families that clinicians are searching for common ground is to characterize the difference in opinion by using "and" rather than "but." This is important, because while the word "but" appears to reject everything in the sentence that comes before it, "and" affirms that there are two reasonable views, both of which the clinician takes seriously. For example, the statement, "I can see you want your father to get better, but he is very sick," could be reframed as, "It sounds like the doctors are saying your father is very sick, and yet you are hopeful that he will get better."

12.2.4 Devising a Strategy Based on Common Ground

Once shared interests are identified, one should be creative in thinking about possible strategies. The resolution of a conflict about treatment decisions often depends on clinicians' willingness to consider alternatives to what they see as the recommended, most medically efficacious treatments. This signals to patients that their perspectives and concerns are valued. The key to talking about different treatment options is to simply list and explain them, including the ideas offered by the patients, along with the advantages and disadvantages of each approach. Patients and families should then be given sufficient time to consider available options before making a critical, life-altering decision.

One possible strategy is a time-limited trial of life-prolonging treatment [6]. For this to help, it is important that they are explicitly structured. The purpose of the trial and the specifics of the utilized treatment need to be explained, and clinicians should identify specific milestones that one would expect to see as evidence of improvement. Additionally, a time frame should be negotiated at the outset.

Despite everyone's best efforts, irreconcilable differences may remain between patients and clinicians. These residual conflicts are often due to contrasting core values, often rooted in social and religious beliefs. In these situations, a clinician may ask oneself how central the issue at hand is to the patient's core values and beliefs. The discomfort and disapproval of the medical team to respecting these values can be addressed by reminding each other of the reasoning behind patients' requests and finding patient-centered goals that everybody can approve, such as optimal symptom control.

12.3 TWO CLINICAL EXAMPLES OF CONFLICT

Two challenging situations that commonly arise in the palliative care setting—requests to "do everything" and patients' and families' beliefs in the possibility of miracles—can lead to conflict. In the following section, we will use these scenarios to demonstrate how the aspects of facts, emotions, and identity contribute to conflict.

12.4 UNDERSTANDING REQUESTS TO "DO EVERYTHING"

When clinicians are discussing treatment preferences with their patients in the context of severe illness, the clinicians may be asked to "do everything." Instead of taking such a request at face value and interpreting it as a desire for every imaginably aggressive treatment, including those that are not medically appropriate, clinicians should use this as the opening to a longer exploration of the patient's views and the emotions which underlie these views [7]. The clinician should explore the patient's understanding of the medical situation, underlying hopes, and how the treatments may achieve these goals. When this is done, one often finds that the interpretation of "doing everything" may range from using every available treatment with even only remote chances of prolonging life, regardless of the effects on their suffering, to providing maximum relief of suffering, even at the cost of shortening life.

It is worthwhile to explore how clinicians may unwittingly contribute to requests to "do everything" through their own language [8]. Clinicians often ask patients and their families whether they would like the medical team to "do everything possible," counterbalanced with the option, "Or would you like us to make you comfortable?" This is usually a well-intended attempt to include patients in their own medical decision-making, but it fails to appreciate the lack of clarity in the phrase, "everything." While this denotes specific processes and interventions to medically trained professionals, nonmedical individuals are forced to interpret it on their own without guidance.

Patients' emotions are often central driving forces behind requests to "do everything." These emotions include fears about becoming sicker, dying, or leaving loved ones. Furthermore, patients may fear abandonment or decreased vigilance on the part of their clinicians if they do not request every possible intervention. Helpful questions to explore emotions include, "What worries you the most?" or "What is the hardest part of all that is going on?"

Serious illness affects the whole family, and the associated familial identities may significantly influence treatment decisions. For example, a patient may request "everything" because he feels that his wife is expecting him to be a "fighter" and not a "quitter." In order to explore contributing family factors, a clinician can ask, "How has your illness affected your family?" or "What worries do you have about your family?"

12.5 UNDERSTANDING BELIEFS IN MIRACLES

A belief in miracles and divine intervention is very common among patients and family members and less common among clinicians [9]. Such beliefs may lead patients and families to believe in the possibility of one surviving a seemingly life-threatening illness. When this hope clashes with the clinicians' factual understanding of the medical reality, the discrepancy in belief systems may lead to conflict.

Instead of judging patients' and families' beliefs as being overly magical or irrational, it may be helpful for clinicians to explore what patients mean when they say they are hoping for a miracle [10, 11]. Believing in a miracle may represent a true belief in a divine intervention that will halt a seeming medical inevitability; more broadly, it may be an expression of hope that an unexpected improvement in the patient's condition may arise. On the other hand, the hope for a miracle is at times an expression of more unsettled underlying emotions such as anger, frustration, or disappointment over the limitations of medicine, as well as denial of impending loss.

Table 12.2 Communication Strategies on How to Respond to Beliefs in Miracles

Strategy	Example
Name it	"I see how important a miracle is to you"
Explore it	"Can you tell me more what a miracle would look like for you?"
Hope for the best, prepare for the worst	"I see how much you want a miracle. I wonder if we can talk about what we should do if this does not happen"
Broaden	"Is there anything else you are hoping for?"

Identity issues also may arise. Religious patients and families may struggle with accepting the advice of clinicians when the advice conflicts with their identities as faithful believers who are not allowed to interfere with what they may see as a divine plan [12]. Conversely, less religiously committed clinicians may be uncomfortable continuing life-sustaining therapies under the notion of a miraculous recovery, as their identities are rooted in science. One way to deal with this is to validate a patient's hope for a miracle and see if the patient is willing to think about the situation should a miracle not occur.

Clinicians may navigate the belief systems of their patients well by avoiding the impulse to refute their beliefs or engage in theological debates. Rather, the patients' beliefs should be validated and then explored. Communication strategies on how to respond to beliefs in miracles are listed in Table 12.2. Involving spiritual counselors who have a deeper understanding of the patient's spiritual beliefs may also be helpful.

12.6 SUMMARY

When facing conflict, clinicians can adapt to a nonjudgmental starting point by asking themselves the humanizing question, "Why is this otherwise reasonable and well-meaning person acting in this challenging and difficult way?" Three aspects are usually involved: (1) disagreements about the facts of the situation, (2) one's emotional reactions to the situation, and (3) how one's viewpoint limits the possible acceptable solutions. Trying to understand conflict along these three aspects can allow for identification of mutually shared goals and values, favoring a resolution of conflict.

REFERENCES

1. Back A, Arnold R, Tulsky J, *Mastering Communication with Seriously Ill Patients*. New York: Cambridge University Press, 2009.
2. Back AL, Arnold RM, Dealing with conflict in the caring for the seriously ill, *JAMA* 2005;**293**(11):1374–1381.
3. Stone D, Patton B, Heen S, *Difficult Conversations*, 10th ed. New York: Penguin Books, 2010.

4. Goold SD, Williams B, Arnold RM, Conflicts regarding decisions to limit treatment, *JAMA* 2000;**283**:909–914.
5. McDonagh JR, Elliott TB, Engelberg RA, et al., Family satisfaction with family conferences about end-of-life care in the intensive care unit: increased proportion of family speech is associated with increased satisfaction, *Crit Care Med* 2004;**32**(7):1484.
6. Quill TE, Holloway R, Time limited trials near the end of life, *JAMA* 2011;**306**(13):1483–1484
7. Quill TE, Arnold RM, Back AL, Discussing treatment preferences with patients who want "every-thing", *Ann Intern Med* 2009;**151**:345–349.
8. Pantilat SZ, Communicating with seriously ill patients—better words to say, *JAMA* 2009;**301**(12):1279–1281.
9. Widera EW, Rosenfeld KE, Fromme EK, Sulmasy DP, Arnold RM, Approaching patients and family members who hope for a miracle, *JPSM* 2011;**42**(1):119–125.
10. Orr RD, Responding to beliefs in miracles, *South Med J* 2007;**100**(12):1263–1267.
11. DeLisser HM, A practical approach to the family that expects miracle, *Chest* 2009; **135**(6):1643–1647.
12. Sulmasy DP, Spiritual issues in the care of dying patients: …it's okay between me and god", *JAMA* 2006;**296**(11):1385–1392.

Section 3

Practice

Chapter 13

Palliative Care Emergencies in Hospitalized Patients

Paul Glare, Yvona Griffo, Alberta Alickaj, and Barbara Egan

13.1 WHAT CONSTITUTES AN EMERGENCY IN PALLIATIVE CARE?

The majority of the care of patients with chronic, incurable, life-limiting illnesses such as cancer is delivered in the ambulatory setting. Very few hospitalizations for these conditions are "elective." Mostly, they are unscheduled admissions for symptoms caused by progression of disease, the side effects of disease-controlling therapy, an acute medical or surgical problem, or a breakdown in the system of care in the community. Sometimes, these problems are true emergencies, such as those shown in Table 13.1. Where they occur in previously healthy patients, they would require an immediate response to prevent loss of life or significant, long-lasting loss of physical or mental health. But when they occur in patients with progressive, eventually fatal illnesses, questions should arise about the kind of response that ought to be provided, and whether it is different to other patients. Sometimes, intervening is appropriate, but as patients get closer to death, the priorities can change, questioning the emergent nature of such situations [1, 2]. Determining the right kind of response is complex and gets to the heart of palliative medicine as a concept.

In the past, the label "palliative care patient" implied a life-threatening illness at a far advanced stage with limited further treatment options and rapidly approaching death. In this situation, prolongation of life is not a realistic aim. In that setting, emergencies are conditions which if left untreated will seriously threaten the quality of life remaining [3]. The aim of responding is to keep the patient safe, comfortable, and with their dignity intact. But nowadays, palliative care is being increasingly upstreamed and integrated with disease-controlling therapies. "Palliative care patients" may now have months or even years to live, a good performance status, and desire to have their life prolonged if possible. In this kind of a model of palliative care, treatment of a medical emergency may be no different to other patients with the same problem.

Hospital-Based Palliative Medicine: A Practical, Evidence-Based Approach, First Edition.
Edited by Steven Pantilat, Wendy Anderson, Matthew Gonzales, and Eric Widera.
© 2015 John Wiley & Sons, Inc. Published 2015 by John Wiley & Sons, Inc.

Table 13.1   Emergencies in Palliative Care

A. Medical problems we don't want to miss (discussed in detail)
   Spinal cord compression
   Pathologic fracture
   Severe hypercalcemia
   Massive hemorrhage
   Superior vena cava syndrome or airway obstruction
   Increased intracranial pressure and coning
   Status epilepticus
   Iatrogenic drug overdoses
B. Other medical emergencies (more part of oncology or general medicine)
   Pulmonary embolus
   Obstructive nephropathy
   Cardiac tamponade
   Tumor lysis syndrome
   Febrile neutropenia
   Hyperviscosity
   Syndrome of inappropriate antidiuretic hormone secretion (SIADH)
   Hypoglycemia
C. Psychosocial emergencies in the hospitalized patients with advanced disease
   Agitated delirium
   Code without a DNR order
   Suicide attempt
   Angry families

Therefore, emergency situations in patients receiving palliative care need to be managed on a case-by-case basis. Management options depend on a complex mix of variables, including the life expectancy, the level of intervention needed, and an assessment of the risks, benefits, side effects, and likely outcome. A three-step decision-making process has been suggested [3]:

- What is the best technical solution to the problem?
- Is this solution appropriate for this patient at this time?
- Does the patient or health-care proxy agree?

Some of the factors influencing these decisions are listed in Table 13.2 [4]. The *stage of disease* and *prognosis* is clearly important, although an intervention should not be dismissed solely on the basis of perceived poor prognosis [3]. For example, internal fixation of a pathological fracture may be advisable for a patient with only weeks to live, as it is challenging to control pain with an unstable hip fracture. The presence of other *comorbidities* and *symptoms* and the *general physical condition of the patient* are also important. A key issue is distinguishing a reversible problem from a terminal event.

The next issue is the *nature of the emergency situation* [3]. What constitutes a real emergency in palliative care? In a patient with advanced disease, it is important

Table 13.2   Factors Influencing the Response to an Emergency
in a Palliative Care Patient [4]

- The stage of disease and prognosis
- Other comorbidities and symptoms
- The general physical condition of the patient
- The nature of the emergency situation
  ◦ Can it be reversed?
  ◦ Should it be reversed?
- The likely effectiveness and toxicity of available treatments
- The wishes of the patient and their carers

Source: Falk S, Fallon M. ABC of Palliative Care. Emergencies. *BMJ*
1997; **315**: 1525–1528. © BMJ.

to differentiate between emergent symptoms, such as a pain crisis or acute breath-lessness, versus an emergent medical condition such as hypercalcemia which may not be symptomatic. Emergent uncontrolled symptoms can and should always be reversed, even if terminal sedation is required. On the other hand, emergent medical conditions need not always be treated.

The likely risks, burdens, and benefits of the emergency treatment need to be considered, but is not always a simple equation. For example, cardiopulmonary resuscitation (CPR) is risky and burdensome. Approximately 50% of patients who code in hospital will achieve a return of spontaneous circulation; however, only 15–20% survive to discharge. But if they do, the neurological outcome is usually good [5]. Unfortunately, those who do not survive to discharge have a poor neurological outcome and are likely to die in ICU on a mechanical ventilator. The survival rates for metastatic cancer patients are approximately half that of the general inpatient population [6].

Even if a minimally invasive, highly effective treatment is available for a medical emergency in a dying patient, should it always be reversed? For example, it may not be necessary to give hydration and bisphosphonates to a patient developing hypercalcemia in the last hours or days of life, as long as the symptoms can be managed by other means [3]. Of course, the wishes of the patient and their carers are central to all these decisions. While this is a given, problems may arise when there is a discord between the hospitalist and the patient/family regarding the burdens and benefits of treating an emergency. This may be particularly problematic for the hospitalist if the patient's usual physician has not addressed these issues previously. The disconnect may work both ways: when the patient/family "want everything", and when they are requesting a hastened death.

An important point to remember with medical emergencies is that many do not arise unexpectedly [3]. As with natural disasters, many medical emergencies are like hurricanes, slowly developing and able to be monitored and planned for, while others are like earthquakes, unpredictable and rapid. This meteorological analogy is especially relevant to palliative care, where discussion of the goals of care (GOC) should cover emergent situations that are both foreseen and unexpected. In fact, the Federal Emergency Management Authority (FEMA) approach to emergencies—"Prepare, Plan, and Mitigate" and "Respond and Recover"—is a useful concept that we will use as a template in this chapter (see Box 13.1). While many of the medical emergencies

---

Box 13.1 *"FEMA" Approach To Palliative Care Emergencies*

1. Emergency Preparedness
Prepare

- Be familiar with the kind of problems that can occur in patients with advanced-stage illness and how they present.
- Keep up-to-date with developments in the minimally invasive options for responding to them.

Plan

- Offer to discuss with the patient and family the treatment options and the risks, burdens, and benefits of each.
- Have a goals-of-care discussion (and/or advance care plan document) regarding how aggressively different kinds of emergencies will be managed, including invasive procedures, resuscitation, and transfer to an intensive care unit [41].
- If aggressive interventions will be offered, develop protocols for assessing and treating patients.
- Make sure good communication and relations are established with the outpatient oncologist and with relevant subspecialties.
- Consult the palliative care team if the psychosocial aspects are complex or the patient and family have limited insight.

Mitigate

- Have a high index of diagnostic suspicion for the development of medical emergencies in individual patients.
- Take prophylactic measures to prevent them.
- Intervene while they are developing so as to ameliorate them.
- Educate the family about the potential problems and warn them of inherent risks.

2. Respond and Recover
Respond

Be competent in responding appropriately to them:
  Treat the symptom—treat the problem—treat the patient and family
Consult the palliative care team for refractory or complex symptoms.

Recover

- If and when the crisis resolves, review with the patient and family what to expect in future and to consider options in various scenarios.
- If difficult to decide whether treatment will succeed, plan to reevaluate with patient/family after few hours to a couple of days.
- If not involved earlier, consultation with the hospital palliative care team may be helpful at this stage.

shown in Table 13.1 are predictable, some are the clinical equivalents of earthquakes, such as pain crises, status epilepticus, and respiratory depression from opioid toxicity.

In these situations, the FEMA principles of Respond and Rescue are applicable, although preparedness principles such as planning, organizing, training, equipping, and evaluating are still important. Because emergencies may not be easy to predict, an overall advanced care plan is important. Close monitoring of patients allows hospitalists to recognize and manage many potential complications before they become emergencies; early recognition, evaluation, and treatment of these potentially serious and at times life-threatening events are important to reduce morbidity and mortality. A useful approach is to remember to "treat the symptom, treat the problem, and treat the patient and family":

> Treating the symptom: A small armamentarium of appropriate medications (e.g., an opioid, a short-acting benzodiazepine, a dopamine antagonist, and an anticholinergic agent) can cover most of pain, dyspnea, and agitation emergencies that may arise at the end of life [7]. Sedation may be required. Many hospitals, including ours, now have an end-of-life order set to improve symptom control, although these are often underutilized [8].

> Treating the problem: If possible and if medically and ethically reasonable.

> Treating the patient and family: Palliative care deals with patients who are suffering from progressive fatal conditions, and death is the expected end. Nevertheless, even if the family is well prepared, the deterioration prior to death often appears to be an emergency to them [7]. In the care of the palliative care emergency, management not only includes ensuring the patient is comfortable but also being concerned with the needs of other patients and relatives observing the event, explaining what is happening and is being done, involving other members of the team, and communicating reassurance to the patient and the relatives as well as to other observers [7].

13.2   TRADITIONAL ONCOLOGIC EMERGENCIES IN PALLIATIVE CARE PATIENTS

13.2.1   Spinal Cord Compression

Spinal cord compression is a major cause of morbidity and suffering in cancer patients. If untreated, it may lead to unrelenting pain, paraplegia, sensory loss, and sphincter dysfunction. Early diagnosis is crucial, as the implementation of treatment before neural injury occurs may allow most patients to maintain neurological function. Compression of the spinal cord or cauda equina compression by a metastatic lesion outside the spinal dura is the most common and is the focus here.

Prepare. Metastatic epidural spinal cord compression (MESCC) is common, occurring in approximately 5% of patients with advanced cancer. In adults, the most common cancers associated with MESCC are prostate, breast, and lung cancer, followed by non-Hodgkin's lymphoma, multiple myeloma, and kidney cancer. It may also be seen in colorectal cancer, sarcomas, and unknown primaries. Although most cases of MESCC develop in patients with known cancer, about 20% of cases are the initial manifestation. The most common site of MESCC is the thoracic spine (60–70%) followed by lumbosacral (30%) and cervical (10%). The major presenting clinical signs and symptoms are pain (90–95%), which can be mechanical bone pain or radicular pain which indicates spinal instability. Motor weakness (60–85%), sensory loss, and bowel and bladder dysfunction (50%) are usually late symptoms. Bisphosphonates or denosumab may reduce skeletal-related events including MESCC [9] and should be administered months before to prevent these complications in vulnerable patients.

Plan. If the patient's prognosis is more than 3–6 months, a full workup and aggressive treatment of MESCC may be appropriate. Selecting the appropriate therapeutic modality is very important and should be done in consultation with a multidisciplinary team including some or all of the following: neurology, neurosurgery or orthopedics, radiation oncology, medical oncology, interventional radiology, anesthesiology, and PMR. In patients with a poor outlook, the plan should be to provide pain relief, excellent nursing care (continued in an SNF or inpatient hospice unit after discharge from hospital), and mobility aids such as a wheelchair.

Mitigate. In patients presenting with escalating back pain, it is very important to identify an impending MESCC before the appearance of neurologic symptoms or signs, in order to improve the clinical outcome. Back pain that is new, progressive, or changing its pattern should raise concern for MESCC, especially if it is worse on recumbency, has a radicular component, is situated in the thoracic region, or is associated with spinal tenderness. Magnetic resonance imaging (MRI) of the total spine, with and without contrast, is the diagnostic procedure of choice. Computed tomography (CT) myelography is indicated in patients who can't have an MRI, for example, with spinal hardware, and does have an advantage in that it permits collection of spinal fluid for cytology and evaluation.

Aggressive supportive care in patients with suspected MESCC is extremely important. Cord compression may present as a pain crisis [10]. Emergency pain control management prior to imaging is necessary to prevent movement artifact and to complete the diagnostic examination. Strategies for managing a pain crisis can be found in Chapter 2 of this book. High-dose corticosteroids, with initial intravenous bolus of dexamethasone dose ranging from 10 to 100 mg, followed by divided q 6 h dosages ranging from 16 to 96 mg daily should also be given when MESCC is suspected [11] and may produce significant clinical improvement even before definitive treatment starts.

Respond. Once an MESCC is confirmed, the choice of the treatment depends on a number of factors including the patient's performance status and overall fitness, the presence or absence of significant spinal fluid flow block and bony vertebral lesions, the degree of spine instability, the primary tumor, the extent of the disease and metastases, and the presence of other complications or medical comorbidities [12]. If the MRI shows epidural disease without significant spinal block, urgent radiation therapy is the treatment of choice, as this provides highly effective palliation for bone pain and will prevent progression in most cases [13]. Highly radiosensitive tumors include lymphoma, myeloma, Ewing sarcoma, seminoma, and neuroblastoma; breast and prostate are less radiosensitive; kidney, colon, lung, and melanoma are relatively radioresistant. There is no general optimal dose and fractionation regimen for MESCC; often 30 Gy in 10 fractions is chosen. Results should start to be seen within a few days of starting radiotherapy. The high-dose corticosteroid therapy should be continued during treatment.

If the MRI shows significant spinal block with cord compression and spinal instability, and the patient is a surgical candidate, lesion-directed surgery and spine stabilization should be considered. Spinal instability is a potential cause of spinal cord damage in addition to the epidural mass and is not affected by radiation therapy. If the patient has a spinal block but is not a surgical candidate, emergency radiation therapy or spinal stereotactic radiosurgery is an option. Chemotherapy is a reasonable treatment option for MESCC when the underlying tumor is chemosensitive. It has been used for both Hodgkin's and non-Hodgkin's lymphoma, breast cancer, germ cell tumors, and neuroblastoma. Hormonal manipulation has also been used in hormone-naïve patient with MESCC from breast and prostate cancer following radiotherapy.

If comfort care is the goal and the patient is unable to undergo emergency radiation treatment or surgery, then corticosteroids and opioids via IV-PCA will be most effective for pain control. In patients with limited life expectancy, regional anesthesia with a continuous epidural spinal catheter or intrathecal pump may be an option.

Recover. If surgery is performed for metastatic MESCC, it is followed by radiation therapy. Several weeks of rehabilitation will also be required following treatment. The outcome depends mainly on two things—the type of cancer and how well it responds to treatment. Treatment of MESCC usually relieves pain, leg weakness, and loss of bladder or bowel control. Radiotherapy controls spinal pain in over 70% of cases [13]. When patients with only minor problems in walking start treatment, they are likely to recover their walking completely. In patients who were unable to walk at the time of surgery or initiating XRT, only 10–20% are likely to regain full mobility [14].

13.2.2   Elevated Intracranial Pressure

Elevated intracranial pressure (EICP) is another potentially devastating neurological complication of cancer, and can occur with both primary brain tumor and cerebral metastases. Intracranial pressure is normally ≤15 mm Hg in adults, and pathologic intracranial hypertension is present at pressures ≥20 mm Hg. Like MESCC, EICP may also present emergently, although this is a much rarer problem than MESCC even in a cancer center. Successful management of patients with EICP requires prompt recognition, therapy directed at both reducing EICP and reversing its underlying cause, and the judicious use of invasive monitoring.

Prepare. Brain metastases are more common cause of EICP than primary brain tumors. The incidence of brain metastases varies by primary tumor site: lung 50%, breast 15–20%, melanoma 10%, and less common with kidney, colorectal, lymphoma, and unknown primary. EICP is caused by vasogenic peritumoral edema and bleeding within necrotic tumor. The symptoms of EICP include headaches, cognitive dysfunction, focal weakness, and seizures, caused by cerebral edema disrupting synaptic transmission and altering neuronal excitability. Unchecked, EICP may result in brain herniation.

Plan. Clinical findings that suggest the need for urgent intervention include worsening headache, vomiting, altered mental status, increasing lethargy and the onset of stupor, unstable vital signs, focal signs such as fixed and dilated pupil(s), or decorticate or decerebrate posturing. Cushing's triad of bradycardia, respiratory depression, and hypertension is an ominous finding, indicative of brainstem compression occurring. As with MESCC, the choice of the treatment of malignant EICP depends on a number of factors including: the patient's performance status and overall fitness, the primary tumor, the extent of the disease and metastases, and the presence of other complications or medical comorbidities. If urgent aggressive intervention is indicated, optimal care requires collaboration between the hospitalist, intensivist, and the neurosurgeon. Brain metastases generally have a poor prognosis so treatment may not be warranted. In patients where the GOC is to allow a natural death, comfort care is the goal and it is reassuring that death from EICP is usually peaceful.

Mitigate. The best therapy for EICP is resection of the tumor. While a decision is being made to pursue this, reduction of intracranial pressure should be begun, and reduction of intracranial pressure and improvement in neurologic symptoms usually begins within hours of commencing glucocorticoids [15]. In patients with severe symptoms, the usual *dexamethasone* regimen consists of a 10 mg loading dose, followed by 4 mg 4 times/day or 8 mg twice daily. There is some evidence that lower doses (1–2 mg 4 times/day) may be as effective and less toxic in patients without impending herniation. Dexamethasone should be stopped in 72–96 h if there is no response. The role of steroids in patients with EICP for comfort care is more controversial. Steroids may have a role if the patient is very symptomatic, but run the risk of unnecessarily prolonging suffering. Opioids may be prescribed if there are bothersome headaches.

Respond. The emergent response to EICP when aggressive treatment is indicated includes resuscitation and reduction of the volume of the intracranial contents. Establishing a secure airway and close attention to blood pressure allow the clinician to identify and treat apnea and hypotension quickly. Standard resuscitation techniques should be instituted as soon as possible, including head elevation, and hyperventilation. In addition to steroids, critically ill patients with unstable vital signs should be given osmotic diuretics such as mannitol (1–1.5 g/kg IV). If appropriate, ventriculostomy is a rapid means of simultaneously diagnosing and treating elevated ICP.

Recover. Patients undergoing aggressive management with neurosurgery ± stereotactic radiosurgery may then go on to have whole brain XRT and/or chemotherapy. Inpatient rehabilitation may then be required for patients with a neurologic deficit. Where a more conservative approach to management has been chosen, keeping the patient sedated decreases ICP by reducing metabolic demand. Fever should be aggressively treated with Tylenol and mechanical cooling, as fever increases brain metabolism thereby increasing and aggravating EICP by increasing the volume of blood in the cranial vault. Seizures can both complicate and contribute to elevated ICP. Anticonvulsant therapy should be instituted if seizures are suspected; there are no randomized trials that have established the superiority of one agent over others. Prophylactic anticonvulsant treatment is generally not recommended for patients with a primary or metastatic brain tumor and without a history of antecedent seizure [16], but may be warranted in some cases which include high-risk mass lesions, such as those within supratentorial cortical locations or lesions adjacent to the cortex.

13.2.3 Status Epilepticus

Status epilepticus (SE), defined as continuous generalized tonic-clonic seizures lasting beyond 5 min without full recovery between seizures, is a life-threatening event and a neurologic emergency. Untreated, it causes multiple metabolic derangements which can produce permanent brain damage if prompt and vigorous treatment is not provided. Other medical complications of SE include aspiration, hypotension, cardiac arrhythmias, rhabdomyolysis, renal failure, hepatic failure, and intracranial hypertension. Immediate treatment with appropriate doses of medications is also critical since uncontrolled SE can become refractory and very difficult to control.

Prepare. Any type of seizure can evolve into SE. In adult palliative care patients, the main causes of SE are brain tumors (primary or metastatic), metabolic derangements (hypoglycemia and electrolyte imbalance), as well as hypoxia, low antiepileptic drug levels, acute cerebrovascular accidents, meningitis, encephalitis, and cerebral abscess. Other causes include global hypoxic–ischemic insult, drug and alcohol abuse or withdrawal, and head trauma. Stroke accounts for almost 50% of acute symptomatic causes of SE in adults and elderly. Primary or metastatic CNS tumors are commonly associated with epilepsy, and seizure is the first presenting symptom in 30–90% of cases. Generalized seizures may occur with a large mass producing increased intracranial pressure.

Plan. In settings where SE is common, such as in the Emergency Room or on the Neurology floor of a cancer center, there should be an algorithm for managing SE that staff members are trained in. If SE is diagnosed or suspected, an emergent neurology consult should be called and an interdisciplinary team including anesthesiology or ICU should be involved, to prepare for intubation and transfer to a neuromonitoring unit.

Mitigate. The diagnosis of generalized tonic-clonic SE is not difficult, and should be easy to differentiate from other conditions. Nonconvulsive (absence) SE may be harder to diagnose and is characterized by stupor, a confused state of altered consciousness and little or no motor activity. It is important to differentiate nonconvulsive SE from pseudostatus or drug-induced coma. Pseudostatus and drug-induced coma lack the typical pattern of EEG activity and evolution seen with SE. A controversial issue is whether all patients with brain metastases should be given anticonvulsants. Patients who present with seizures require anticonvulsants; however, prophylactic anticonvulsants did not protect against subsequent seizures. Furthermore, antiepileptics stimulate the cytochrome P450 enzyme, enhancing the metabolism of some chemotherapy agents, rendering them less effective. Anticonvulsants also enhance metabolism of corticosteroids, thus reducing control of cerebral edema. They also frequently cause drug interactions associated with life-threatening side effects such as Stevens–Johnson syndrome. Therefore, prophylactic anticonvulsants are not recommended for patients with underlying brain metastases or other structural brain lesions. Patients with brain metastases from melanoma may be an exception to the general recommendation against prophylactic anticonvulsants, given their higher prevalence of seizures.

Respond. Treatment should be begun immediately when diagnosing SE. Maintain airway, breathing, and circulation, obtain finger stick to assess for hypoglycemia, and give benzodiazepines. Maintain Airway patency by positioning patient's head (backward head tilt with chin lifted up), Breathing by giving supplemental oxygen by nasal cannula or mask and Circulation by fluid support. Minimize injury by moving the patient to a safe environment to prevent falls or head injury. Obtain IV access and draw blood samples for serum chemistry, glucose level, hematology studies, toxicology screen and antiepileptic drug levels. Begin continuous vital signs and ECG monitoring. The Memorial Sloan Kettering Cancer (MSKCC) algorithm for managing SE is shown in Box 13.2.

Recover. Continue ECG, EEG, and vital signs monitoring; ventilatory assistance; and vasopressors as needed. Order neuroimaging (head CT followed by MRI later). An LP may be warranted if infection is suspected. Identifying the underlying etiology of SE is crucial for a proper further management of SE. Many etiologies such as intracranial infections, hypoglycemia, and other metabolic abnormalities, inappropriate anticonvulsant levels, stroke, and CNS primary tumors or metastases are treatable. Treatment of alcohol or benzodiazepine withdrawal or drug overdose is essential for generalized tonic-clonic SE. Treating the underlying cause, and not just the generalized SE itself, is critical in these cases and influences outcome. Management of the complications of convulsive SE involves understanding and managing the physiological consequences of prolonged tonic-clonic seizures and involvement of the multidisciplinary team. Longer duration of the sedation and coma is associated with increased morbidity and mortality. A multitude of medical consequences emerges after SE. Hyperthermia may persist and contribute to further brain damage, cardiac arrhythmias and ischemic changes as well as hyperglycemia may result from elevated epinephrine, and acidosis may result from accumulation of lactate, renal failure from rhabdomyolysis, and compromised respiratory status from

Box 13.2   *The MSKCC Algorithm for Managing Status Epilepticus*

- Administer an IV benzodiazepine such as lorazepam 4 mg IV or 0.1 mg/kg IV or diazepam 5 mg IV or 0.2 mg/kg IV over 2 min and repeat in 5 min after first dose.
- Give thiamine 100 mg IV.
- If hypoglycemic (less than 70 mg/dl), give 50 ml of dextrose 50 IV.
- If bacterial meningitis is suspected, start emergently ceftriaxone, vancomycin, and ampicillin. Start acyclovir if HSV encephalitis is suspected.
- If SE persists or diazepam was used to stop SE, administer fosphenytoin 20 mg/kg IV at 50 mg/min. Monitor ECG and vital signs.
- If SE still persists:
  - Repeat additional dose of fosphenytoin 10 mg/kg to total dose of 30 mg/kg.
  - Give phenobarbital 20 mg/kg IV at 50–100 mg/min, and intubate since risk of apnea or hypopnea is great when phenobarbital is given after benzodiazepine and transfer to ICU or NOU.
  - Start midazolam IV load 0.2 mg/kg and repeat boluses 0.2–0.4 mg/kg every 5 min until seizures stop up to maximum loading dose of 2 mg/kg.
  - Alternatively, use propofol IV load 1 mg/kg; repeat 1–2 mg kg boluses every 3–5 min until seizures stop up to maximum loading dose 10 mg/kg.
  - Use thiopental 5–15 mg/kg IV bolus, followed by 0.5–3 mg/kg/h drip.

aspiration pneumonia. Addressing GOC and organizing family meetings regarding prognosis and overall outcomes is very critical in the palliative care setting.

13.2.4 Pathological Fractures of Long Bones

Pathological fractures may affect both the axial and appendicular skeleton. Often an osteolytic bone metastasis has been identified as at risk of fracturing but treatment is deferred for as long as possible, so emergency preparedness is very important. Pathological fracture of vertebrae may lead to MESCC. This section focuses on fracture of long bones.

Prepare. In palliative care patients, fractures of long bones may occur due to bone metastases, osteoporosis, or trauma (falls). Nearly every malignant tumor can metastasize to bone and may be associated with a pathological fracture, but the most common are breast, lung, prostate, and myeloma. The most common site of fracture is in the femur, but any long bone is at risk. Characteristics include sudden increase of pain, spontaneously or after minimal trauma; swelling and deformity; altered mobility or other loss of function; shock; and altered mental status [4].

Plan. As with other emergencies, the choice of treatment in the palliative care patients depends on the primary tumor, the extent of disease, the prognosis, the general fitness of the patient and presence of other complications. If intervention is planned, a variety of specialties may be involved and should function as an interdisciplinary team, including orthopedics, radiation oncology, anesthesiology, and PMR.

Mitigate. If imaging shows cortical thinning, prophylactic fixation may be considered. Radiation therapy will provide pain relief, control the underlying tumor, and prevent further osteolysis. Bisphosphonates or denosumab may also reduce skeletal events, but need to be administered for months before these outcomes are seen.

Respond. Patients with a pathological fracture of a long bone often present with a pain crisis (see Chapter 2). Once the patient is made comfortable, a splint or padding should be applied and the diagnosis confirmed radiologically. Surgical treatment falls between internal or external surgical fixation, and may be the one way of ensuring adequate pain relief even in a patient with far advanced disease. If the pathological fracture is the first presentation of metastatic disease, a biopsy to confirm histological diagnosis should also be done.

Recover. Postoperative XRT helps to prevent loosening of any internal fixation. Several weeks of rehabilitation will also be required, a factor which needs to be kept in mind when deciding on the treatment plan. If comfort care is the goal, a PCA will be most effective for rapid control of incident pain caused by limb movement. In patients whose prognosis is very poor (days), regional anesthesia with a continuous block of the involved nerves can play a role.

13.2.5   Major Airway Obstruction and Superior Vena Cava Obstruction

Dyspnea may occur emergently in a dying patient and its management is discussed elsewhere. When patients become acutely short of breath, the key is to distinguish between those who have a reversible, treatable problem such as pneumonia, a pleural effusion, or pulmonary embolus, from those whose breathlessness is an irreversible part of the dying process. If the dying patient is acutely dyspneic and much stressed, this is a case for palliative sedation (see section on terminal agitation). Two specific oncologic emergencies that are associated with breathlessness and are discussed in more detail here: major airway obstruction (MAO, defined as from the larynx to the lobar bronchi) and superior vena cava obstruction (SVCO).

Prepare. MAO is high risk in head and neck cancers, lung cancer, and mediastinal masses. If a patient has airway narrowing and becomes acutely obstructed, simple causes such as sputum retention or kinking of a tracheostomy tube need to be excluded. SVCO is most common in lung cancer and lymphoma and results from extrinsic pressure by mediastinal tumor and less commonly from direct invasion of the vessel wall or intraluminal tumor thrombus. SVCO may also be a complication of a central line or other intravascular devices.

Plan. MAO should be anticipated as early as possible, so that GOC can be discussed, because the option is between a burdensome, invasive intervention (tracheostomy, airway stenting, laser therapy, or XRT), and comfort care. With SVCO, the obstruction to venous drainage usually occurs over weeks or months, also allowing time to plan the most appropriate approach. Symptoms and signs include tachypnea and breathlessness (due to laryngeal edema or tracheal/bronchial compression); headache, classically worse on stooping, or feelings of pressure in the head and face; visual changes or engorged conjunctivae with periorbital edema; dizziness; cyanosis; nonpulsatile and dilated neck veins; dilated collateral veins in the arms and chest with a dusky color to the skin in the chest, arms and face; and edema of the hands and arms. Papilledema is a late feature. Occasionally, the obstruction occurs rapidly over days and needs urgent treatment. If this is the first presentation of cancer, a tissue diagnosis, often done by image-guided needle biopsy, is typically appropriate.

Mitigate. SVCO generally has a gradual onset of symptoms including hoarseness secondary to vocal cord edema, headache secondary to cerebral edema, cough, and dyspnea and has the hallmark signs of facial and upper extremity edema, distention of arm veins, and dilated collateral veins over the chest wall. Elevate the patient's head and avoid venipuncture and IV catheter placement in the upper extremities. Steroids (dexamethasone 6–10 mg 2–4 times/day) can be commenced while the treatment plan is being formulated.

Respond. Generally in the setting of palliative care, the diagnosis is known. In acute MAO, tracheostomy or rigid bronchoscopy is indicated if the patient is "full code." In SVCO, immediate relief of symptoms such as dyspnea and anxiety through pharmacological, practical, and psychological methods is necessary. Opioids and possibly benzodiazepines are indicated. Initiation of high-dose dexamethasone can be useful in SVCO.

If SVCO presents emergently in yet unknown/undiagnosed disease, treatment with steroids may need to be tempered in order to obtain a tissue diagnosis. If the airway obstruction presents very acutely, tracheotomy may be needed. For SVCO, thrombolytic therapy is indicated if it is catheter associated. If SVCO presents very acutely, oxygen, opioids, and benzodiazepines will effectively palliate the patient. If the patient is actively dying and very distressed, stronger sedation with phenobarbital or propofol may be indicated.

Recover. If patients survive the emergent management of SVCO and are seeking aggressive treatment, laser therapy, cryotherapy, brachytherapy, and bronchial stents may have a role. For SVCO, 16 mg/day of dexamethasone should be continued initially for 5 days and then stopped if not effective or gradually tailed off if effective as other treatments take effect. Stenting of the superior vena cava with or without thrombolysis should be considered. The outcome of SVCO needs to be considered along with the history of the underlying cancer; however, as a prognostic indicator, only 15–20% of patients will survive for a year. Treatment will provide effective palliation of symptoms in more than 60% of patients with a median duration of 3 months.

13.2.6 Hypercalcemia

Malignancy is the most common cause of hypercalcemia in hospitalized patients, and hypercalcemia of malignancy (HCM) is the most common life-threatening metabolic disorder in cancer patients (others include hyponatremia due to SIADH, tumor lysis syndrome, acute renal failure, and hepatic failure). Severe HCM (>14 mg/dl) is a medical emergency because of the risk of cardiac arrhythmias. Less severe HCM is not emergent but warrants treatment if it is causing symptoms such as delirium, which can compromise dignity. As discussed in the Introduction (section 13.1), treating HCM may not always be appropriate in palliative care, as it can provide a peaceful "metabolic" death and its symptoms can be palliated by other means.

Prepare. HCM occurs in about 20–30% of cancer patients, so a high index of suspicion is necessary. The incidence of HCM varies with the type of malignancy, being most common in breast, lung, and multiple myeloma. Symptoms are often proportional to the rate of development of elevated serum calcium levels, that is, a slow rise may be accommodated more easily than a rapid rise. Additionally, age and comorbidities influence the severity of symptoms. Depending on the rate of rise in the serum calcium level, symptoms are not usually troublesome until over 12.0 mg/dl. Patients with renal impairment and patients with rapidly advancing disease are susceptible to a rapid rise. Symptoms of mild–moderate HCM (12.0–14.0 mg/dl) include anorexia, nausea, vomiting, constipation, thirst, and polyuria. These changes are often subtle and diagnosis can often be delayed. The symptoms of severe HCM include severe dehydration, drowsiness, confusion, coma, neurologic symptoms, and cardiac arrhythmias and are often distressing to the patient and carers. An ionized serum calcium should be ordered for any patient being investigated for delirium.

Plan. The discovery of a raised serum calcium per se is not an indication to treat, particularly in the terminal phase where treatment can impose unnecessary burden without benefit. Treatment is only necessary if symptoms of HCM are causing distress or have done so in the past, and there is a good prospect of response. Treatment of moderate–severe HCM can dramatically improve quality of life even when life expectancy is limited, although treatment may be inappropriate if the patient is near to death.

Mitigate. If HCM is suspected and the patient is experiencing symptoms but does not have a raised calcium level, check the level again after 1 week. If the decision is made by the patient not to have treatment or it is deemed inappropriate to treat, the symptoms should be managed appropriately through the terminal phase of illness.

Respond. If the decision has been made to treat the HCM, volume expansion is needed (200–500 ml/h 0.9% saline) before treatment with agents such as bisphosphonates, the amount of fluid and rate given depending on the clinical and cardiovascular status of the patient and the concentrations of urea and electrolytes (after rehydration). Diuretics (furosemide 20–40 mg IV) can also increase the renal excretion of calcium and may be needed to manage the hypervolemia caused by aggressive fluid resuscitation;

however, furosemide should never be given alone without aggressive IV hydration. Once the patient is rehydrated, bisphosphonates are also indicated, zoledronate being superior to pamidronate [17]. The initial dose of zoledronate is 4–8 mg IV over 15 min, dependent on the ionized calcium level. Lower doses and slower infusion may be necessary in renal disease (creatinine >3.0 mg/dl). In patients who do not respond or relapse after 4 mg, 8 mg can be given. Common side effects include transient pyrexia (acetaminophen prior to administration may prevent this) and influenza-like symptoms. Osteonecrosis of the jaw is a recognized but rare complication only seen after repeated infusions. Calcitonin is no longer used to any extent, although it may be indicated in severe HCM (>14 mg/dl) as it works faster than zoledronate. Corticosteroids are probably useful in the management of tumors which are responsive to their cytostatic effects (myeloma, lymphoma and some breast cancers). Denosumab is not used in the treatment of HCM.

Recover. Although the serum calcium level will fluctuate up and down for the first 48 h following a bisphosphonate infusion, in 80% of cases, it will return to normal within a week and last 1–3 weeks. Some symptoms, particularly confusion, may lag behind the normalization of the calcium levels. Another dose of bisphosphonate can be given after a week if the initial response is inadequate. Recurrence of HCM can be prevented by controlling the underlying malignancy if possible; maintenance treatment with bisphosphonates may also be necessary, as determined by serial monitoring of serum calcium every 3 weeks. It is also useful to limit the dietary calcium intake, increase weight-bearing, and replete phosphorus orally. Oral bisphosphonates are considered more suitable for maintenance therapy but have the disadvantage of being poorly absorbed. Hypocalcaemia is a side effect to be considered and sometimes calcium supplementation is eventually required if the serum calcium drops below the normal range. HCM is a poor prognostic sign in most advanced cancers, with a median survival of typically 1 month in patients with solid tumors on best supportive care [18]. The outlook can be better if patients are still on chemotherapy or have breast cancer or a hematologic malignancy, so treatment of HCM may buy time for further antitumor treatment, if available.

13.3   OTHER EMERGENCIES IN THE HOSPITALIZED PALLIATIVE CARE PATIENT

13.3.1   Acute Massive Hemorrhage

Patients with advanced cancer and other life-limiting illnesses (e.g., liver failure) can have hemorrhagic complications which can be very traumatic for patients, family, and staff. Major causes include tumor invasion of vessels, thrombocytopenia due to marrow failure, treatment-related complications (NSAIDS, low platelets, mucositis, GVHD), coagulopathies due to comorbid liver disease, DIC, and acquired factor deficiencies or inhibitors. Examples of acute massive hemorrhage (AMH) include a carotid "blowout," hematemesis and melena, or a massive hemoptysis. These may be a terminal event.

Prepare. Acute hemorrhage occurs in 6–10% of patients with cancer. Although the conditions that can lead to it are relatively common, AMH as a terminal event is relatively rare [19]. Hemorrhage is common in head and neck cancers (erosion into a major vessel, with up to 40% mortality), lung cancer (hemoptysis in 20%, with 3% fatal), vascular tumors (RCC, melanoma), GI (gastric, rectal, stromal) tumors with chronic bleeding which may occasionally be massive, and hematologic malignancies associated with thrombocytopenia and/or DIC. In patients who are at risk for hemorrhagic events, consideration should be given to stopping anticoagulants, weighed against the potential benefits of anticoagulants in cancer patients who have had or are at risk of having thromboembolic events.

Plan. Minor self-limiting episodes of bleeding may precede an acute event. It is important to plan and anticipate the probability of AMH and have a strategy for dealing with it that is communicated early and that the patient and their family members are comfortable with. While it is important to prepare the patient and caregiver early on what do in the event of an AMH, this needs to be balanced with the potential for causing unnecessary anxiety related to "sitting on a time bomb". Crisis Orders: When there is an identified risk of AMH and death is inevitable, it is wise to have a crisis order for sedation readily available to allow the patient to be unaware of the anxiety and distress associated with AMH; such orders must include immediately available and rapidly acting. The patient, family, and staff members need education on the purpose of a crisis order, that is, to give sufficient rapidly acting medication to deeply sedate the patient and prevent distress while dying—it is not designed to terminate the life of the patient. Practical considerations include having dark-colored towels on hand, bowls, and facecloths. The code status should be discussed, documented, and communicated. A patient at very high risk for AMH should not be left alone. If aggressive intervention is planned, then the maintenance of adequate IV access and the early involvement of relevant subspecialists (such as thoracic surgeons, interventional radiologists, gastroenterologists, etc.) are warranted.

Mitigate. Smaller, self-limiting (and therefore nonfatal) hemorrhage can be managed using first aid, with application of pressure dressings to accessible bleeding sites. Adrenalin 1:1000 soaked dressings can also be used topically.

Respond. If AMH does occur, the patient should be put in the recovery position and kept comfortable and warm. They should be repositioned as needed to maintain the patency of the airway. If more aggressive treatment is planned, possible appropriate responses include packing, compression dressing, administration of blood products (PRBCs, platelets, FFP), vitamin K, vasopressors, surgery, etc. If the patient is dying, direct pressure should be applied to any bleeding area; dark-colored towels are best. The patient will usually lose consciousness rapidly, but medication should be given by the central intravenous route if possible, due to the peripheral shutdown in shock. If a patient is opioid naïve, 10 mg of morphine together with a benzodiazepine such as midazolam 10 mg or clonazepam 1.0 mg will usually be sufficient initially and can be repeated if necessary at 10 min intervals until distress is relieved. If the patient is already on opioids, an opioid bolus dose double the usual breakthrough dose together with a sedative drug is appropriate.

Recover. If patient survives an episode of AMH, prevention of recurrence is important. Options include endoscopy for hemoptysis or hematemesis, radiotherapy, interventional radiological thromboembolic techniques and tranexamic acid. Tranexamic acid 1 gm 3 times a day can often be effective, though care needs to be taken in the presence of urinary tract bleeding where clotting and ureteric obstruction could be precipitated. It can be made by a pharmacist into a liquid to be used as a topical agent on persistently oozing lesions. Sucralfate combined with a proton pump inhibitor can often be effective for persistently oozing gastric mucosa.

13.3.2 Acute Respiratory Depression ("Overnarcotization") due to IV Opioids

Respiratory depression is the most feared side effect of opioids, and is related to central nervous system (CNS) toxicity or secondary to pulmonary edema. Fortunately, tolerance to their respiratory depressant effects develops quite rapidly with chronic opioid administration, making respiratory depression a rare event in cancer patients whose opioid dose has been titrated gradually against their pain. However, opioids do cause respiratory depression and coma in overdosage, and this may occur in the hospital when opioids are being rapidly titrated to manage a pain crisis. Opioid-induced respiratory depression may also occur if the pain is suddenly eliminated or diminished, following a therapeutic procedure, and the opioid dose is not reduced.

Prepare. The CNS side effects of opioids are generally dose related, although other factors such as dementia, metabolic or cerebrovascular encephalopathy, brain neoplasm, or concomitant use of CNS depressants may make an individual patient more sensitive. Specific precautions for respiratory depression should be used in patients with underlying pulmonary disease. When respiratory depression occurs, it is always accompanied by sedation. Initiation of opioid therapy or significant dose escalation commonly induces sedation that persists until tolerance to this effect develops, usually in days to weeks. When sedation is used as clinical indicator of CNS depression by opioids and appropriate steps are taken (see Mitigate section below), respiratory depression is rare. Other systemic manifestations of opioid overdose include hypoventilation, hypotension, bradycardia, hypothermia, miosis, and cool, clammy skin.

Plan. Respiratory depression in patients on chronic opioid therapy is reversed by administration of the opioid antagonist, naloxone. Improvement of ventilation after naloxone should not be taken as a proof that respiratory depression was caused by the opioid alone, since naloxone improves ventilation even when other underlying cardiac or pulmonary process is the primary cause of the respiratory depression. Naloxone may precipitate withdrawal symptoms or a pain crisis and should be administered only when strongly indicated. Naloxone has a fast onset of action (1–2 min) and also short duration of action (45 min). A low-dose naloxone infusion or repeated incremental dosing should be considered for severe respiratory depression induced by long-acting opioids. Short-term intubation should be planned for if there is a high risk of aspiration or respiratory arrest and involve the interdisciplinary team, including the anesthesiologist and the intensivist if intubation is indicated.

Mitigate. Opioid-induced respiratory depression may be preventable if opioid-naïve patients or patients on chronic opioid therapy are closely monitored. Sedation is used as a clinical indicator of emerging CNS toxicity and if appropriate steps (such as dose reduction or opioid rotation) are taken immediately, an emergency may be prevented. If the patient has bradypnea with respiratory rate not less than 8/min and is easily aroused and the peak plasma level of the last opioid dose has already been reached, the opioid dose should be withheld and patient monitored until improvement is seen. If the patient develops severe hypoventilation with respiratory rate below 8/min and cannot be aroused, IV naloxone should be administered regardless of the associated factors contributing to respiratory distress.

Respond. Awaken patient and encourage breathing. Apply oxygen via nasal cannula or mask. Withhold next opioid dosing (stop IV-PCA) until breathing improves; reduce subsequent opioid dosing by 25–50%.

If the respiratory rate is below 8/min, assisted respiration by oxygen bag or mask may be needed, and give naloxone immediately. The MSKCC algorithm for using naloxone is shown in Box 13.3.

Recover. If a patient has an episode of opioid-induced respiratory depression, careful screening for underlying pulmonary pathophysiology and a review of precautions to be taken when using opioids in these patients may prevent undesired respiratory-related events recurring. Opioids are similar in their prevalence of predictable and expected side effects, but there are marked individual variability in these effects, so cautious rotation from one opioid to another should be considered. Equianalgesic doses should be reduced to 25–50% of the calculated dose (or 15–25% when switching to methadone) due to incomplete cross-tolerance.

13.3.3   The Patient Who "Codes" Without a Goals-of-Care Discussion Having Taken Place

Modern hospitals treat patients of advancing age and complexity with increasingly complicated and invasive therapies. Patients may become rapidly unwell, and depending on the severity of the physiological derangement they are experiencing, this may lead to a code, RRT call, or ICU consult if the deterioration is life-threatening. This scenario can become an emergency if the dying patient has not had a

Box 13.3	*MSKCC Algorithm for Using Naloxone to Manage Overnarcotization*

- Awaken patient if possible and encourage breathing.
- Apply oxygen via nasal cannula or mask.
- Withhold next opioid dosing (stop IV-PCA) until breathing improves.
- Reduce subsequent opioid dosing by 50–25%.
- If the respiratory rate is below 8/min, assist respiration by oxygen bag or mask as needed.

  In comatose patients, short-term intubation may be prudent to prevent aspiration and further medical complications.

  Give immediately diluted dose of naloxone (Narcan 1 ml in 9 ml of normal saline) 0.04 ml IV push over 15 s in repeated doses every 1–3 min as needed and monitor if ventilation improves.

  ○ To reduce the risk of severe withdrawal from opioids, always use diluted naloxone (1:10) in doses titrated to respiratory rate and improved ventilation and level of consciousness.

  ○ Do not give bolus dose of undiluted naloxone as severe pain crisis and severe withdrawal symptoms may ensue.

  Consider starting a low dose of diluted naloxone infusion 0.02 mg/kg or repeated incremental dosing, especially if patient was using long-acting opioids or opioids with long-life plasma levels (methadone, levorphanol, etc.).

GOC discussion or they have had one but the patient and family insist on "doing everything" [20].

Prepare. The mortality in acute care hospitals is approximately 2–3%, so identifying who is at risk of high in-hospital mortality is important to insure as many of these discussions as possible take place preemptively. Surprisingly, there have been few studies of the predictive factors for death following admission to the hospital in individual cancer patients [21, 22], although the period preceding cardiac arrest, unplanned admission to the ICU, and unexpected death is typically foretold by derangements in the patient's vital signs, laboratory results, or the development of new clinical problems [23]. Unfortunately, these signs are inconsistently recognized by ward nurses and physicians, leading to delay in appropriate triage and care. Some of the reasons these discussions do not occur include the following: the team may not have recognized or may not accept that "the patient is dying"; they may not have had sufficient time or are not comfortable or skilled in having such discussions; an unwillingness of the family or usual clinicians to accept an ACD or administration of comfort care, despite the presence of advanced comorbidity and an irreversible new illness because of personal and religious reasons or because of the investment the usual clinicians may have had in the patient's care; acute or unexpected deterioration; awaiting family meeting; actively treating the patient for a reversible condition; not knowing the patient well enough; and resuscitation status not yet discussed by the usual physician.

Plan. As discussed in the Introduction, preemptive and proactive GOC discussions which involve the patient and their surrogate in the decision-making process should be held as early as possible in the admission if the risk of intrahospital mortality is considered to be high. Extra education and training in GOC discussions should be provided for staff in areas where a high proportion of codes, ICU consults, or RRT calls occur.

Mitigate. A system of documenting ACD has been shown to reduce codes/ICU consults/RRT calls. In one study, patients who receive facilitated advanced care planning including documentation were more likely to have their end-of-life wishes known and followed than those who did not [24]. Moreover, family members suffered less stress, anxiety, and depression when they participated in the facilitated planning, and there was no difference in mortality when patients documented their ACD.

Respond. Depending on the gravity of the situation, a code, RRT call, or ICU consult will occur. If a code is called on a patient who is terminal and is then canceled when the ICU team arrives, this creates considerable stress among the staff and is a waste of health-care resources without good justification. In the case of RRT calls, it has been reported that in approximately ¼ of calls, the RRT felt that institution of a Do Not Resuscitate (DNR) order was appropriate and in about 5% of cases, the RRT actually implemented a new DNR order during the call [25].

Recover. If the patient survives a code, obtaining a DNR order may prevent another episode, but is only the beginning of the process of ensuring a good death for the patient. A family meeting needs to be called at which time all the treatment efforts that go beyond the usual ward level care need to be addressed (such as ICU admission, intubation, ventilation or vasopressor support, etc.) and whether or not they will be provided. It needs to be made clear in good communications to the family (and junior house staff and some nurses) that DNR does not mean Do Not Treat. Oxygen, intravenous fluid, antibiotics, etc. are not part of "Resuscitation" and their loved one will continue to receive them [26].

13.3.4 Family Emergencies on the General Medical Floor

In palliative care, the patient and family are considered the unit of care [27]. Being the family caregiver (FCG) for a patient with an advanced, life-limiting illness is an extremely stressful process. Many FCG feel poorly prepared for the task [28] and may be less able to accept impending death than dying patients can [29]. Because many admissions of patients with advanced disease are precipitated by some kind of crisis, hospitalists need to understand that they are very stressful for the family as well as the patient, and that families vary in how they cope with these stressful situations. Families who do not cope may present with a psychosocial emergency, and the hospitalist should be skilled in how to deal with these. Depression and anxiety are common in FCG of patients with cancer and may be more severe than in cancer patients themselves [30]. Depression in FCG may be associated with increased suicidal ideation, and many FCG have reported contemplating suicide [31].

Prepare. Families vary in how they cope with stressful situations, influenced by their adaptability and cohesiveness [32]. Maladaptive coping may be exhibited in various ways and should be watched out for. Behaviors may include conflict among family members, dissatisfaction with care, or with depression and anxiety. It has been estimated that half the families of palliative care patients are dissatisfied with some aspect of the patient's care and that approximately 5% develop conflict with staff [33]. Many FCG contemplate suicide, with 20% of FCG in one survey reporting suicidal ideation and 3% attempting suicide during the previous year [34].

Plan. Staff members should be trained in how to identify maladaptive coping by families and what kind of interventions are available. Situations that could cause harm to the FCG or others require an intervention before a crisis occurs. If a floor has a lot of distressed families, a "crisis prevention plan" may be developed, outlining each staff person's role before and during a crisis situation. All members of the team meet to formulate the plan, using the available resources (social work, psychiatry, etc.). Staff members must work together as a team in a crisis situation. A team coordinator may be appointed to facilitate the process during development and planning and in a crisis situation. This should be the person on the team who has been found to work well with staff in difficult situations and is interested in coordinating the effort.

Mitigate. If there is conflict between the FCG and staff, the complaint should be investigated. If it is unreasonable, the FCG should be educated. If the conflict does not resolve then counseling can be offered concomitant with other interventions for maladaptive coping. If the problem is depression and anxiety in the FCG or conflict between family members, then conflict resolution and psychosocial interventions such as support groups, CBT, and pharmacotherapy can be offered.

Respond. Sometimes, FCG stress can boil over, creating a psychosocial emergency, in the worst cases resulting in FCG threatening or attempting harm to oneself, to other family members, or to staff. Terrible incidents—such as the one at Johns Hopkins Hospital in 2010 involving a distraught FCG who pulled a gun, shot and wounded a physician, and then killed the patient and himself in the patient's room—indicate how serious this issue can be. While some of these incidents are predictable and can be prepared for, other times they occur without warning. If a family member becomes violent or a weapon is produced, the hospital's Disaster Plan needs to be activated. If there is no violence or weapon, page Security, Social Work, and Psychiatry and the primary Attending to come to the floor emergently.

Recover. Unsuccessful crisis intervention may lead to complicated grief or posttraumatic stress disorder of the family members or caregivers. The common reactions arising include panic or fear, being upset or depressed, feeling overwhelmed or exhausted, or being angry or frustrated, which may require psychiatric intervention. On the other hand, successful crisis intervention can contribute to a good death for the patient and personal growth in caregivers and staff [35].

13.4   SUMMARY AND CONCLUSION

Most care of patients with cancer is ambulatory. Very few admissions are elective and most are "emergent" in patients with advanced disease, advancing age, and much medical complexity and who are receiving increasingly complicated and invasive therapies. These patients may become rapidly unwell, and medical emergencies and other psychosocial crises are common in hospitalized patients with advanced disease. Many of them are manifestations of dying. Deciding how to correctly respond to these kinds of problems is a complex clinical and bioethical challenge that needs to take into account the disease, the patient's overall situation, and the goals and wishes of them and their family. While some of these situations arise truly emergently, many have been developing for some time, making it possible to put in place an action plan to be dealt with them when they arise. We have found that the FEMA mantra of Prepare, Plan, and Mitigate and Respond and Recover may be a useful way for the hospitalist and other clinicians to think about how to approach these problems to obtain the optimal outcome for the individual palliative care patient and their family. Good communication between the patient's usual physicians and the hospitalist is needed to ensure the emergency is handled appropriately. Calling a palliative care consult should be considered early on for more complex cases.

REFERENCES

1. Nauck F, Alt-Epping B, Crises in palliative care—a comprehensive approach, *Lancet Oncol* 2008;**9**:1086–1091.
2. Schrijvers D, van Fraeyenhove F, Emergencies in palliative care, *Cancer J* 2010;**16**:514–520.
3. Care Management Guidelines: Emergencies in Palliative Care. Dept of Health & Human Services, Tasmania, Australia, 2009.
4. Falk S, Fallon M, ABC of palliative care. Emergencies, *BMJ* 1997;**315**:1525–1528.
5. Ehlenbach WJ, Barnato AE, Curtis JR, et al., Epidemiologic study of in-hospital cardiopulmonary resuscitation in the elderly, *N Engl J Med* 2009;**361**:22–31.
6. Reisfield GM, Wallace SK, Munsell MF, et al., Survival in cancer patients undergoing in-hospital cardiopulmonary resuscitation: a meta-analysis, *Resuscitation* 2006;**71**:152–160.
7. Smith AM, Emergencies in palliative care, *Ann Acad Med Singapore* 1994;**23**:186–190.
8. Walling AM, Ettner SL, Barry T, et al., Missed opportunities: use of an end-of-life symptom management order protocol among inpatients dying expected deaths, *J Palliat Med* 2011;**14**:407–412.
9. Gralow JR, Biermann JS, Farooki A, et al., NCCN Task Force Report: bone health in cancer care, *J Natl Compr Canc Netw* 2009;**7**(Suppl 3):S1–S32; quiz S33–S35.

10. Moryl N, Coyle N, Foley KM, Managing an acute pain crisis in a patient with advanced cancer: "this is as much of a crisis as a code", *JAMA* 2008;**299**:1457–1467.
11. Loblaw DA, Perry J, Chambers A, et al., Systematic review of the diagnosis and management of malignant extradural spinal cord compression: the Cancer Care Ontario Practice Guidelines Initiative's Neuro-Oncology Disease Site Group, *J Clin Oncol* 2005;**23**:2028–2037.
12. Laufer I, Rubin DG, Lis E, et al., The NOMS framework: approach to the treatment of spinal metastatic tumors, *Oncologist* 2013;**18**:744–751.
13. Gerszten PC, Mendel E, Yamada Y, Radiotherapy and radiosurgery for metastatic spine disease: what are the options, indications, and outcomes? *Spine (Phila Pa 1976)* 2009;**34**:S78–S92.
14. Chaichana KL, Woodworth GF, Sciubba DM, et al., Predictors of ambulatory function after decompressive surgery for metastatic epidural spinal cord compression, *Neurosurgery* 2008;**62**:683–692; discussion 683–692.
15. Alberti E, Hartmann A, Schutz HJ, et al., The effect of large doses of dexamethasone on the cerebrospinal fluid pressure in patients with supratentorial tumors, *J Neurol* 1978;**217**:173–181.
16. Mikkelsen T, Paleologos NA, Robinson PD, et al., The role of prophylactic anticonvulsants in the management of brain metastases: a systematic review and evidence-based clinical practice guideline, *J Neurooncol* 2010;**96**:97–102.
17. Major P, Lortholary A, Hon J, et al., Zoledronic acid is superior to pamidronate in the treatment of hypercalcemia of malignancy: a pooled analysis of two randomized, controlled clinical trials, *J Clin Oncol* 2001;**19**:558–567.
18. Ralston SH, Gallacher SJ, Patel U, et al., Cancer-associated hypercalcemia: morbidity and mortality. Clinical experience in 126 treated patients, *Ann Intern Med* 1990;**112**:499–504.
19. Prommer E, Management of bleeding in the terminally ill patient, *Hematology* 2005;**10**:167–175.
20. Quill TE, Arnold R, Back AL, Discussing treatment preferences with patients who want "everything", *Ann Intern Med* 2009;**151**:345–349.
21. Bozcuk H, Koyuncu E, Yildiz M, et al., A simple and accurate prediction model to estimate the intra-hospital mortality risk of hospitalised cancer patients, *Int J Clin Pract* 2004;**58**:1014–1019.
22. Hui D, Kilgore K, Fellman B, et al., Development and cross-validation of the in-hospital mortality prediction in advanced cancer patients score: a preliminary study, *J Palliat Med* 2012;**15**:902–909.
23. Jones D, Moran J, Winters B, et al., The rapid response system and end-of-life care, *Curr Opin Crit Care*, 2013;**19**:616–23.
24. Detering KM, Hancock AD, Reade MC, et al., The impact of advance care planning on end of life care in elderly patients: randomised controlled trial, *BMJ* 2010;**340**:c1345.
25. Parr MJ, Hadfield JH, Flabouris A, et al., The Medical Emergency Team: 12 month analysis of reasons for activation, immediate outcome and not-for-resuscitation orders, *Resuscitation* 2001;**50**:39–44.
26. Tsang JY, The DNR order: what does it mean? *Clin Med Insights Circ Respir Pulm Med* 2010;**4**:15–23.
27. World Health Organization. *Cancer Pain Relief*. Geneva: World Health Organization, 1986.
28. Rabow MW, Hauser JM, Adams J, Supporting family caregivers at the end of life: "they don't know what they don't know", *JAMA* 2004;**291**:483–491.
29. Tin LP, Crisis in palliative care, Newsletter of the Hong Kong Society of Palliative Medicine, Sep. 2009, pp. 13–14.
30. Edwards B, Clarke V, The psychological impact of a cancer diagnosis on families: the influence of family functioning and patients' illness characteristics on depression and anxiety, *Psychooncology* 2004;**13**:562–576.
31. Stenberg U, Ruland CM, Miaskowski C, Review of the literature on the effects of caring for a patient with cancer, *Psychooncology* 2010;**19**:1013–1025.
32. Loscalzo M, Zabora J, Care of the cancer patient: response of family and staff. In Bruera E, Portenoy R, editors. *Topics in Palliative Care*. New York: Oxford University Press, 1998, pp. 209–246.

33. Jenkins CA, Bruera E, Conflict between family and staff: diagnosis, management and prevention. In Bruera E, Portenoy R, editors. *Topics in Palliative Care*. New York: Oxford University Press, vol. 2, 1998:311–26.
34. Park B, Kim SY, Shin JY, et al., Suicidal ideation and suicide attempts in anxious or depressed family caregivers of patients with cancer: a nationwide survey in Korea, *PLoS One* 2013;**8**:e60230.
35. Palliative Care Guidelines: Emergencies in Palliative Care, Version 2. NHS Lothian, Scotland, 2010.

Chapter 14

Withdrawing Life-Sustaining Interventions

James M. Risser and Howard Epstein

14.1 ETHICAL CONSIDERATIONS

It is the physician's duty to preserve life and relieve suffering. These dual obligations sometimes conflict, most frequently at the end of life. The principle of patient autonomy generally requires the physician to respect the decision of a patient or their surrogate decision maker to withhold or withdraw treatment they believe will not help them achieve their goals of care [1]. Life-sustaining treatment by definition serves to prolong quantity of life without reversing the underlying disease process(es) or necessarily improving the quality of life. Because approximately one-third of all deaths in the United States occur in an acute care hospital and 22% of all deaths occur in or subsequent to an ICU admission, it is incumbent upon today's hospitalist to understand the three ethical principles relating to the withdrawal of life-sustaining treatment [2, 3]:

1. *Withholding and withdrawing life support are equivalent.* Although clinicians and family members are often psychologically more comfortable withholding treatments than withdrawing them, likely due to the passive nature of the former and the seemingly more active nature of the latter, there is no ethical or legal distinction between the two [1, 4]. As with any medical intervention, the benefits and burdens must be weighed. When a patient has not responded to an adequate trial of a particular intervention, the physician is not obligated to continue [5, 6]. Indeed, continued intervention may only serve to prolong the dying process and potentially exacerbate the patient's suffering.

2. *Acknowledging and allowing natural death is ethically and legally distinct from killing.* Through numerous legal precedents of the U.S. judicial system— including landmark cases such as Quinlan, Conroy, and Cruzan—the withholding or withdrawal of life-sustaining interventions is consistent with

Hospital-Based Palliative Medicine: A Practical, Evidence-Based Approach, First Edition.
Edited by Steven Pantilat, Wendy Anderson, Matthew Gonzales, and Eric Widera.
© 2015 John Wiley & Sons, Inc. Published 2015 by John Wiley & Sons, Inc.

the ethical principles of autonomy and nonmaleficence. In other words, it may be better to not do something rather than risk doing more harm [1, 4]. The concepts of physician-assisted suicide, legally permissible in only two U.S. states (Oregon and Washington), and euthanasia are beyond the context of this discussion.

3. *The doctrine of double effect.* This philosophical and legally recognized principle is used to draw an ethical and moral distinction between an intended consequence of a particular action and a merely foreseen result of an action [4]. The words of former U.S. Supreme Court Justice William Rehnquist perhaps best summarize this doctrine as follows: "It is widely recognized that the provision of pain medication is ethically and professionally acceptable even when the treatment may hasten the patient's death if the medication is intended to alleviate pain and severe discomfort, not to cause death" [7]. Thus, once it has been decided to pursue comfort as the primary treatment goal, concerns regarding the use of pain and other symptom-alleviating medications become secondary to the primary intent of providing comfort.

14.2   MEDICAL-LEGAL CONSIDERATIONS

In order to alleviate pain and other symptoms at the end of life or during the withdrawal of life-sustaining treatments, it is often necessary to provide large and sometimes rapidly increasing dosages of opioids and other medications. It is critical to clearly express the intent of such orders in verbal communication to the patient's family and hospital staff and via written documentation in the medical record. This intention is evident when the physician consistently demonstrates ongoing assessment of the patient's condition along with the titration of medications in accordance with accepted clinical practice [4].

14.3   COMMUNICATION AND THE CRITICAL ROLE OF THE FAMILY

The literature is replete with the essential role of surrogate decision makers and family in the shared medical decision-making process and is covered elsewhere in this book. The decision-making process to withhold or withdraw life-sustaining therapies is no different; however, the magnitude of the decisions and the emotional, psychological, spiritual and religious, and even financial ramifications may be quite profound and especially long lasting.

The ability to conduct effective family care conferences to address decisions to withhold or withdraw life-sustaining treatments is an especially crucial skill, reflected by the fact that as many as 95% of critically ill patients are unable to make their own decisions due to the effects of their illness or medications [4]. As many as half the family members in ICU care conferences have been found to have important misunderstandings about the diagnosis, treatments, or prognosis of the critically ill patient [8].

Effective communication about end-of-life care in the ICU may enhance the quality of care and reduce symptoms of anxiety, depression, and posttraumatic stress disorder among family members [9]. To best accomplish an effective care conference, it is considered best practice to do so in a structured, interdisciplinary team fashion (see Chapter 8) [10]. It is also helpful to employ tools and a consistent approach to improving end-of-life communications in the ICU that are evidence based, follow expert recommendations, and provide a basis for continuous learning and improvement[11, 12] (see Table 14.1).

Although there is considerable debate over whether physicians should routinely provide their personal recommendations to surrogates during end-of-life decisions, it

Table 14.1   Strategies for Improving End-of-Life Communication in the Intensive Care Unit (ICU)

1. Communication skills training for clinicians
2. ICU family conference early in ICU course
Evidence-based recommendations for conducting family conference:
Find a private location.
Increase proportion of time spent listening to family.
Use "VALUE" mnemonic during family conferences.
Value statements made by family members.
Acknowledge emotions.
Listen to family members.
Understand who the patient is as a person.
Elicit questions from family members.
Identify commonly missed opportunities.
Listen and respond to family members.
Acknowledge and address family emotions.
Explore and focus on patient values and treatment preferences.
Affirm nonabandonment of patient and family.
Assure family that the patient will not suffer.
Provide explicit support for decisions made by the family.
Additional expert opinion recommendations for conducting family conference:
Advance planning for the discussion among the clinical team
Identify family and clinician participants who should be involved.
Focus on the goals and values of the patient.
Use an open, flexible process.
Anticipate possible issues and outcomes of the discussion.
Give families support and time.
3. Interdisciplinary team rounds
4. Availability of palliative care and/or ethics consultation
5. Development of a supportive ICU culture for ethical practice and communication

Source: Truog RD, Campbell ML, Curtis R, et al. Recommendations for end-of-life care in the intensive care unit: a consensus statement by the American College of Critical Care Medicine. *Crit Care Med* 2008; 36: 953–963. © Lippincott Williams & Wilkins.

seems prudent to ask family members first and then view the recommendation as a starting point for shared deliberations about how to act in the best interests of the patient [13].

Furthermore, the relative immediacy of death and especially the cultural beliefs and practices surrounding death require particular sensitivity and vigilance. The use of trained medical interpreters should be mandatory during such care conferences and strong consideration should be given to the use of social services, chaplaincy, and specialty palliative care services, if available.

Although family presence during CPR has been associated with positive results on psychological variables and does not interfere with medical efforts, increase stress in the health-care team, or result in medicolegal conflict [14], research on the effects of having family and/or loved ones present during the withdrawal of life-sustaining treatments is lacking. It is our opinion that this option be discussed and the decision, as with most others, should be arrived at jointly with regard to the potential or perceived benefits and burdens on the patient and family, with adequate education, preparation, and support throughout the process, as described by Marr and Weissman:

> Families may choose to be present during the procedure or prefer to wait outside the room and then be brought in as soon as the patient is comfortable. If the family wishes to be present for the process, a space should be made available to them and their comfort attended to. Families may hope to be able to speak with their loved one after extubation but should be prepared that this may not be possible. Patients who are cognitively intact prior to extubation may have "unfinished business" and feel that there are people to whom they need to say goodbye to or people who need to say goodbye to them. If possible, it is very important that these wishes be accommodated. The room can be transformed into a "sacred space" by allowing families to personalize it as much as possible. [15]

Finally, remember to have procedures and structure in place to provide bereavement support to family and caregivers, including members of the care team.

14.4   VENTILATOR WITHDRAWAL

The withdrawal of mechanical ventilation is typically the final step in withdrawal of life-sustaining support in the intensive care unit. While discontinuing intravenous fluids, vasopressors, dialysis, antibiotics, and other medications are often part of the discussion and process regarding stopping life-prolonging treatments, it is the removal of ventilator support that can prove to be the most difficult emotional step for families. There are a number of reasons why the process can be particularly anxiety provoking:

1. Withdrawal of the mechanical ventilation tends to be more of an immediate determinant of death.

2. Many families fear that patients will suffer an acute exacerbation of dyspnea and other distressing symptoms once ventilator support has been removed.

3. Patients on ventilators are often (but not always) unable to participate actively in the final decision to withdraw mechanical ventilation—leaving families in distress about the proper timing of removing the last piece of life support.

Withdrawal of mechanical ventilation is therefore to be considered only one part in the continuum of end-of-life counseling for patients and families in the ICU. The process starts with discussions of goals of care. When it is decided that further intensive care is no longer meeting the goals of ventilator-dependent patients, discussing withdrawal to allow natural death is appropriate. It is then important to walk families (and patients if lucid) through the process and mechanics of ventilator withdrawal. Providing information about what to expect before, during and after the ventilator is withdrawn is crucial to providing a more peaceful death experience for both the patient and the family.

We recommend starting by gauging expectations and understanding of the withdrawal process. After hearing family and patient's concerns and insights, it is reasonable to discuss expected outcomes—and specifically discuss prognosis for survival once the ventilator is removed and how the dying process actually looks as it progresses.

In one study, the median survival time from withdrawal of mechanical ventilation to death was 0.93 h. The proportion of patients who died within 24 h of terminal withdrawal was 93.2% [16]. Thus, estimating expected survival in terms of several minutes to several hours is likely to be accurate in the majority of cases. However, there will always be outliers. Some patients may die in seconds and a very small minority may not die at all. As such, appreciating the nuances of each individual situation is important. There are general predictors of time to death and they can serve as a guide to clinicians and families about expected outcomes. Predictors associated with *shorter time to death include*:

1. Number of organ failures
2. Use of vasopressors
3. Use of intravenous fluids
4. Certain demographic data (younger patients, men, and nonwhites display shorter times to death) [16]

For some families, more concrete and exact prognostication may not be as important as it will be for other families. For those families with complicated dynamics (unresolved anger issues, poor support networks, resentment of the medical establishment, etc.), incorrectly estimating prognosis may create distrust during an already stressful period. Sometimes, if the patient lives longer than predicted, this can cause the family to seriously question whether withdrawal of life-sustaining treatments was the right thing to do in the first place. We recommend telling families that estimation of prognosis is neither an exact science nor is it a guarantee, but it is our best opinion given the information at hand. Managing expectations before the withdrawal and allowing for the option to reevaluate after the withdrawal is a crucial messaging piece.

Patients and families should be prepared for what choices they have and what they are going to see happen during and after the period of ventilator withdrawal.

Patients and families can decide whether they would like the endotracheal (ET) tube left in to have the ventilator disconnected or whether they would prefer the entire apparatus be removed (see Section 14.4.1). Describe the entire withdrawal procedure in clear and simple terms; avoid jargon such as ET tube, weaning trail, and T-piece, if possible. Discuss the role of low-flow supplemental oxygen and medications for symptom control. Assure them that the patient's comfort is of primary concern. Explain that labored breathing, agitation, and some signs of pain could occur but that the care team will do everything they can to manage those symptoms proactively and effectively with medications. Reassure them that placing the patient back on the ventilator will likely not control these symptoms and will prolong the dying process. Indicate that the patient will probably have to be kept asleep to control their symptoms effectively. Educate the family on the signs of active dying that can include noisy breathing ("the death rattle"), periods of not breathing ("apnea"), irregular final breaths ("agonal breaths"), and skin changes ("mottling") and that these signs are not painful—they are a normal part of the process.

14.4.1   Options for Ventilator Withdrawal

1. *Immediate Extubation*: The endotracheal tube is removed after appropriate suctioning. Humidified air or oxygen is administered to prevent the airway from drying. Comfort medications are administered. This is the preferred approach for conscious patients with lower volume secretions and no suspicion of/evidence for airway compromise.

2. *Terminal Weaning*: Ventilator settings are decreased as tolerated to minimal support over 30–60 min. This can be performed more rapidly as apparent comfort dictates. The ventilator rate, positive end expiratory pressure (PEEP), and oxygen levels are decreased while the ET tube is left in place. If the patient survives, the ET tube is then removed for ongoing control of symptoms. For some patients with concern over upper airway patency, some families may opt to leave the ET tube in place and a Briggs T-piece is placed [17].

The decision to pursue a terminal weaning process and to leave the ET tube in place for comfort cares is based on family preference and patient circumstances. It's important to note, however, that terminal weaning may actually prolong the dying process. It's also worth pointing out that many survivors of critical illness recall that the ET tube itself and the associated suctioning involved with maintaining it was a source of distress unto itself. Thus, an argument can be made to remove artificial airways on comfort grounds in the withdrawal of life-sustaining treatments. Acknowledging all this, we encourage clinicians to make a clear recommendation to families as to what they think the best plan of care is based on their own assessment of the most secure way to keep a patient comfortable as ventilator support is removed.

14.4.2 Medications in the Management of Terminal Extubation

Opioids are considered the mainstay of treatment in treating air hunger and pain in the period around ventilator withdrawal. Most protocols include the use of an opioid as the primary vehicle of dyspnea and pain management. Opioids have a number of well-documented physiologic effects that unload the cardiopulmonary system, cause symptomatic relief, and are often considered neutral with regard to the tendency to hasten death [18].

Some key points to remember when administering medications for comfort in the setting of ventilator withdrawal are as follows:

1. Use the IV route. The oral and subcutaneous route is generally inadequate for the rapid titration necessary in the ICU setting.

2. Administer an IV bolus dose and begin an IV continuous infusion 30 min *before* removal of the ET tube or terminal wean.

3. Starting doses are recommended in the following section (14.5), but realize that you may need to up titrate (to over 200–300% of the starting dose) quickly to achieve symptom relief, especially after removal of the ET tube.

4. The amount of drug necessary is determined not by the amount of milligrams used, but by the comfort effect created. Specific doses are less important than symptom control. Drugs are titrated to control labored respirations (targeting a respiratory rate of <30) with a goal of eradicating any facial grimacing or moaning if possible.

5. Have additional medication ready to administer in bolus form to treat unresolved distress. Bolus dosing (e.g., 5–10 mg of morphine IV push q 5–10 min) is used to *achieve* relief; uptitrating the continuous infusion is used to *maintain* relief. *This underscores a key point: drip titration is a slow and inadequate way of addressing uncontrolled symptoms; bolus administration is the appropriate initial step in achieving symptom control.*

Morphine is recommended as the agent of choice due to its efficacy, low cost, familiarity to the health-care team, and potentially beneficial euphoric effects. It does, however, have a higher association with urticaria, pruritus, and flushing. Fentanyl and hydromorphone are also reasonable choices [4].

Benzodiazepines are considered as important adjunctive medications to opioids in the control of anxiety associated with dyspnea. They should not be used as sole agent of comfort for a patient undergoing terminal extubation as they have no analgesic properties. Their benefits in this setting derive from their sedative, anxiolytic, hypnotic, and amnesic effects [4].

Haloperidol is considered the drug of choice for agitated delirium in critically ill patients. Haloperidol reaches maximal effect 30 min after IV administration. IV doses of haloperidol can be doubled every 30 min to achieve effect. Single adult dose of more than 20 mg is rarely needed or recommended [4].

Paralytics do not have role in the treatment of discomfort associated with terminal extubation. The paralysis induced can mask signs of distress that the patient would otherwise normally be able to register. In general, if paralytics have been given before care goals have shifted to exclusively comfort-based treatment, waiting for the effects of the paralytics to wear off before performing ventilator withdrawal is recommended. However, the benefits of continuing life support should be balanced with the burden that continued mechanical ventilation imposes on the patient and family. If it is felt that waiting for resolution of paralysis causes an unacceptable delay and actually generates more emotional and or physical distress, it is reasonable to proceed with ventilator withdrawal more expeditiously. If this is the case, extra care should then be taken to assure that the patient is comfortable as they may not manifest physical signs of discomfort as readily [4].

Propofol is an intravenous anesthetic used commonly in ICU settings to sedate critically ill patients. The use of propofol has several advantages, including rapid onset and onset of effect, allowing for ease of titration [4].

Barbiturates and *ketamine* can be used but typically are reserved for patients who are refractory or intolerant to more standard agents [4].

14.5 MEDICATION PROTOCOLS

1. *Morphine Plus Midazolam*: Preferred for patients with decreased level of consciousness and without high tolerance due to previous prolonged exposure to opioids and benzodiazepines.

   Bolus: Morphine 2–10 mg and midazolam 1–2 mg

   Infusion: Morphine 50% of the bolus dose in mg/h and midazolam 2–4 mg every 4 h scheduled or 1 mg/h [19]

   Keep in mind that these are starting doses of medication for naïve patients. Patients already on opioids or benzodiazepines may require higher doses.

2. *Propofol*: Appropriate for the more alert patients who are expected to have respiratory distress after extubation.

   Bolus: 1–2 mg/kg
   Infusion 1–2 mg/kg/h [19]

14.6 ICU POLICIES TO SUPPORT FAMILIES

It is important to create an environment that is supportive of families undergoing the difficult process of life-sustaining care withdrawal for their loved one. A calm, peaceful environment can be facilitated by making sure that a family know what to expect and ensuring systematic pharmacologic and procedural policies that minimize the appearance of distress to their loved one. To that end, we recommend removing physical restraints and other unnecessary medical paraphernalia to return the patient to a more natural and nontethered state. We recommend turning off all monitors and alarms, assuring families that this does not help tell us when a patient is going to die—but rather creates more chaos in the room and distracts from the patient. Families should be encouraged to speak with and hold their family members if they feel comfortable doing so. Having trained medical staff with extensive experience readily available to answer questions is critical. Routine palliative care consultations should be the norm to provide additional support and information. Encourage families to make arrangements for special music or personalized rituals as they see fit.

14.7 WITHDRAWAL OF OTHER LIFE-SUSTAINING INTERVENTIONS

14.7.1 Noninvasive Ventilation

The use of noninvasive positive pressure ventilation (NIPPV), such as bi-level positive airway pressure (BiPAP) devices, has become commonplace in the hospital. Such devices are typically used to stabilize patients in respiratory distress/failure as a measure to avoid intubation While considered "noninvasive," these treatments can incur a significant impediment to comfort given the need to create a tight facial seal and can lead to claustrophobia and skin breakdown. For those patients who do not desire intubation, failure of NIPPV often represents a life-ending situation. Ideally, NIPPV is intended to be a bridge to improvement, not a bridge to death. It is reasonable to offer a trail of continuous NIPPV to patients who want to avoid intubation, but if that trial extends beyond 24–48 h, reevaluation of whether the treatment is prolonging life versus prolonging death is reasonable. If NIPPV removal is appropriate, we recommend managing this in fashion similar to a terminal extubation, where the patient is started on bolus and IV medications and titrating those medications up as needed as NIPPV settings are titrated down to minimal support. Once the patient is comfortable on minimal settings, the NIPPV can be removed [20].

14.7.2 Withdrawal of Dialysis

As with any life-sustaining procedure, it is ethically acceptable to discontinue dialysis when it no longer meets the goals of treatment. In a non-ICU setting, withdrawal of dialysis typically leads to death within several days to a week or two. In critical care settings, dialysis is often one of the multiple life-sustaining treatments being stopped (along with vasopressors, antibiotics, and mechanical ventilation), so the timeline to death is often much shorter [21, 22].

14.7.3 Automated Internal Defibrillators

If a patient is transitioning to comfort care, it is important to be cognizant of the presence of implanted defibrillators. In addition to being painful for the patient, it can be emotionally devastating for a family member to witness their loved one receive multiple shocks when comfort has been agreed upon as the goal of care. We recommend deactivating all AICD's in patients who are transitioning to comfort cares. Representatives from device companies should be contacted to deprogram the devices as soon as possible. Reassure family that the device does not have to be physically removed to be deactivated. If immediate deactivation is required, placing a magnet over the device will temporarily suspend defibrillation therapy and inhibit shocks for as long as the magnet remains over the implanted device.

REFERENCES

1. AMA's Code of Medical Ethics, Section 2.0: Opinions on Social Policy Issues, Opinion 2.20 Withholding or Withdrawing Life-Sustaining Medical Treatment. Issued December 1984 as Opinion 2.18, Withholding or Withdrawing Life-Prolonging Medical Treatment, and Opinion 2.19, Withholding or Withdrawing Life-Prolonging Medical Treatment—Patients' Preferences. In 1989, these Opinions were renumbered 2.20 and 2.21, respectively. Updated June 1994 based on the reports "Decisions Near the End of Life" and "Decisions to Forego Life-Sustaining Treatment for Incompetent Patients," both adopted June 1991 (Decisions Near the End of Life. *JAMA* 1992;**267**:2229–2233), and updated June 1996.
2. Hall MJ, Levant S, DeFrances CJ, Trends in Inpatient Hospital Deaths: National Hospital Discharge Survey, 2000–2010. *NCHS Data Brief No 118.* Hyattsville: National Center for Health Statistics, 2013.
3. Angus DC, Barnato AE, Linde-Zwirble WT, et al., Use of intensive care at the end of life in the United States: an epidemiologic study, *Crit Care Med* 2004;**32**:638–643.
4. Truog RD, Campbell ML, Curtis R, et al., Recommendations for end-of-life care in the intensive care unit: a consensus statement by the American College of Critical Care Medicine, *Crit Care Med* 2008; **36**:953–963.
5. AMA's Code of Medical Ethics, Section 2.0: Opinions on Social Policy Issues, Opinion 2.035—Futile Care. Available at http://www.ama-assn.org/ama/pub/physician-resources/medical-ethics/about-ethics-group/ethics-resource-center/end-of-life-care/ama-policy-end-of-life-care.page? Accessed October, 23, 2014.
6. Luce JM, Physicians do not have a responsibility to provide futile of unreasonable care if a patient or family insists, *Crit Care Med* 1995;**23**:760–766.
7. Vacco v. Quill 117 S. Ct 2293. 1997.
8. Azoulay E, Chevret S, Leleu G, et al., Half the families of intensive care unit patients experience inadequate communication with physicians, *Crit Care Med* 2000;**28**(8):3044–3049.
9. Lautrette A, Darmon M, Megarbane B, et al., A communication strategy and brochure for relatives of patients dying in the ICU, *N Engl J Med* 2007;**356**:469–478.
10. Ambuel B and Weissman DE, Moderating an end-of-life family conference, 2nd ed. Fast Facts and Concepts. Available at http://www.eperc.mcw.edu/EPERC/FastFactsIndex/ff_016.htm. Accessed on August 16, 2005.
11. IP-SDM Model, as included in: Kryworuchko J, et al., *Am J Hosp Palliat Care* 2012;**29**:37.
12. Delgado EM, Callahan A, Paganelli G, et al., Multidisciplinary family meetings in the ICU facilitate end-of-life decision making, *Am J Hosp Palliat Care* August/September 2009;**26**:295–302.
13. White DB, Evans LR, Bautista CA, et al., Are physicians' recommendations to limit life support beneficial or burdensome? *Am J Respir Crit Care Med* 2009;**180**:320–325.
14. Jabre P, Belpomme V, Azoulay E, et al., Family presence during cardiopulmonary resuscitation, *New Engl J Med* 2013;**368**(11):1008–1018.
15. Marr L, Weissman D, Withdrawal of ventilatory support from the dying adult patient, *J Support Oncol,* 2004;**2**:283–288.
16. Cooke, Colin R. MD, et al., Predictors of time to death after terminal withdrawal of mechanical ventilation in the ICU, *Chest* August 2010;**138**(2):289–297.

17. Charles Von Gunten, David Weissman, *Ventilator Withdrawal Protocol*, 2nd ed. Fast Facts #33. End of Life/Palliative Education Resource Center (EPERC). http://www.eperc.mcw.edu/EPERC.htm.
18. Bakker J, Jansen TC, Lima A, Kompanje EJO, Why opioids and sedatives may prolong rather than hasten death after ventilator withdrawal in critically ill patients, *Am J Hosp Palliat Care*, April/May 2008;**25**(2):152–154.
19. Von Gunten C, Weissman D, *Symptom Control for Ventilator Withdrawal in the Dying Patient*, 2nd ed. Fast Facts #34. End of Life/Palliative Education Resource Center (EPERC). http://www.eperc.mcw.edu/EPERC.htm.
20. Yeow, Mei-Ean, et al., *Using non-Invasive ventilation at the End of Life*. Fast Facts #230. End of Life/Palliative Education Resource Center (EPERC). http://www.eperc.mcw.edu/EPERC.htm.
21. Davidson S, Rosielle D, *Withdrawal of Dialysis: Decision-Making*. Fast Facts #207. End of Life/Palliative Education Resource Center (EPERC). http://www.eperc.mcw.edu/EPERC.htm.
22. Davidson S, Roseille D, *Clinical Care Following Withdrawal of Dialysis*. Fast Facts #208. End of Life/Palliative Education Resource Center (EPERC). http://www.eperc.mcw.edu/EPERC.htm.

ADDITIONAL RESOURCES

AMA's Code of Medical Ethics, Section 2.0: Opinions on Social Policy Issues; http://www.ama-assn.org/ama/pub/physician-resources/medical-ethics/code-medical-ethics.page? Accessed on July 28, 2014.
End of Life/Palliative Education Resource Center (EPERC): Fast facts; http://www.eperc.mcw.edu/EPERC?docid=67983. Accessed on July 28, 2014.
UpToDate: Ethics in the Intensive Care Unit: Withholding and withdrawing ventilatory support in the ICU.

Chapter 15

Artificial Nutrition and Hydration in Patients with Serious Illness

Thomas T. Reid

15.1 INTRODUCTION

Artificial nutrition and hydration (ANH)—provided either enterally (enteral nutrition (EN)) or parenterally (parenteral nutrition (PN))—is a common short-term intervention to support patients with reversible causes of nutritional deficiency resulting from a temporary inability to eat. Its risks and benefits are less clear for patients with serious chronic illness—particularly those near the end of their lives.

While outcome data in these populations should inform shared decision-making, it is critical to recognize and address the symbolic importance and emotional valence of food and feeding. More often than not, these emotional factors are more important to patients and families than even the most iron-clad data. As in other areas of palliative medicine, discussing artificial nutrition relies on excellent communication that focuses on uncovering assumptions and addressing family concerns. Ultimately, though, ANH is a medical intervention and medical providers have the final responsibility for delivering or withholding it.

15.2 EN

15.2.1 Introduction

Options. EN refers to artificial nutrition delivered directly to the GI tract via catheter. Gastric tubes (G-tubes) and jejunal tubes (J-tubes) pass directly through the abdominal and stomach walls and are secured inside and out with bumpers to

Hospital-Based Palliative Medicine: A Practical, Evidence-Based Approach, First Edition.
Edited by Steven Pantilat, Wendy Anderson, Matthew Gonzales, and Eric Widera.
© 2015 John Wiley & Sons, Inc. Published 2015 by John Wiley & Sons, Inc.

prevent dislodgement. Depending upon the clinical circumstances and the expertise of available providers, a variety of techniques may be used including upper endoscopy, radiologic visualization, and direct surgical placement.

Nasogastric tubes (NGTs) are inserted through the nose and terminate in the stomach. As compared with G-tubes, there is no difference in mortality, complications in the first month, or aspiration pneumonia at 6 months [1, 2]. Even so, placing a percutaneous tube is recommended if enteral access is needed for more than 30 days because of a greater incidence of recurrent displacements resulting in treatment interruptions. Though not a medical indication for placement, many skilled nursing facilities will only accept EN patients with G-tubes.

Demographics/Prevalence. Over 200,000 gastrostomy tubes are placed annually in the United States [3]. Nearly 4 out of every 1000 patients admitted to a hospital have a G-tube placed and rates continue to rise [4]. Fifty-four of every thousand patients with dementia in U.S. nursing homes have gastrostomy tubes placed annually, and high rates of transition between healthcare settings are associated with greater incidence of tube placement [5].

Risks. Serious procedural complications associated with G-tube placement (death, aspiration, hemorrhage, perforation, organ injury) are generally rare (<1%) in otherwise healthy patients but may be as high as 10% in cancer patients and other seriously ill inpatients [6, 7].

Medical complications after tube placement are common (overall long-term incidence is 32–70%; see Table 15.1). Equally and sometimes more important are a variety of psychosocial and functional problems associated with providing artificial nutrition by tube (see Table 15.1) [8]. Many of these problems are most acute in patients with dementia, up to 70% of whom require various forms of restraint to prevent tube dislodgement. EN also medicalizes the act of ingestion, reducing or eliminating the pleasure derived from eating and changing mealtimes from a social to a procedural activity.

Table 15.1 Common Problems with G-Tube Placement and ANH

Medical Problems	Psychosocial Problems
Tube clogging (45%)	Need for restraints
Diarrhea (10–20%)	Need for tube reinsertion
Peptic ulcer disease (15%)	Medicalization of eating
Infection (3–18%)	Increased anxiety
Gastrointestinal bleeding	Combative behaviors
Peristomal leakage	Decreased socialization
Ileus	Need to clear clogged tube
Tube dislodgement	
Increased skin breakdown	

15.2.2   Disease-Specific Evidence

15.2.3   Cancer

CANCER ANOREXIA–CACHEXIA SYNDROME. Nearly 80% of patients who die from cancer develop the cancer anorexia–cachexia syndrome (CACS)—a progressive wasting of muscle and fat accompanied by anorexia, weakness, fatigue, and other signs of metabolic failure [9]. Because CACS is a dysmetabolic state that causes the body to favor catabolism over anabolism, both enteral and parenteral nutritional support are not effective at reversing it. Trials of various supplements and other interventions are ongoing but at present there are no clearly effective treatments.

METASTATIC CANCER. Short-term EN may be helpful when needed to support surgery (should be started 10–14 days before surgery and is helpful even if surgery has to be delayed) if a patient is already malnourished or expected to consume less than 60% of their estimated energy expenditure for greater than 10 days [10]. It should not be used routinely for patients undergoing radiation, chemotherapy, or stem cell transplant [10]. Thirty-day mortality after percutaneous endoscopic gastrostomy (PEG) placement has been associated with an American Society of Anesthesiology (ASA) score ≥4, elevated WBC count, and advanced tumor stage [11]. Patients who are losing weight due to insufficient nutritional intake and have failed other nutritional interventions may benefit from EN to help *maintain* function or a currently acceptable quality of life (QOL). Patients with short prognoses and already low QOL usually do not benefit from gastrostomy, as additional nutrition generally does not reverse cancer cachexia and no data support improved survival or QOL with tube feeding. In practice, it is often difficult to distinguish these populations, making a careful, goal-directed discussion of risks and benefits especially important.

HEAD AND NECK CANCER. In addition to the CACS common to many cancers, head and neck cancer (HNC) patients are particularly at risk for anatomic obstruction and the side effects of the standard chemoradiation treatments: dysphagia, odynophagia, dysgeusia, xerostomia, tissue necrosis, and infections [12]. Additionally, several risk factors associated with HNC (e.g., low socioeconomic status, male gender, older age, and the heavy use of alcohol and tobacco) are also associated with poor diet and intake at baseline. At present, between 60 and 100% of treated HNC patients receive enteral feeding [13]. Patients remain dependent on G-tubes for a median of between 21 weeks and 7.1 months, with 10–30% of tubes still in place after 1 year [12, 13]. Though G-tubes are associated with poorer QOL in many diseases, some recent data suggest that this may not be the case for HNC patients [14].

While these factors lead some experts to recommend prophylactic G-tube placement, a Cochrane review concluded that there is insufficient evidence to support the practice and G-tubes may result in greater dysphagia after radiation [12, 15]. Finally, when EN is indicated for HNC patients, NGTs and G-tubes appear to be equally effective [16].

Advanced Dementia. Extensive observational data (no randomized clinical trials have been published) show no benefit—and in some cases potential harm—to providing ANH to patients with advanced dementia.

MORTALITY. A Cochrane review and several subsequent studies showed either no difference in or increased mortality with G-tube placement [17–19]. Additionally, 6-month mortality was no better for nursing home patients with dementia admitted to hospitals with high versus low rates of feeding tube placement [20]. For U.S. nursing home residents with advanced dementia, placing feeding tubes sooner after the onset of dysphagia does not change survival [21].

QOL AND FUNCTION. QOL is difficult to assess in patients with advanced dementia, but numerous factors (see previous discussion) suggest that G-tube insertion is more likely to degrade than improve it. Surrogates of nursing home patients with advanced dementia may be more satisfied with end-of-life care when feeding tubes are not present [22]. No data support improved function in patients with dementia receiving ANH.

ASPIRATION AND PRESSURE ULCERS. G-tubes do not prevent or reduce and may actually increase oral secretions, aspiration, and pressure ulcers [17]. Neuroleptics also increase aspiration risk (OR 3.1) in patients with dementia, while thicker liquid consistency and cervical spine mobilization may decrease it [23, 24]. Pressure ulcers may also be caused or exacerbated by decreased activity associated with being connected to a catheter pump (tethering).

Dysphagic Stroke. Half of dysphagic stroke patients will die or recover effective swallow function within 2 weeks, and there is no increase in long-term survival or decrease in complications associated with initiating ANH within the first week after a stroke [25, 26]. These data and other studies showing benefit to delaying G-tube placement (discussed elsewhere) strongly suggest it is preferable to delay G-tube placement in dysphagic stroke patients for at least a week. If consistent with their goals of care (GOC), stroke patients with persistent dysphagia should receive G-tubes, which may be associated with lower mortality and are associated with fewer complications/treatment failures and improved nutrition as compared with NGTs in this population [25, 26]. Outcomes for dysphagic stroke patients in whom a G-tube is placed are described in Table 15.2 [27]. Eventual tube removal is strongly correlated with the absence of aspiration (OR 11) or pharyngeal trigger delay (OR 15) on video-fluoroscopic swallow studies performed at the time of tube insertion [28].

As alternatives or supplements to ANH, acupuncture and behavioral interventions (e.g., swallow therapy, modified diets, positioning) may reduce aspiration in dysphagic stroke patients [25].

In one study, among patients who suffered hemorrhagic strokes, those who received a G-tube were less likely to return home (7% vs. 19%) [29]. Though patients who did not receive a G-tube had higher short-term mortality (median survival 57 days vs. 266 days), those who survived to discharge without a G-tube ultimately lived longer (1 year mortality 35% vs. 49%).

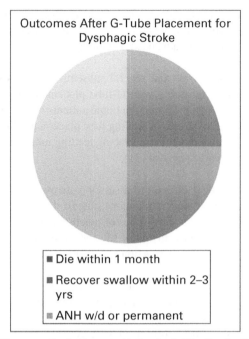

Figure 15.1   What Happens to Stroke Patients with Dysphagia Who Receive G-Tubes? A quarter of stroke patients who receive PEG tubes die within a month and another quarter regain enough swallowing ability to have the tube removed within 2–3 years. In the remaining half of patients, enteral feeding is withdrawn or becomes essentially permanent.

ALS. Good nutrition is linked to survival in ALS [30]. Though no randomized controlled trials (RCTs) were available for analysis, a recent Cochrane review found weak to moderate evidence of survival and nutrition benefits from ANH [31]. Though there is ongoing debate over early versus late tube insertion, most studies do not show increased mortality or procedural complications related to decreased lung function or ventilatory support, suggesting that there may be no medical downside to delaying insertion. Evidence-based guidelines from the American Academy of Neurology support using ANH via G-tube when this is consistent with a patient's GOC [30].

15.2.4   Other Factors

Aspiration. NG and PEG tube feeds, including techniques such as continuous pump feeding [32], do not reduce the risk of aspiration or pneumonia and may even increase it [17]. A meta-analysis of 11 RCTs in the ICU did not show any difference in aspiration rates for postpyloric (duodenal or jejunal) feeds as compared with gastric feeds, and the gastric group had far fewer problems with feeding tube placement or blockage (RR 0.13) [33]. It is unclear if these data may be extrapolated to other populations.

Waiting Period. Limited data suggest that a waiting period prior to hospital placement of a G-tube may improve outcomes [34, 35]. Inpatients who had a G-tube placed were 7 times more likely to die within 30 days (4% vs. 29%) than community nursing home patients and twice as likely to die than matched inpatient controls. Additionally instituting a required 1-month waiting period reduced 30-day mortality by 40% from the time of G-tube request and 87% from the time of insertion.

15.3   PN

15.3.1   Introduction

PN is the provision of some or all essential macro- and micronutrients via intravenous infusion. Once started, it requires close monitoring of blood glucose, electrolytes, and prealbumin as well as occasional checks of trace elements.

Risks. Aside from mechanical risks associated with central line placement and maintenance, the main risks of PN are infections and metabolic complications. Patients using lines to provide TPN are 4 times more likely to develop line infections (5/1000 catheter days), which are more likely to be fungemic and are associated with very high mortality (12–25% per episode) [36]. Cholecystitis may occur in as many as 4% of patients, mostly after 3 months. Metabolic complications center on the liver and bone, increase over time, and include liver function abnormalities, hyperglycemia, steatosis, and refeeding syndrome—collectively leading to eventual end-stage liver disease (~50%) and/or metabolic bone disease (40–100%) over a period of years.

As with G-tubes, PN also tethers the patient to an IV pump, which may reduce independence and indirectly lead to complications associated with limited movement such as pressure ulcers and general functional decline.

When to Consider. Even more so than with EN, a discussion of PN should be driven by a patient's GOC. Additionally, with rare exceptions, PN should only be considered for patients who lack a functional gut. EN stimulates gut function, maintains the mucosal barrier, and improves immunity.

In palliative care contexts, PN is most commonly considered for patients with HNC or malignant bowel obstruction. No RCTs met inclusion criteria in a Cochrane review of the effects of medically assisted nutrition on QOL and length of life in palliative care patients, but lower-quality data do suggest a survival benefit over the days to a couple of months that would be expected as the best case for patients who receive no supplementation or IVF alone [37].

Table 15.3 summarizes the conditions under which it is reasonable to recommend destination PN to palliative care patients.

15.3.2   Disease-Specific Evidence

Cancer. Outside of short-term support (e.g., chemo-/radiation-induced mucositis), PN has little benefit and is potentially harmful for well-nourished cancer patients, particularly during bone marrow transplantation, where it is associated with a higher incidence of infections and longer hospital stays [38].

Table 15.2   When Should PN Be Recommended for Palliative Care Patients?

Criterion	Notes
Meets patient's goals of care	Discuss goals first, and then determine if PN might meet them
EN not feasible	If all other criteria are met, consider EN
Current QOL/function acceptable to patient	PN may preserve existing function but is unlikely to improve it
Risks (medical and psychosocial) acceptable to patient	Emphasize infection, hospitalization, and tethering
Prognosis >1–2 months	Is the patient more likely to die of disease than malnutrition? If all other criteria are met, consider IVF alone

For patients with serious illness and limited prognosis, it is reasonable to recommend PN when *all of the earlier mentioned* criteria are met.

PN in conjunction with chemotherapy may have a modest mortality benefit (5 weeks) after venting gastrostomy for malignant bowel obstruction in gynecologic cancers [39]. Whether this is true for other cancer types and chemotherapy regimens is unclear and must be weighed against the concern that immunosuppressive regimens might increase the risk of infectious complications associated with PN. Of note, study patients had a particularly high rate of G-tube complications requiring medical intervention (56%). No other data provide insight into the common practice of providing PN to malnourished cancer patients with no enteral route. Finally, though it is a common concern, there is no evidence that PN stimulates tumor growth in a clinically significant fashion [10].

Organ Failure, Dementia, and HIV. PN for patients with severe heart, lung, and liver failure has either not been studied or is not recommended based on existing evidence. Data and expert opinion are mixed regarding the value of PN given as a supplement during hemodialysis (intradialytic PN). Though it has not been studied directly, PN use in patients with severe neurocognitive impairment (including dementia) is likely to have greater risk and less benefit than EN for the same indications (see aforementioned text for discussion). Home TPN does not affect survival or rehospitalization for advanced HIV/AIDS patients [40]. Given the paucity of data, discussions in these conditions should focus on function, risks, and how (if at all) PN would meet a patient's goals.

15.4 ARTIFICIAL HYDRATION ONLY?

When indicated, artificial hydration with isotonic fluids alone may be delivered intravenously, subcutaneously (hypodermoclysis), or per rectum (proctoclysis). In the hospice setting, 1–2 liters boluses may be delivered—including at home—every 1–2 days.

Table 15.3 Surrogate Decision-Making

Triggers for Discussion	Common Expectations of Benefit	Reasons for Refusal
Weight loss	Improved nutrition (96%)	Poor QOL
Worsening nutrition	Better health (93%)	Food refusal
Feeding difficulty	Prolonged life (90%)	Advance healthcare directive
Swallowing difficulty	Improved QOL (87%)	
Food refusal	Fewer eating problems (83%)	
	Greater comfort (79%)	
	Less choking (79%)	
	Less hunger/thirst (70%)	

A Cochrane review of the effects of artificial hydration on the QOL and length of life of palliative care patients uncovered mixed results for sedation and myoclonus but multiple signs of third spacing (edema, ascites, pleural effusion) and no improvement in patients' ability to communicate, agitation/hyperactive delirium, myoclonus, or bedsores—findings confirmed by a recent update of the main study reporting them [41, 42]. While the study also showed greater signs of dehydration in the group not receiving IVF, attention to oral care is thought to alleviate any associated suffering. Published since the Cochrane review, a high-quality blinded RCT compared IVF administration of 1000 ml/day versus 100 ml/day in hospice-enrolled advanced cancer patients with reduced oral intake and signs of dehydration [43]. There was no difference in survival or improvement of the sum of four dehydration symptoms (fatigue, myoclonus, sedation, and hallucinations) at either 4 or 7 days between the two groups. Nighttime delirium was worse in the placebo group at 7 days.

Overall, these findings reinforce the need for individualized, goal-driven decision-making. As noted in Table 15.3, artificial hydration may be best used for patients with limited prognoses but otherwise good QOL. When artificial hydration is provided, the clinician should discuss the potential for discomfort associated with fluid overload and be alert for signs that it is developing.

15.5 DECISION-MAKING AROUND ANH

15.5.1 Cultural, Religious, Psychological, and Emotional Factors

Food and eating carry deep significance in all cultures and for many individuals. Serious psychological distress is associated with reduced interest in eating, a limited capacity to digest food, fatigue, and altered body image [44]. Interestingly, families are more worried about anorexia than patients and do not feel staff are worried enough [44]. Families, and especially spouses, also frequently view intake as a measure of disease progression, often confusing cause and effect [44]. While these beliefs can complicate conversations with providers, the family's insistence on ANH resulting from them also creates relational problems with and generates loneliness, helplessness, and guilt in patients [44]. Cultural factors may override these patterns. For example, families with a Hindu cultural background may view reduced consumption as a sign of death rather than a cause [44]. Finally, while mainstream teachings of most major religions allow for flexibility in end-of-life decision-making, it is always important to ask about how individual spiritual and religious beliefs relate to decisions regarding ANH. Even for religious individuals, religion may or may not play a central role in their decision-making. In all cases, psychological, social, religious, and cultural factors are best understood as potential patterns that may or may not be expressed in a particular patient–family unit.

15.5.2   Starvation and Dehydration

As noted earlier, nearly every family worries that their loved one will "starve to death" or suffer from thirst without adequate nutrition and hydration. Among terminally ill, mentally aware patients admitted to a comfort care unit who received only small amounts of food and water (given at the request of the patient) 63% never experienced hunger, and initial hunger in nearly all the other patients (34%) eventually disappeared [45]. A ketogenic state is associated with reduced hunger, and healthy fasting subjects report a short initial period of hunger followed by a marked reduction [46]. Carbohydrate loads in this setting may actually stimulate intense hunger. Studies of fasting individuals often describe euphoria, and rat studies have demonstrated endorphin-mediated analgesia after 24 h without food. Physiologically, fasting reduces cortisol secretion and increases the inactivation of thyroxine. Finally, fasting patients experience fewer of the most troublesome end-of-life symptoms, notably respiratory secretions, coughing, nausea, vomiting, and diarrhea.

While there is no sure way to know if severely cognitively impaired patients suffer from fasting at the end of life, the available evidence suggests that, at worst, significant hunger likely persists for only a few days. For many of these patients, fasting may actually keep them more comfortable. Regardless of the data, "starvation" is an emotional issue. Ultimately, these concerns should always be addressed in the broader context of the patient's illness trajectory and the risks/benefits of possible interventions.

15.5.3   Patient Decision-Making

In pursuing discussions of ANH, it is helpful to anticipate common patient reactions. The most common reasons given by patients for favoring ANH are preserving life, the palliation of symptoms, not abandoning the struggle against illness, and feelings of anxiety [44]. The most common reasons patients wish to decline ANH are to avoid becoming a burden, to avoid prolonging suffering, and a fear of dependence. Interestingly, data show both that physician beliefs regarding the efficacy of ANH vary widely and that they may be the most influential single factor in the final decision, highlighting the critical role a hospitalist can play in the shared decision-making process.

15.5.4   Surrogates

Because many seriously ill patients lack decision-making capacity, conversations regarding ANH are often held with surrogates. The most common triggers of discussions of ANH with surrogates are changes in a patient's condition such as weight loss, nutritional status, difficulties with feeding (including swallowing), and food refusal [47].

Surrogate Decision-Making. Surrogates may take many factors into account when making decisions about ANH (see Table 15.3). In general, they understand the benefits more than the risks, and fewer than half eventually believe the intervention improved the patient's QOL [48]. Of surrogates who chose G-tube placement, only 10% knew the patient's explicit wishes, and 25% would have consented to placement even if they knew the patient had expressed a contrary preference [49].

QOL is often cited as the most important factor in decision-making and may be interpreted in numerous ways. In evaluating the impact of ANH on a patient's QOL, surrogates typically consider "freedom from" (pain, discomfort, interference with the dying process) and "freedom to" (eat despite the risk, enjoy the social activity of eating) [47]. Using this terminology may help the clinician to frame the discussion.

Surrogate Expectations of Benefit. Surrogate expectations of benefit from G-tube placement for ANH reflect an optimism not generally supported by the data (see Table 15.3) [50]. Both patients and surrogates view hydration alone as providing hope for improved QOL and comfort [51]. Families also expect reduced fatigue, increased alertness and energy, reduced pain, and improved effectiveness of pain medications. They may also view fluids in a holistic way as replenishing mind, body, and spirit.

15.6   DISCUSSING ANH AT EOL

15.6.1   Alternatives

Any discussion of ANH should include an exploration of alternate approaches that may meet the patient's GOC equally or more effectively.

15.6.2   Oral Feeding

Before discussing ANH, it is important to ensure that all effective modifications to oral feeding have been attempted. A recent meta-analysis reviewing the benefits of oral feeding options in patients with dementia found "sparse but consistent" evidence showing no effect on function, cognition, or mortality for people with moderate to severe dementia [52]. The authors did find low- to moderate-quality evidence that several methods did lead to weight gain (0.5–2.0 kg of weight gain over 1–6 months), though given the other findings it is unclear if this result has any clinical relevance.

Specific evidence-based interventions may include altering the texture, cohesiveness, viscosity, temperature, and density of food; changing the patient's posture while eating; denture adjustment or addressing other dental concerns; and medication adjustment [53]. These results show oral feeding to be at least as effective and possibly more effective than G-tube nutrition at meeting many of the goals for which a tube is commonly considered. It should also be noted that tube and oral feeding are not mutually exclusive. Indeed, all tube-fed patients should receive oral care and many also receive varying amounts of food by mouth.

15.6.3   Comfort Feeding

Comfort feeding is distinct from regular oral feeding in that its primary purpose is to maximize a patient's QOL rather than endpoints such as weight or caloric/nutritional intake. More so than tube feeding, comfort feeding also encourages human contact and interaction, perhaps making it a better way to demonstrate care and compassion for a patient.

15.7   LAW AND ETHICS

15.7.1   Law

Choosing to forego life-sustaining medical treatment is a clearly established legal right in the United States [8]. Federal courts have been clear that ANH is a medical treatment under this definition and that surrogates may speak for a patient without capacity. In the absence of an advance directive, courts have also ruled that there must be only one official decision-maker, though the processes by which a surrogate is selected and the strength of evidence she or he must present documenting the patient's preferences vary from state to state. Twenty states and the District of Columbia impose more stringent requirements on withholding and/or withdrawing ANH [54]. In states where the evidentiary threshold for discontinuing tube feeds is set quite high, it is therefore especially critical to ask surrogates to thoroughly examine patients' goals before tube feeds are initiated.

15.7.2   Ethics

Long-term artificial nutrition remains an area of ethical controversy, especially when medical indications for its use are less clear. Though withdrawing any form of life-sustaining intervention is emotionally challenging, the ethical case for withdrawing interventions is generally stronger than that for withholding them, as there is usually evidence of their specific failure to address the patient's goals [55].

Other arguments specific to ANH from those who oppose withholding or withdrawing it include concern for starvation, fear that withholding ANH in potentially appropriate cases may make it easier to do so in less appropriate situations ("slippery slope"), and the perception that EN is "ordinary care" [56]. In this last view, tube feeding is seen as fulfilling a duty to care for and support the helpless. However, if the goal of feeding is to demonstrate compassion, the acts of offering food and helping a patient to eat are more likely to achieve that end than the more "medicalized" process of administering tube feeds. Also, unlike regular food, ANH is not a basic intervention that can be administered by anyone [55]. Furthermore, evidence (see previous text) suggests that dying patients probably do not suffer from reduced or absent intake. The slippery slope argument is unconvincing because it requires the clinician to impose suffering on a real patient out of concern for future theoretical patients, and is probably better addressed by developing formal safeguards against abuse. There is, in any case, no evidence that withholding ANH has had this effect.

Arguments against ANH include the assertions that it prolongs dying ("force feeding") and that withholding it does not seem to cause suffering while both the tubes/catheters themselves and the act of providing ANH may do so. In patients in the terminal phase of their disease, some also worry about the potential psychological harm of false hope when a G-tube is placed [8].

Though respect for patient autonomy (either directly or through their surrogate) is a central principle of modern medicine, ultimately providers are not obligated to provide treatments they do not feel will benefit their patients. If a patient or surrogate persists in demanding such a treatment, the clinician does have a responsibility to facilitate a second opinion or transfer of care to another provider.

15.8 PRINCIPLES AND TOOLS FOR THE ANH CONVERSATION

15.8.1 Use Goals to Provide Structure

In a family meeting to discuss tube placement, a busy medical team may understandably want to focus on the decision at hand. ANH, however, is rarely urgent and represents a long-term commitment. Taking into account any larger goals that have already been expressed (e.g., extend life except where it would cause discomfort), first start with the problem (e.g., not eating, aspirating), then elicit the family's goals and worries related to that problem (e.g., starvation, choking), and finally discuss alternatives—which may or may not include ANH—that best address those goals and worries. Uncovering family concerns up front allows a skillful clinician to address the questions that matter most to the family as well as to frame the discussion as a whole in a way that makes sense to them. In particular, a framing that focuses on what has been and *will* be done, rather than what will *not* be done, can help to highlight past achievements and avoid a false "care" versus "no care" dichotomy that sometimes arises around ANH decisions. Here, a detailed description of hand feeding or other alternatives may help a family to see that they or the staff of a facility can and will still care for their loved one. If everyone is clear about what decisions were made, at the end of the meeting summarize what the family chose rather than what they did not.

15.8.2   Anticipate and Explore Assumptions

Sometimes patients and surrogates may make decisions about ANH that do not seem to meet their expressed goals. Other times cultural and linguistic differences between the provider and family may make it hard to follow their reasoning. Nearly all families worry about "starvation" and "dehydration." When something "feels funny" about an ANH conversation, it is often because of these differences in unspoken assumptions. Politely exploring reasoning by asking "why do you feel that _____?" is a good way to uncover assumptions the clinician may not share. A genuine desire to understand how a patient or family member thinks and what she or he believes is usually appreciated.

15.8.3   Provide Information in Context

Address the major factors impeding clear, goal-driven decision-making around ANH: anxiety regarding the meaning of decreased intake, poor knowledge of risks and benefits, external pressure, and a low level of awareness of imminent death [44]. As noted earlier, data show that surrogates are more aware of the benefits of gastrostomy than the risks. Explicitly share the hope for a good outcome while also outlining short- and long-term risks and downsides that may not be apparent. Where relevant to the disease process or stage of illness, explain how the body may not benefit from and could even be harmed by nutrition and hydration. For cancer patients, it may be helpful to discuss the CACS. Finally, conversations about ANH should take place in the context of a clear understanding of prognosis and the natural history of the patient's disease.

15.8.4   Emphasize Artificiality

While avoiding jargon is usually desirable, replacing the words "tube feeding" with "artificial nutrition" may help to emphasize the medical nature of ANH as an intervention distinct from eating.

15.8.5   Set Limits at the Outset

ANH is often considered when outcomes are in doubt. Medical interventions have a certain inertia, and though most ethicists do not draw a distinction, many families find stopping ANH to be harder than withholding it initially. For a decision to initiate ANH to be truly goal driven, it should include a discussion of when to stop. The reasons (as expressed by the patient or surrogate) for starting the therapy are a good starting point. Also discuss a timeframe after which the effectiveness of the ANH in meeting the expressed goals will be reassessed. This is referred to as a time-limited trial. Depending on the likelihood of success, this date can be presented as a default stopping point or just a check-in.

15.8.6   Suggest a Waiting Period

As there may be increased mortality associated with urgent G-tube procedures and high-quality evidence demonstrates no difference in 30-day complications between NG and G-tubes, consider suggesting a 30-day delay in G-tube placement. A delay allows the decision-makers time to adjust to what may be a new medical situation and removes the environmental pressure to "get things done" that often exists in the hospital setting.

15.8.7   Consider Using Decision Aids

In a large, multicenter trial, use of a print decision aid to discuss feeding alternatives with the surrogates of nursing home patients with advanced dementia resulted in less decisional conflict, better knowledge (particularly of the risks of tube feeding), more feeding-related communication with providers, better adherence to dysphagia care standards such as dysphagia diets, and less weight loss [57].

15.8.8   Ask for Help

Gastrostomy placement and tube feeding are part of the knowledge base of many specialties and disciplines. Consulting with other team members can provide critical insight into a family's thinking and will help to provide a consistent message. Whenever possible, nurses should be an active part of the decision-making process as they are the most frequent point of contact for the patient and family [44]. Where questions of disease natural history or special procedural concerns (e.g., pulmonary compromise or abnormal abdominal anatomy) exist, consultation with the relevant subspecialists may be helpful. Where cultural or religious concerns are paramount, consider consulting a chaplain reaching out to members of those communities.

REFERENCES

1. Gomes CA, R, Jr., Lustosa SAS, Matos D, Andriolo RB, Waisberg DR, Waisberg J. Percutaneous endoscopic gastrostomy versus nasogastric tube feeding for adults with swallowing disturbances, *Cochrane Database Syst Rev* 2010;CD008096.
2. American Gastroenterological Association Medical Position Statement: guidelines for the use of enteral nutrition, *Gastroenterology* 1995;**108**:1280–1281.
3. Duszak R, Mabry MR, National trends in gastrointestinal access procedures: an analysis of Medicare services provided by radiologists and other specialists, *J Vasc Interv Radiol* 2003;**14**:1031–1036.
4. Mendiratta P, Tilford JM, Prodhan P, Curseen K, Azhar G, Wei JY, Trends in percutaneous endoscopic gastrostomy placement in the Elderly From 1993 to 2003, *Am J Alzheimers Dis Other Demen* 2012;**27**:609–613.
5. Teno JM, Mitchell SL, Skinner J, et al., Churning: the association between health care transitions and feeding tube insertion for nursing home residents with advanced cognitive impairment, *J Palliat Med* 2009;**12**:359–362.
6. Schrag SP, Sharma R, Jaik NP, et al., Complications related to percutaneous endoscopic gastrostomy (PEG) tubes. A comprehensive clinical review, *J Gastrointestin Liver Dis* 2007;**16**:407–418.

 7. Keung EZ, Liu X, Nuzhad A, Rabinowits G, Patel V, In-hospital and long-term outcomes after percutaneous endoscopic gastrostomy in patients with malignancy, *J Am Coll Surg* 2012;**215**:777–786.
 8. Heuberger R, Artificial nutrition and hydration at the end of life, *J Nutr Elder* 2010;**29**:347–385.
 9. Evans WJ, Morley JE, Argilés J, et al., Cachexia: a new definition, *Clin Nutr* 2008;**27**:793–799.
10. Bozzetti F, Arends J, Lundholm K, Micklewright A, Zurcher G, Muscaritoli M, ESPEN Guidelines on Parenteral Nutrition: non-surgical oncology, *Clin Nutr* 2009;**28**:445–454.
11. Richards DM, Tanikella R, Arora G, Guha S, Dekovich AA, Percutaneous endoscopic gastrostomy in cancer patients: predict ors of 30-day complications, 30-day mortality, and overall mortality, *Dig Dis Sci* 2013;**58**:768–776.
12. Locher JL, Bonner JA, Carroll WR, et al., Prophylactic percutaneous endoscopic gastrostomy tube placement in treatment of head and neck cancer: a comprehensive review and call for evidence-based medicine, *JPEN J Parenter Enteral Nutr* 2011;**35**:365–374.
13. Paleri V, Patterson J, Use of gastrostomy in head and neck cancer: a systematic review to identify areas for future research, *Clin Otolaryngol* 2010;**35**:177–189.
14. Osborne JB, Collin LA, Posluns EC, Stokes EJ, Vandenbussche KA, The Experience of head and neck cancer patients with a percutaneous endoscopic gastrostomy tube at a Canadian Cancer Center, *Nutr Clin Pract* 2012;**27**:661–668.
15. Langmore S, Krisciunas GP, Miloro KV, Evans SR, Cheng DM, Does PEG use cause dysphagia in head and neck cancer patients? *Dysphagia* 2011;**27**:251–259.
16. Nugent B1, Lewis S, O'Sullivan JM, Enteral feeding methods for nutritional management in patients with head and neck cancers being treated with radiotherapy and/or chemotherapy, *Cochrane Database Syst Rev* 2012;1–20:CD007904.
17. Sampson E, Candy B, Jones L, Enteral tube feeding for older people with advanced dementia, *Cochrane Database Syst Rev* 2009;**2**:CD007209.
18. Higaki F, Yokota O, Ohishi M, Ohishi, Factors predictive of survival after percutaneous endoscopic gastrostomy in the elderly: is dementia really a risk factor? *Am J Gastroenterol* 2008;**103**:1011–1016.
19. Gaines DI, Durkalski V, Patel A, DeLegge MH, Dementia and cognitive impairment are not associated with earlier mortality after percutaneous endoscopic gastrostomy, *JPEN J Parenter Enteral Nutr* 2008;**33**:62–66.
20. Cai S, Gozalo PL, Mitchell SL, et al., Do patients with advanced cognitive impairment admitted to hospitals with higher rates of feeding tube insertion have improved survival? *J Pain Symptom Manage* 2013;**45**:524–533.
21. Teno JM, Gozalo PL, Mitchell SL, et al., Does feeding tube insertion and its timing improve survival? *J Am Geriatr Soc* 2012;**60**:1918–1921.
22. Engel SE, Kiely DK, Mitchell SL, Satisfaction with end-of-life care for nursing home residents with advanced dementia, *J Am Geriatr Soc* 2006;**54**:1567–1572.
23. Wada H, Nakajoh K, Satoh-Nakagawa T, et al., Risk factors of aspiration pneumonia in Alzheimer's disease patients, *Gerontology* 2001;**47**:271–276.
24. Alagiakrishnan K., Bhanji RA, Kurian M, Archives of gerontology and geriatrics, *Arch Gerontol Geriatr* 2012;**56**:1–9.
25. Geeganage C, Beavan J, Ellender S, Bath PMW, Interventions for dysphagia and nutritional support in acute and subacute stroke (Review), *Cochrane Database Syst Rev* 2011;1–134.
26. Koretz RL, Avenell A, Lipman TO, Braunschweig CL, Milne AC, Does enteral nutrition affect clinical outcome? A systematic review of the randomized trials, *Am J Gastroenterol* 2007;**102**:412–429.
27. Skelly RH, Are we using percutaneous endoscopic gastrostomy appropriately in the elderly? *Curr Opin Clin Nutr Metab Care* 2002;**5**:35–42.
28. Yi Y, Yang EJ, Kim J, Kim WJ, Min Y, Paik NJ, Predictive factors for removal of percutaneous endoscopic gastrostomy tube in post-stroke dysphagia, *J Rehabil Med* 2012;**44**:922–925.
29. Skolarus LE, Morgenstern LB, Zahuranec DB, Burke JF, Langa KM, Iwashyna TJ, Acute care and long-term mortality among elderly patients with intracerebral hemorrhage who undergo chronic life-sustaining procedures, *J Stroke Cerebrovasc Dis* 2013;**22**:15–21.
30. Miller RG, Jackson CE, Kasarskis EJ, et al., Practice Parameter update: the care of the patient with amyotrophic lateral sclerosis: drug, nutritional, and respiratory therapies (an evidence-based review):

Report of the Quality Standards Subcommittee of the American Academy of Neurology, *Neurology* 2009;**73**:1218–1226.

31. Katzberg HD, Benatar M, Enteral tube feeding for amyotrophic lateral sclerosis/motor neuron disease, *Cochrane Database Syst Rev* 2011;CD004030.

32. Lee JS, Kwok T, Chui PY, et al., Can continuous pump feeding reduce the incidence of pneumonia in nasogastric tube-fed patients? A randomized controlled trial, *Clin Nutr* 2010;**29**:453–458.

33. Ho KM1, Dobb GJ, Webb SA, A comparison of early gastric and post-pyloric feeding in critically ill patients: a meta-analysis, *Intensive Care Med* 2006;**32**:639–649.

34. Abuksis G, Mor M, Segal N, et al., Percutaneous endoscopic gastrostomy: high mortality rates in hospitalized patients, *Am J Gastroenterol* 2000;**95**:128–132.

35. Abuksis G, Outcome of percutaneous endoscopic gastrostomy (PEG): comparison of two policies in a 4-year experience, *Clin Nutr* 2004;**23**:341–346.

36. Kulick D, Deen D, Specialized nutrition support, *Am Fam Physician* 2011;**83**:173–183.

37. Good P, Cavenagh J, Mather M, Ravenscroft P, Medically assisted nutrition for palliative care in adult patients, *Cochrane Database Syst Rev* 2008;CD006274.

38. Murray SM, Pindoria S, Nutrition support for bone marrow transplant patients, *Cochrane Database Syst Rev*, 2009;CD002920.

39. Diver E, O'Connor O, Garrett L, et al., Gynecologic Oncology, *Gynecol Oncol* 2013;**129**:332–335.

40. Young T, Busgeeth K, Home-based care for reducing morbidity and mortality in people infected with HIV/AIDS, *Cochrane Database Syst Rev*2010;CD005417.

41. Good P, Cavenagh J, Mather M, Ravenscroft P, Medically assisted hydration for palliative care patients, *Cochrane Database Syst Rev* 2008;CD006273.

42. Nakajima N, Hata Y, Kusumuto K, A clinical study on the influence of hydration volume on the signs of terminally ill cancer patients with abdominal malignancies, *J Palliat Med* 2013;**16**:185–189.

43. Bruera E, Hui D, Dalal S, et al., Parenteral hydration in patients with advanced cancer: a multicenter, double-blind, placebo-controlled randomized trial, *J Clin Oncol* 2012;**31**:111–118.

44. Río MI, Shand B, Bonati P, et al., Hydration and nutrition at the end of life: a systematic review of emotional impact, perceptions, and decision-making among patients, family, and health care staff, *Psycho-Oncology* 2011;**21**:913–921.

45. McCann RM, Hall WJ, Groth-Juncker A, Comfort care for terminally ill patients. The appropriate use of nutrition and hydration, *JAMA* 1994;**272**:1263–1266.

46. Winter SM, Terminal nutrition: framing the debate for the withdrawal of nutritional support in terminally ill patients, *Am J Med* 2013;**109**:723–726.

47. Clarke G, Harrison K, Holland A, Kuhn I, Barclay S, Malaga G, Ed. How are treatment decisions made about artificial nutrition for individuals at risk of lacking capacity? A systematic literature review, *PLoS ONE* 2013;**8**:e61475.

48. Mitchell SL, Berkowitz RE, Lawson FM, Lipsitz LA, A cross-national survey of tube-feeding decisions in cognitively impaired older persons, *J Am Geriatr Soc* 2000;**48**:391–397.

49. Berger JT, Hida S, Chen H, Friedel D, Grendell J, Grendell, Surrogate consent for percutaneous endoscopic gastrostomy, *Arch Intern Med* 2011;**171**:178–179.

50. Carey T, Hanson L, Garrett JM, et al., Expectations and outcomes of gastric feeding tubes, *Am J Med* 2006;**119**:527.e11–527.e16.

51. Cohen MZ, Torres-Vigil I, Burbach BE, de la Rosa A, Bruera E, The meaning of parenteral hydration to family caregivers and patients with advanced cancer receiving hospice care, *J Pain Symptom manage* 2012;**43**:855–865.

52. Hanson LC, Ersek M, Gilliam R, Carey TS, Oral feeding options for people with dementia: a systematic review, *J Am Geriatr Soc* 2011;**59**:463–472.

53. Palecek EJ, Teno JM, Casarett DJ, Hanson LC, Rhodes RL, Mitchell SL, Comfort feeding only: a proposal to bring clarity to decision-making regarding difficulty with eating for persons with advanced dementia, *J Am Geriatr Soc* 2010;**58**:580–584.

54. Sieger CE, Arnold JF, Ahronheim JC, Refusing artificial nutrition and hydration: does statutory law send the wrong message? *J Am Geriatr Soc* 2002;**50**:544–550.

55. Casarett D, Kapo J, Caplan A, Appropriate use of artificial nutrition and hydration--fundamental principles and recommendations, *N Engl J Med* 2005;**353**:2607–2612.
56. Lo B, *Resolving Ethical Dilemmas: A Guide for Clinicians.* 4th edn. Philadelphia, PA: Lippincott Williams & Wilkins, 2009.
57. Hanson LC, Carey TS, Caprio AJ, et al., improving decision-making for feeding options in advanced dementia: a randomized, controlled trial, *J Am Geriatr Soc* 2011;**59**: 2009–2016.

ONLINE RESOURCES

- American Society for Parenteral and Enteral Nutrition (ASPEN)
  http://www.nutritioncare.org/ (accessed on July 28, 2014)
- European Society for Clinical Nutrition and Metabolism (ESPEN)
  http://www.espen.org/ (accessed on July 28, 2014)
- EPERC Fast Facts #84, #133, and #190
  http://www.eperc.mcw.edu/EPERC/FastFactsandConcepts (accessed on July 28, 2014)

Chapter 16

Last Days of Life: Care for the Patient and Family

Jason Morrow

16.1 INTRODUCTION: CARE DURING THE LAST DAYS OF LIFE

The last days of life provide an opportunity for physicians to promote comfort, peacefulness, dignity, healing, and closure. In the hospital setting, this opportunity is beset with many challenges and sources of distress for patients who seek relief and answers in an often strange and tumultuous environment and for providers who strive to provide safe and effective care while navigating the complexities of tertiary care.

Amidst the flurries of tests, procedures, uncertainties, and handoffs, hospitalists are capable coordinators of clinical care. They are like guides in a foreign land, familiar with pathways and pitfalls, speaking the native tongue, striving to offer guidance, protection, advocacy, and, ultimately, safe and efficient discharge from the hospital. Patients and families, then, are travelers who rely on their guides implicitly, sometimes desperately, for hope that their journey in this strange land will yield rescue and recovery. Yet, when the journey ends in the hospital, hospitalists must find new strategies for offering hope and guidance. Hospitalists may find this final phase as foreign and stressful as do families. The purpose of this chapter is to identify and explore practical and effective strategies for hospitalists who strive to improve patient and family experiences at the end of life. For a list of helpful online resources that include specific conditions and patient populations, see the web resources at the end of this chapter.

Death is an increasingly common hospital event, not because health systems fail to deliver effective treatments but because our population is aging and hospitals remain a bastion of hope. The over-65 population is expected to double from about 35 to 72 million from 2012 to 2030. This growing population faces a high prevalence of cancer and chronic illness, including coronary disease, hypertension, diabetes, COPD, and osteoarthritis, each of which potentially carries a high symptom burden, such as pain, depression, and disability, and a high risk of an acute episode requiring

Hospital-Based Palliative Medicine: A Practical, Evidence-Based Approach, First Edition.
Edited by Steven Pantilat, Wendy Anderson, Matthew Gonzales, and Eric Widera.
© 2015 John Wiley & Sons, Inc. Published 2015 by John Wiley & Sons, Inc.

hospitalization. Many of these patients will die in the hospital. As of 2007, about 1.4 million out of 2.4 million deaths in the United States, or 57%, occurred in the hospital setting. And while chronically ill patients are increasingly experiencing their last days in nursing homes, nearly 30% of both young and old will continue to die in the hospital.

For many people, admission to the hospital represents an implicit and potential confrontation with mortality. Yet the specter of death remains shrouded in uncertainty, hope, and denial and is usually not acknowledged—much less accepted—until a trial of acute or intensive care has failed. Hospital physicians, then, are increasingly expected to fight for life against long odds, to harness vast resources and brandish the latest technology, while at the same time minimizing suffering and preparing families for loss.

Hospital Medicine may be the fastest growing medical specialty in history, and hospitalists are increasingly relied upon to coordinate end-of-life care. While some dying patients may be cared for by intensivists, surgeons, or palliative care specialists, and some may be discharged with hospice services, many of these patients will spend their final days under the care of a hospitalist. Whether in the community or academic setting, in collaboration with nurse practitioners, physician assistants, or physicians-in-training, hospitalists can represent the professional ideals of trust and nonabandonment and must therefore endeavor to master the necessary skills to support families, manage symptoms, and create a peaceful environment.

The first step hospitalists can take toward ensuring a minimally traumatic and potentially meaningful death is to recognize the opportunity for maximizing comfort measures as soon as possible. In many cases, physicians recognize the inexorable process of impending death based on a physiologic or clinical process, such as severe brain injury, malignant arrhythmias, or withdrawal of ventilator support in a patient with decompensated respiratory failure. It is this ability to prognosticate and anticipate the most appropriate focus of clinical care that creates a unique opportunity to guide and support families whose desperation expands as their options dwindle (see Chapter 11: Estimating Prognosis).

The setting of withheld or withdrawn life-sustaining measures is a special context with unique professional challenges (see Chapter 14: Withdrawing Life-Sustaining Measures). First, hospitalists may feel that their clinical services are of little value, as is suggested by the unfortunate tropes "withdrawal of care" and "there's nothing we can do" and the sad reality that death is imminent. Withdrawal of life support, however, does not entail the retreat of the physician. To the contrary, there are many important clinical skills that a hospitalist can bring to bear in a patient's last days, the first of which is vigilance for those moments when a family needs a physician to offer a clear and firm commitment to employing every means necessary to ensure patient comfort and promote healthy grieving.

Vigilance entails a further responsibility to remain sensitive to the emotional lives of families. Families who have either requested or consented to withdrawal of life support and allowing natural death are likely to experience dizzying emotions that are tied to the complex process of medical decision-making. For many cancer patients who are dying in the MICU, a veritable army of patients, families, oncologists, and other clinicians have prayed and fought for a cure until that penultimate moment when a downcast clinician breaks the news that death is near. Feelings of shock, guilt, anger, and angst—as well as family tensions—can rise quickly and dominate the conversation. Intense emotions may be kept in check in order to render a decision that life support should be withheld or withdrawn, and a quick transition to "comfort measures only" may proceed. But the hospitalist who then hopes to deliver on that promise of comfort must be sensitive to the intense feelings arising prior to or during the decision-making process that linger and require competent and compassionate engagement. Emotional support is an iterative process.

When a decision is made to forgo life support, families in some way start to believe or accept that the end is near. Alternatively, the context in which no decision to limit care is made, when life-sustaining measures are pursued until the moment of death, is in some ways emotionally simpler. While feelings of guilt are a natural part of grieving, trying "everything" can be a natural antidote for feelings of accountability for death in the hospital. Decision-making among patients, families, and physicians can be heavily influenced by possible feelings of regret, inadequacy, or powerlessness. Thus, whether or not life support is deliberately withheld or withdrawn near the end of life, the hospitalist should liberally and concisely remind family members that disease and trauma are the underlying causes of death, that heroic measures and life support are always trials limited by the risk of harm and suffering, and that sometimes respect for autonomy and patient preferences means letting go before we feel ready.

Hospitalists are well aware that just because death is imminent doesn't mean that all family members, or even other clinicians, recognize this. In this case, the best possible care of the patient, or the maximization of comfort, may have to be implemented stepwise in order to patiently accommodate the beliefs and preferences of the family. For example, in a debilitated elderly patient with metastatic cancer, a time-limited trial of hemodialysis can be offered with an agreed-upon understanding that if hypotension, delirium, or signs of severe pain or anxiety persist, then symptoms will be managed promptly and hemodialysis will be either discontinued or reconsidered during an interdisciplinary family meeting in the days ahead.

A helpful strategy for communicating in this context is to offer the family a clear description of what the road to recovery looks like and what bad news looks like. Be specific. Provide the family with baseline lab values, vital signs, or treatment goals, and then describe the milestones needed, say for the next family meeting, to suggest whether or not the patient is on the road to recovery. This will set the stage for a possible transition to an exclusive focus on comfort measures.

In addition to emotional vigilance and sensitivity, how else can hospitalists effectively attend to the needs of families who have, moments or days prior, let go of the hope for rescue and recovery and who now face a dying process they long feared? Three strategies can be brought to bear, manifested in the phases of doctor–family communication at the end of life. First, as decisions are made and the specter of death is acknowledged, hospitalists should focus on an ongoing commitment to provide timely and empathic communication, addressing common concerns while drawing on key phrases and resources for healthy grieving. Second, as comfort measures are implemented, core strategies include signposting and delivery of expert symptom management and supportive care. The third strategy entails respectful follow-through, including competent pronouncement of death, provision of postmortem care, and initiating a plan for bereavement.

16.2 LAST DAYS: EMPATHIC COMMUNICATION AND INTERDISCIPLINARY CARE

Empathic communication during a decision-making process or a time-limited trial of medical therapy is easier and more effective when involved clinicians give clear and consistent information and when an interdisciplinary team is involved.

The hospitalist is most effective in his or her role when an interdisciplinary team is available to help families at every step during decision-making and grieving processes. If a case involves difficult prognostication, complex family dynamics, or transfer across clinical units, then interdisciplinary members of a specialized Palliative Medicine Team, if available, can provide both expert guidance and continuity of care. The earlier these team members can assess and establish rapport with patients and families, the better. Other advantages of services provided by a team of Palliative Medicine specialists include the dynamics of efficiency and of interprofessional support that come with a team that routinely collaborates on clinical care.

Some hospitalists personally find empathic communication at the end of life to be a daunting task. There may be no substitute for experience, practice, and exposure to exemplary role models, but having supportive phrases, recommendations, and resources handy can help any clinician communicate with proficiency (see Chapter 7: General Principles and Core Skills in Communication).

16.3 LAST DAYS: SIGNPOSTING AND SYMPTOM MANAGEMENT

One of the most effective ways to help a family prepare for death is to provide signposts for the journey ahead. Signposting should begin with a tactful invitation such as, "Would you like me to share some signs and symptoms that you can expect to see?" Some family members may not be emotionally ready to hear details, and for them an informational handout or brochure can be offered for reading at their own pace. Several valuable resources exist including "Hard Choices for Loving People" which is available in both English and Spanish.

For family members who accept the invitation to talk, a simple explanation of the normal signs of dying can be reassuring. A discussion of signs of possible suffering can also be fruitful because some family members will find it empowering and meaningful to participate in the plan of care. One way to approach this subject is to advise family members that since they know the patient better than the clinical staff, and since they are likely better at interpreting the patient's facial expressions, body language, and verbal cues, their role in assessing patient comfort is vital. To that end, hospitalists should bring the patient's nurse and family together to identify signs or symptoms that should be reported to the nurse, physician, or other clinicians for further assessment. Of course in this context the family should be counseled on their options for participating in bedside care, including oral care, verbal reassurance, massage, and ensuring a peaceful environment among family visitors.

When the invitation to signpost is accepted, hospitalists can describe the signs of dying both as a general account of how the body shuts down and as a specific account of how particular disease trajectories will likely unfold. One way to describe the final hours and days of life is to explain how the human body can be expected to undergo a series of changes that reflect a decline in cellular metabolic activity and energy among various interrelated organ systems. Another is to emphasize that dying is both a part of life and, like other transitions such as birth and marriage, an opportunity to engage in rituals that demonstrate respect, honor, and a value for life and love in their many forms. Relatedly, it is important to inquire about families' spiritual beliefs so that the hospitalist's framing of the dying process can accommodate expectations such as the release of the patient's spirit or soul.

Perhaps the most familiar signs of dying are those that relate to the neurologic symptoms of fatigue, somnolence, and decreased alertness. These signs may be caused directly by neurologic injury in the case of stroke or traumatic brain injury or indirectly in case of cerebral hyper/hyponatremia or hypoperfusion associated with sepsis, heart failure, or dehydration. Other organ involvement will accelerate neurologic dysfunction: uremia due to renal failure, hyperbilirubinemia due to hepatic malignancy, or hypoxemia/hypercarbia due to respiratory failure. In each case, neurocellular demand for energy outstrips the available supply resulting in impairment of cortical function and central activation or awareness. In counseling families on the signs of neurologic decline, hospitalists should emphasize that the descent into unresponsiveness is a natural and expected consequence of the body and organs shutting down.

One of the most common questions among families with regard to decreased responsiveness is: "Can she hear me?" It is important to recognize that this question often reflects a personal hope to connect or say goodbye. The answer to this question, therefore, can provide a unique opportunity to promote healing and closure. The hospitalist may reply with something like: "I am not sure if she can hear us. In fact, I could not explain it based on my understanding of her brain injury, but I always assume that my patients can hear me. And I also know that your voice is more recognizable than mine, so I recommend that you speak to her, say the things that are important like 'I love you' and 'I know you love me', and, when other family members are in the room, just chat with one another—share memories or stories—so that your voices can offer familiarity and comfort."

Another common question related to the patient's level of alertness in the last hours of life is: "Should I stay at the bedside?" If death is imminent, it may be prudent to encourage bedside vigilance if the family wishes to be present at the moment of death. A private room with no limits on visitor hours and with a sleeper sofa or futon can be extremely useful in this regard.

On the other hand, sometimes the timing of the dying process is difficult to predict, and family members experience stress and fatigue related to hypervigilance.

In this case, the hospitalist may recommend that family members take shifts so they can sleep and take care of their own mental and physical health. And it may be helpful to advise family members in advance that sometimes patients will only take their last breaths when family is not there to witness, as if doing so is a purposeful, protective act. This observation may serve as a narrative construct that relieves guilt.

One of the other most familiar signs of dying relates to changes in breathing patterns and sounds. As the body shuts down, fluid shifts may result in pulmonary edema, organ dysfunction or hypoperfusion may cause metabolic acidosis, and increased intracerebral pressure or brainstem injury may impair the respiratory centers of the brain. In each of these cases, breathing patterns at the end of life are likely to include periods of rapid shallow breathing as well as apnea spells. Families should be advised that changes in respiration are normal signs of dying and not necessarily a sign of pain or suffocation, whether rapid breathing or apnea follows a crescendo–decrescendo pattern (Cheyne–Stokes respirations) or else a clustered–intermittent pattern (Biot's respirations).

One of the challenges of maximizing patient comfort in the final hours of life relates to the patient's inability to communicate pain while at the same time possibly demonstrating a rapid breathing pattern that, in other circumstances, might indicate pain or distress. For this reason, it is standard of care to provide either a low-dose infusion or hourly, as-needed doses of opioids. An effective and ethically sound strategy for administering opioids in the tachypneic and unresponsive dying patient is to titrate opioids to a respiratory rate range. For example, to ensure that pain is controlled while avoiding the unnecessary risk of hastening death, a hospitalist could place a nursing order to administer low-dose, concentrated, sublingual morphine for a respiratory rate greater than 30 and to withhold opioids for a respiratory rate less than 8. Development of a comfort care order set for nurses and physicians that includes pharmacologic options for symptom management and protocols for tailoring bedside care to a patient's needs at the end of life—including a focus on oral hygiene and limitations on vital signs and bloodwork—is a powerful strategy for standardizing and improving care in the last days of life. A link to a sample comfort care order set is provided in the web resources section of this chapter.

For many patients, a declining respiratory rate such as four breaths per minute is a telltale sign that death is likely to occur with minutes, not hours. Similarly, when pulmonary excursion or air movement is limited and respirations consist of "mandibular" or "guppy" breathing, death is almost certainly at hand.

Another respiratory sign of impending death is commonly known as the "death rattle." This audible, gurgling sound usually indicates that secretions have accumulated in the retropharynx or trachea where air movement creates a resonating sound. This sound is more disturbing to families than it is to the moribund patient. Warning in advance will mitigate this potentially unnerving experience, as will routine oral care, which can be intimately provided by inclined family members. Management can be aided—perhaps modestly—by discontinuing unnecessary fluids, whether enteral or parental, as soon as possible in the course of identifying comfort as the primary goal of care and by employing pharmacologic agents such as ophthalmic atropine given sublingually or parenteral glycopyrrolate.

Table 16.1   Signs and Symptoms of Impending Death and Estimated Prognosis

	Hours Prior to Death	
Sign	Mean ± SD	Median
Retained respiratory secretions audible (death rattle)	57 ± 82	23
Respirations with mandibular movement (jaw movement increases with breathing)	7.6 ± 18	2.5
Cyanosis of extremities	5.1 ± 11	1
No radial pulse	2.6 ± 4.2	1

Source: Adapted from Morita et al. (1998). © SAGE.

Other common signs of impending death that hospitalists can include in sign-posting are those that arise from hemodynamic changes associated with hypovolemia or multiorgan dysfunction. Anuria usually occurs within the final days of life. Myclonus may follow from acidosis or electrolyte disturbances. As blood pressure drops, perhaps approaching 60/40 mm Hg, radial pulses may become thready, limbs may feel cool, and mottling—lacy, irregular patches of discoloration—may appear. These signs usually indicate that the patient is within hours of dying. Common signs of impending death are listed in Table 16.1 along with their usual associated prognosis.

16.4 LAST DAYS: AN APPROACH TO PRONOUNCING DEATH

Pronouncing death is an awesome responsibility. Most clinicians remember their first encounter with death and issuing a pronouncement. For many, the act serves as a sobering ritual that signifies consummation of physicianhood. Over a career, the fear some physicians may experience related to pronouncing death diminishes, but for most physicians, encounters with patients in the moments after death continue to inspire a sense of humility and solemnity. Successful performance of this intrinsically sad ritual can bring closure, finality, and a sense of confidence in the totality of the doctor–patient relationship, attesting to a scope that encompasses the entirety of human existence. For this reason, physicians should attend to the essential elements of pronouncing death as well as avoidable pitfalls.

As with other aspects of clinical care, perhaps the most important strategy for arriving at accurate diagnoses and offering helpful recommendations to patients and families is to diligently gather evidence from available resources. On some occasions, the physician who pronounces death and certifies or determines the cause of death is the physician who is present in the final moments. Perhaps this person will be the patient's surgeon if the person dies in surgery or in the postoperative period. Perhaps this will be an on-call hospitalist or intensivist. Or perhaps it will be a first responder. In each of these circumstances, bearing witness to the final moments of a person's life imparts an element of first-person testimony to the pronouncement process.

To a family member, such testimony may make the death pronouncement more personal and meaningful. Many family members especially wonder if the dying patient suffered or showed signs of suffering in their final moments. And the physician who provides first-person testimony may be specially positioned to offer condolences and reassurance of a peaceful passing.

A common pitfall among pronouncing physicians is speculating about the causes of death to family members prior to gathering evidence. If the pronouncing physician was not present for the moment of death, then he or she will need to discuss those final moments with the physician or other clinicians who were present. It will be important to characterize relevant clinical history and circumstances and physiological changes. Signs of sepsis, cardiovascular decline, respiratory insufficiency, or changes in mental status will need to be documented, as will specific interventions in the last moments or days. Providers who were present for the changes in the patient's status or for relevant clinical interventions will need to be identified, including the bedside nurses, code team, family members, and other providers.

The pronouncing physician may need to speak with a patient's primary care physician, attending physician, oncologist, surgeon, or other specialist to obtain further evidence about the penultimate causes of the patient's death. If these providers are not available for consultation, then a careful review of the medical record will be essential. All of these efforts will help the pronouncing physician to develop accurate determination of and documentation of the causes of death, and they will enhance the physician's ability to accurately field questions from the patient's family.

16.5   LAST DAYS: DOCUMENTING AND DISCLOSING DEATH

Death assessment gives rise to two unique acts of communication, the written death note or summary and disclosure to the family and involved clinicians. Expectations for a note depend on the involvement of the pronouncing physician. If the physician witnessed the death or participated in the final clinical management, whether the scene involved a failed attempt at resuscitation or a successful delivery of comfort measures, then the written record will require a characterization of events including chronology and physiologic signs. The pronouncing physician should either verify that other clinicians who contributed to clinical management have personally documented their role or, alternatively, assume responsibility for documenting the other clinicians testimony including reference to the time of the clinical conversation.

The required elements of a death summary or death note include identification of the pronouncing physician, the process by which he or she came to be involved in the pronouncement, a brief statement on the causes of death, description of the signs of death, documentation of sources of clinically relevant information, and a record of family members and clinicians who have or who have not been notified. The essential elements of a death note are listed in Table 16.2.

One common source of confusion among physicians, especially those providing cross-coverage at night, is the role of the pronouncing physician in providing a death note that is also a death summary, or a note that includes a summary of the patient's admission and hospital course. Some cross-covering physicians will have the time, ability, and interest to offer a more robust death note that can function as a hospital summary. In that case, members of the primary team may later document their own assessment of the hospital course if they feel additional information is needed. When a cross-covering physician does not provide a clinical summary, the physician should confirm that another provider will do so. Hospitalist programs may anticipate confusion over documentation of clinical summaries and develop an agreed-upon protocol for ensuring communication and collaboration among cross-covering and attending physicians.

Table 16.2   Elements of a Death Note

Time and date of note

Name and ID of patient: confirm wristband or other patient identifier

Name and role of note writer

Process of involvement: "Called by patient's nurse at *time* after patient found unresponsive at *time*. Arrived to find patient unresponsive at *time*." Or "Patient found unresponsive at *time*, attempted resuscitation documented separately by myself or Dr. X at *time*, and *time* of death declared at *time*."

Physical exam indicating death has occurred:
   Unresponsive to voice or touch: painful stimuli are not indicated in this setting
   Fixed and dilated pupils
   Absent carotid pulse
   Absent respirations and radial pulse for 2 min using visual exam, stethoscope, and palpation
   Pale and waxy skin changes

Individuals present at the time of death including family and staff

Key family members or clinicians who have and have not yet been notified
   Whether circumstances of death warranted contacting ME
   Due to accident, trauma, suicide, homicide, violence, disaster, poisoning, or suspicious circumstances
   Patients who are in police custody, jail, or prison
   Deaths during surgery or anesthetic procedures
   Deaths associated with epidemic
   Unattended or unwitnessed death

Outcome of conversation with ME: if ME case, then autopsy will be arranged by ME and patient's nursing staff should be notified. If not an ME case, then full and limited autopsy should be offered to family. If family request autopsy, patient's nurse should be notified.

Clinical summary if possible: if a clinical summary is not provided, then the time and method of communication of the need to provide this summary to another provider should be referenced
   Family requests regarding handling of the body and remains

Obvious family psychosocial needs requiring further attention by a chaplain, social worker, or other providers

---

The second key act of communication involves disclosure to involved clinicians and the patient's family. Notifying the patient's outpatient and inpatient providers may require a tactful email, phone call, voicemail, or other missive. If these providers are inpatient consultants or members of the primary inpatient team, timely notification is essential as an act of professional courtesy and to permit those providers the opportunity to express condolences. Timely notification can also prevent embarrassment the next time the provider speaks with the family. Again, hospitalist programs may consider establishing institutional or team protocols for cross-cover communication, including easy access to attending and consulting physician contact information.

Taking the time to perform a delicate, respectful, and thorough physical exam in the presence of family is itself a ritualistic form of compassionate communication. Gravitas and complete attention to the task at hand can be therapeutic features of this encounter with patients' families. Asking the patient's charge nurse to help maintain a quiet environment on the clinical unit, and then turning off one's pager and cell phone, can set the stage for a respectful assessment and pronouncement.

Strategies for communication when pronouncing death should take into account whether the death is expected and welcome or unexpected and shocking. Unexpected deaths require careful attention to the environment in which the news is delivered. When possible, both the physician and family should be seated either in the patient's room or in another space that is unlikely to be interrupted by other families or hospital staff.

Pronouncing physicians should introduce themselves and their role in the plan of care including their relationship with the primary team, and they should clarify the names and relationships of family members. Out of respect for patient autonomy and privacy, the patient's medical power of attorney or surrogate decision-maker should be notified first and permission should be obtained before notifying other family members.

Many physicians worry about making mistakes or unintentionally offending a family member. The keys to an effective encounter are to maintain ordinary civility, to be patient, and to be attentive. Shaking hands with family members, when culturally appropriate, can be a kind gesture. Be sure to have adequate seating, tissues, and available support staff. A medically proficient interpreter for families who do not speak English or a spiritual provider when requested can make all of the difference for delivering news effectively. A "warning shot" such as "I want to share with you the results of my physical exam," "Your husband has been fighting bravely for some time—today something very serious happened to his heart," or simply "I'm afraid I have some bad news for you" will help the family make emotional preparations. A clear, simple, jargon-free statement that the patient has died should be made. It is acceptable to redescribe the patient's death as "passing" or "moving on" but at some point a concise statement indicating the patient's time of death will help avoid confusion.

A brief summary of clinical events leading to death ("We believe that he passed out due to sudden bleeding and swelling in the brain") and of the nature of death pronouncement ("I'm very sorry but I carefully checked your father's heartbeat for two min and confirmed that he died") may be helpful for families who are surprised by the news. When appropriate, reporting that the death was peaceful and without suffering or noting that the presence of family was meaningful may be reassuring to the family. A period of silence may occur in which case the physician should patiently wait to see what comments or questions emerge. There is no need to fill empty space with speech in an emotional moment. At the same time, empathic statements such as "I am so sorry for your loss" or "You love her so much—this must be so hard" may be comforting.

Many family members will experience acute grief and a series of intense emotions including anger, sadness, disbelief, and guilt. The physician should permit expressions of these feelings, even if family members focus on medical errors or complaints about the hospital or its staff. The physician should humbly reassure the family that questions or concerns about medical management will be answered as thoroughly and promptly as possible. Writing down specific questions and the family member's contact information will demonstrate a willingness to follow through. Questions about the patient's death and the events that follow in the hospital and beyond should be fielded calmly and plainly. It may be helpful to prepare the family for their grief by observing that waves of intense feelings are normal and that healthy grieving requires permitting oneself to experience these feelings while occasionally trusting others to listen and to help.

Occasionally, physicians will notify family members of a patient's death over the telephone. In this case, it is crucial that the family member not be driving a vehicle. It is also preferable if the family member is not alone. Thus, after identifying oneself and clarifying the identity of the family member, it may be appropriate to ask the family member to pull over or come directly and safely to the hospital. It is always best to deliver news in person. At the same time, withholding serious information can be stressful for both the physician and the family. It may be useful to report that the patient has "changed" or to say "I need to speak to you in person—when can you be here?" If the family member is unable to visit soon, then both parties should first confirm one another's location and contact information, and then full disclosure over the telephone will be appropriate. Some family members will want full disclosure and inquire about visiting the body. In this case a specific plan should be proposed and, if necessary, a clinician should be identified for family follow up. When death is expected as in the case of a comatose patient receiving comfort measures only, it will be helpful to clarify in advance whom to contact at night for such phone calls.

If the patient or family has not already expressed preferences related to organ donation, then the physician should expect some questions about this practice. Questions should be answered honestly, and further inquiry should be directed to the local organ procurement organization (OPO). In general, treating or pronouncing physicians should not initiate a conversation about organ donation because doing so can confuse the roles and goals of the physician. An alternative is to contact the local OPO and ask their representative to contact the family.

One of the more awkward moments in the conversations that follow from pronouncing death is the invitation to refer the patient for autopsy. If it is a medical examiner (ME) case, then the family should be informed that an autopsy is required. The family can speak with the ME's office directly for further questions. The physician should explain that autopsies are performed carefully and respectfully by medical professionals for the purpose of understanding the causes of death and illuminating the patient's medical condition.

If it is not an ME case, then a full or limited autopsy should be routinely offered. One strategy for broaching this topic is to offer, "I know it is painful to think about, but some people choose an autopsy because families need to know what happened or to know more about possible inherited conditions or because the patient had a sense of altruism or a spirit of scientific inquiry. Autopsies help doctors better understand how to diagnose and treat all sorts of medical conditions. Is this something you or your loved one would want?"

FURTHER READING

1. Auerbach AD, Pantilat SZ, End-of-life care in a voluntary hospitalist model: effects on communication, processes of care, and patient symptoms, *Am J Med* May 15, 2004;**116**(10):669–675.
2. Field MJ, Cassel CK, editors. *Approaching Death: Improving Care at the End of Life*. Washington, DC: National Academy Press, 1997.
3. LeGrand SB, Walsh D, Comfort measures: practical care of the dying cancer patient, *Am J Hosp Pall Med* 2010 Nov;**27**(7):488–493.
4. Morita T, Ichiki T, Tsunoda J, Inoue S, Chihara S, A prospective study on the dying process of terminally ill cancer patients, *Am J Hosp Palliat Care* 1998 July–Aug;**15**(4):217–222.
5. Wee BL, Coleman PG, Hiller R, The sound of death rattle II: how do relatives interpret the sound? *Palliat Med* 2006 Apr;**20**(3):177–181.

WEB RESOURCES

Online Resources for Hospitalists to Help Families Coping with Death and Dying

American Cancer Society		
End of life + handouts	http://www.cancer.org/treatment/ nearingtheendoflife/ nearingtheendoflife/index (accessed on 28 July, 2014)	Answers to common questions about end-of-life care for families
Financial coping with a loss handout	http://www.cancer.org/acs/groups/ content/@editorial/documents/ document/ copingfinanciallywiththelossof.pdf (accessed on 28 July, 2014)	Financial tips and pitfalls for families
Grief + handout	http://www.cancer.org/treatment/ treatmentsandsideeffects/ emotionalsideeffects/griefandloss/index (accessed on 28 July, 2014)	Focuses on grief experienced with the recent or impending loss of a loved one

Hospice care	http://www.cancer.org/treatment/ findingandpayingfortreatment/ choosingyourtreatmentteam/hospicecare/ index (accessed on 28 July, 2014)	Describes hospice care and the services they provide to patients and their families
FMLA	http://www.cancer.org/treatment/ findingandpayingfortreatment/ understandingfinancialandlegalmatters/ family-and-medical-leave-act (accessed on 28 July, 2014)	Answers to common questions about FMLA
Alzheimer's		
7 stages of Alzheimer's	http://www.alz.org/alzheimers_disease_ stages_of_alzheimers.asp (accessed on 28 July, 2014) http://www.alz.org/national/documents/ topicsheet_stages.pdf (accessed on 28 July, 2014)	What to expect in each stage of Alzheimer's, for families: handout and brochure
Late-stage caregiving	http://www.alz.org/care/alzheimers-late-end-stage-caregiving.asp (accessed on 28 July, 2014) http://www.alz.org/national/documents/ brochure_latestage.pdf (accessed on 28 July, 2014)	How to be a late-stage Alzheimer's caregiver: handout and brochure
VA		
Burial and memorial benefits	www.cem.va.gov (accessed on 28 July, 2014)	VA-specific burial information
Caregiver support	www.caregiver.va.gov (accessed on 28 July, 2014)	VA-specific caregiver support resource
Other Resources		
National Hospice and Palliative Care Organization	http://www.caringinfo.org/files/public/ brochures/ UnderstandingtheDyingProces.pdf (accessed on 28 July, 2014)	Physical signs of dying for families
FMLA	http://www.dol.gov/whd/fmla/index.htm (accessed on 28 July, 2014)	Official website for FMLA
Hospice education	http://www.hospicenet.org/ (accessed on 28 July, 2014) http://www.hospicenet.org/html/ caregivers.html (accessed on 28 July, 2014)	Accessible website about end-of-life care: explanation for hospice, resources/ links for caregivers
Grief	http://www.aarp.org/home-family/ caregiving/grief-and-loss/ (accessed on 28 July, 2014)	AARP website on grief and loss
"Five Wishes"	http://www.agingwithdignity.org/ five-wishes.php (accessed on 28 July, 2014)	A website describing the "Five Wishes" end-of-life conversation guide

"Hard Choices"/"Decisiones Dificiles?"	http://www.hnehealth.nsw.gov.au/__data/assets/pdf_file/0016/54250/HardChoices.pdf (accessed on 28 July, 2014) http://hankdunn.com/wp-content/uploads/2012/06/Hard_choices_5th_Edition_Spanish_sample.pdf (accessed on 28 July, 2014) http://hankdunn.com/purchase/book-titles/ (accessed on 28 July, 2014)	Comprehensive booklet on end-of-life care for families: English pdf file, sample Spanish pdf file, link to order from publisher
Handbook for Mortals	http://www.growthhouse.org/mortals/mor0.html (accessed on 28 July, 2014)	Link to online version of a classic, practical book on end-of-life care for caregivers
Society for Hospital Medicine comfort care order set	http://www.hospitalmedicine.org/sig/palliativecare/comfort care order set.pdf (accessed on 28 July, 2014)	Link to an example of comfort care order set

Chapter 17

Palliative Care after Discharge: Services for the Seriously Ill in the Home and Community

Amy M. Corcoran, Neha J. Darrah, and Nina R. O'Connor

17.1 INTRODUCTION

Hospitalized patients requiring palliative care after discharge have a variety of options to choose from. In order to match your patient/family needs with services, it is valuable to know the benefits and limitations of the various programs. Hospice is the most comprehensive and well-known postacute palliative care program, yet many programs are limited to patients preferring only comfort care with a prognosis of 6 months or less, which makes it less applicable to many seriously ill patients. Most other palliative care programs are devised to meet the needs of those with life-limiting illness in their community. Hospitalists are instrumental in initiating and facilitating palliative care referrals for patients postacute care discharge. Unfortunately, physicians often refer patients to palliative care and hospice too late in their disease course. The CARING criteria, a set of clinically relevant criteria with a high sensitivity and specificity for identifying patients with a high likelihood of mortality at 1 year, can help identify patients who would benefit from a palliative care approach. The criteria include primary cancer diagnosis, nursing home residence, greater than 2 admissions for chronic illness to the hospital in the past year, ICU admission with multisystem organ failure, and fulfillment of greater than >2 noncancer hospice guidelines [1]. Another way to frame thinking about prognosis is to ask yourself, "Is the patient sick enough that dying this year would not be a surprise?" [2]. Palliative care postdischarge should be considered for all patients who meet one of these criteria.

Hospital-Based Palliative Medicine: A Practical, Evidence-Based Approach, First Edition.
Edited by Steven Pantilat, Wendy Anderson, Matthew Gonzales, and Eric Widera.

17.2   HOSPICE

Hospice originated in England and the philosophy of providing holistic care to the dying spread to the United States roughly in the 1970s when Dr Florence Wald and others formed Hospice, Inc. of New Haven, Connecticut, the first hospice [3]. The National Hospice and Palliative Care Organization (NHPCO) defines hospice as "The model for quality compassionate care for people facing a life-limiting illness, hospice provides expert medical care, pain management, and emotional and spiritual support expressly tailored to the patient's needs and wishes. Support is provided to the patient's loved ones as well [4]." In the 1980s, the U.S. Congress passed the Medicare Hospice Benefit (MHB). Today, anyone who is eligible for Medicare Part A, has a prognosis of 6 months or less should their disease run a natural course as certified by two physicians (one referring physician and one hospice physician), and agrees with the hospice philosophy may enroll in MHB [5]. Table 17.1 highlights the

Table 17.1   Medicare Hospice Benefit Rights and Eligibility Requirements [5]

To qualify for hospice services under Medicare, patients must:	Be eligible for Medicare Part A Be certified as terminally ill by: 1. The patient's own physician 2. A physician from the hospice Defined as likely prognosis of 6 months or less if disease follows expected course Elect the Medicare Hospice Benefit Waive rights to Medicare payment for nonhospice services related to the terminal diagnosis Choose one hospice to coordinate and deliver all care
To provide care for patients under Medicare, hospices must:	Provide care that includes multiple members of the interdisciplinary team (physician, nurse, social worker, chaplain, pharmacist) Provide hospice aide services to include personal care and light housekeeping Provide medication related to pain and symptom management for the terminal diagnosis (at no cost to patient) Provide necessary medical equipment Provide bereavement counseling for 1 year following the patient's death Reassess each patient's eligibility for hospice after 90 days, 180 days, and every 60 days thereafter
While on hospice, patients are entitled to:	Choose their own attending physician or nurse practitioner and continue to see that provider for the terminal diagnosis Continue to receive nonhospice care for unrelated conditions Change hospices once per benefit period Revoke hospice at any time with resumption of regular Medicare benefits (must be done in writing)

MHB eligibility requirements. The MHB reimbursement structure is a per diem capitated structure under which the hospice receives a predetermined amount of money each day to provide all of the services necessary to care for the patient and family. While many private insurance companies also cover hospice care, most of these programs model their benefits after the MHB; therefore, we will focus on the MHB in this chapter.

Hospice care is provided by an interdisciplinary team at home, residential communities, nursing home communities, hospitals, and inpatient units. The hospice interdisciplinary team is made up of nurses, social workers, chaplains, physicians, bereavement specialists, nursing aides, and therapists who specialize in physical, occupational, or nutritional issues. Each discipline adds their unique expertise in caring for the patient and family. The hospice team meets at least every other week to discuss the plan of care for each patient and family. Hospice offers a 24/7 emergency contact number which is usually staffed by a nurse to assist with any symptom emergencies that may arise. Finally, one of the most important benefits is the 13-month postdeath bereavement support offered to the patient's family.

When patients elect hospice services, the hospice assumes responsibility for management of all care related to their terminal diagnosis. Patients waive their right to payment for nonhospice services related to this diagnosis though, as described in the following, patients can revoke the benefit at any time if their goals of care change. All testing and treatment is coordinated by the hospice and paid for by the hospice out of their per diem payment. As a result, testing is usually limited to simple tests that would change management of symptoms or enhance comfort. Because hospice programs receive a capitated payment for each patient they treat and focus these resources on support in the home or inpatient facility, treatment usually excludes expensive therapies like transfusions, chemotherapy, and radiation (but individual hospices may cover exceptions when clearly palliative in nature). Patients who opt for rehospitalization related to their terminal diagnosis must come off hospice so that the hospice is not financially responsible for the hospitalization. In contrast, hospice patients may continue to receive standard care for all diagnoses other than their terminal diagnosis. For example, a patient who elects hospice care for pancreatic cancer can be hospitalized and treated for a hip fracture or can continue to receive dialysis if it is unrelated to the hospice diagnosis [5, 6]. When questions arise around which patients may be eligible for hospice and what treatments they might be able to receive, we recommend speaking with the hospice agency's medical director. Many agencies provide treatments not traditionally provided by hospice on a case-by-case basis, and these experienced medical directors will provide advice about how hospice might be able to meet the patient's specific goals.

If their treatment goals change, patients can revoke hospice at any time. Their regular Medicare or insurance benefits then resume immediately. Patients can also reelect hospice services at any time, even if they have been on hospice in the past. While it is obviously not preferable to start and stop hospice, it can be reassuring to patients that election of hospice is not an irreversible decision.

17.2.1   Hospice Levels of Care

Four levels of care are offered under MHB (Table 17.2) [4–7]. The majority of patients receive hospice care at the routine level of care. This level of care is provided in the patient's home, assisted-living facility, or long-term care facility. The frequency of hospice staff visits depends upon the patient's clinical status and plan of care and may range from one registered nurse visit per week to daily contact from a home hospice aide plus multiple visits from the nurse, social worker, and chaplain. Families should not expect more than an hour or two of services, however; family or paid caregivers must provide any required care the rest of the time. Patients on routine level of care may be declining, but their symptoms can be managed in a home or nursing home setting.

For patients with symptoms that cannot be managed in the home or nursing home, hospice programs offer general inpatient level of care. This may be offered in a dedicated inpatient hospice center or through contracts with a hospital or nursing home. Patients at this level of care typically need frequent medication adjustments and titrations. The need for IV medications may also justify inpatient care. Inpatient hospice is not appropriate for patients with stable symptoms who lack the social support to go home; these patients should be placed in long-term care facility with hospice services. If an inpatient hospice patient's symptoms stabilize, that patient must be transitioned to routine level of care in a different setting.

Table 17.2   Hospice Levels of Care [4, 5]

Level of Care	Setting	Criteria	Duration of Care
Routine level of care	Home, assisted-living, long-term care, residential	Eligible for hospice based on prognosis <6 months, stable symptoms	Indefinite
General inpatient care	Hospice inpatient center, hospital, nursing home	Uncontrolled symptoms, need for frequent medication adjustments and/or IV medications, complex care that cannot be provided in any other setting	No limit but generally short term, 1 week or less
Respite care	Hospice inpatient center, nursing home	Need for caregiver rest	Up to 5 days at a time
Continuous home care	Home, assisted-living, residential	Uncontrolled symptoms, caregiver breakdown, crisis	Short term, typically 1–2 days

Respite level of care is offered as a benefit for caregivers. Hospice patients with stable symptoms can periodically receive up to 5 days of care in a nursing facility or hospice facility to allow for caregiver rest. This benefit can also be used if a hospice patient's caregiver is sick or needs to travel.

Finally, continuous home care is offered for brief periods of crisis (usually uncontrolled symptoms or caregiver breakdown) when a patient is either unable or unwilling to transfer to an inpatient setting. Hospice staff stays in the patient's home with at least half the time covered by a registered nurse or licensed practical nurse. The remaining time may be provided by a hospice aide. Hospices may not always have available staff to provide continuous home care on short notice.

Hospices receive different per diem payments based on the level of care provided. Since general inpatient level of care is paid at a significantly higher per diem than routine level of care, there is increasing regulatory scrutiny to ensure that inpatient care is justified [8].

17.2.2   Hospice for Those Residing in Nursing Homes

The nursing home provides 24h room and board, personal care, and nursing care, while hospice provides interdisciplinary symptom management and emotional and spiritual support and covers cost of terminal illness. MHB is provided under routine level of care to those residing in nursing homes. The room and board is paid for by the patient, family, charity, or Medicaid in some states. This model requires exquisite collaboration between the interdisciplinary teams via a systematic communication approach, knowledge of nursing home regulatory environment, and shared care planning [9, 10].

17.2.3   Hospice for Specific Diagnoses

Hospice was originally developed for cancer diagnoses in which prognostication is generally predictable. Hospice is now widely accepted for noncancer diagnoses, but prognostication in these chronic illnesses can be much more challenging. Specific eligibility guidelines have been developed by Local Coverage Determination (LCD) Medicare intermediaries for noncancer diagnoses which may vary by region. These are truly meant as guidelines and do not replace the clinician's judgment regarding prognosis of 6 months or less. Because it is difficult for many clinicians to say with certainty that a patient will die within 6 months, we often recommend patients be considered for hospice if their clinicians "would not be surprised" by the patient's death within the next 6 months.

Chronic obstructive pulmonary disease (COPD) and congestive heart failure (CHF) are chronic illnesses characterized by slow decline punctuated by exacerbations. It can be difficult to determine during an exacerbation whether a patient will return to their previous level of functioning. Guidelines exist to help clinicians identify which patients should be considered for hospice (Table 17.3). Caution must be exercised with these specific diagnoses due to the difficulty in prognostication.

Table 17.3 Hospice Care for Patients with COPD and CHF [11–14]

	COPD	CHF
Criteria to support hospice referral[a]	• Disabling dyspnea at rest • Poor response to bronchodilators • Decreased functional capacity • FEV1 < 30% • Increased office visits, ER visits, and hospitalizations • $pO_2 < 55$ mm Hg or O_2 sat <88% at rest • $pCO_2 > 50$ mm Hg	• NYHA Class IV symptoms (i.e., dyspnea at rest) • Symptoms despite optimal medical regimen • Ejection fraction ≤20% • Treatment resistant dysrhythmias • History of cardiac-related syncope or cardiac arrest
Medications to continue on hospice as long as tolerated	• Inhaled steroids[b] • Inhaled beta-agonists[b] • Inhaled anticholinergics[b] • Oral steroids	• Diuretics • Oral potassium • Beta-blockers[c] • ACE inhibitors[c] • Nitrates[c]
Medications to consider discontinuing	• Inhalers once patient lacks respiratory strength to use; substitute nebulized forms • Theophylline[b]	• Statins • Amiodarone[d] • Aspirin
Medications to consider adding	• Opioid for dyspnea • Benzodiazepine for anxiety	• Opioid for dyspnea • Benzodiazepine for anxiety

[a]Eligibility ultimately depends upon the clinician's judgment about prognosis and may take into account comorbid conditions. Patients are not required to meet all the above criteria.
[b]Hospices vary in their ability to provide costly, brand-name inhalers. Some hospices will substitute shorter-acting or nebulized medications.
[c]May eventually discontinue due to hypotension.
[d]Consider toxicity versus benefit for symptoms.

In addition, many of the medications used to treat COPD and CHF should be continued after referral to hospice in light of their palliative as well as curative effects (Table 17.3).

Another slowly progressive, life-limiting illness is the neurodegenerative diseases, especially Alzheimer's disease. The challenge to care for those with end-stage dementia and to properly prognosticate has been a focus of research over the past decade. Currently, the Centers for Medicare and Medicaid Services (CMS) utilizes the FAST tool [15] as a guideline for prognostication and looks for those with end-stage dementia who are specifically bedbound with additional weight loss, skin breakdown, progressive dysphagia, and/or recurrent infections. A hospitalization may trigger a discussion regarding hospice. When families are facing progressive dysphagia that is leading to recurrent aspiration pneumonia and weight loss with comfort feeding as the primary goal, hospice may be most appropriate.

17.2.4   Discharging a Patient to Hospice

Discharge from the hospital can be a vulnerable time for patients. This is particularly true for patients being discharged to hospice. One strategy for ensuring a safe discharge is the use of a standardized discharge checklist. In 2005, the Society of Hospital Medicine's Hospital Quality and Patient Safety Committee developed a discharge checklist for the older adult which provided guidance on medication education, effective discharge summary writing, patient instructions, providers, follow-up plan, medication list, and resuscitation status [16]. This checklist can be modified for patients being discharged to hospice (Table 17.4). Three special considerations for patients being discharged to hospice include identifying the patient's hospice attending, performing thorough medication reconciliations, and determining self-care responsibilities.

When patients enroll in hospice, two physicians must certify that the patient has a life expectancy of 6 months or less if the illness runs its normal course. One of these physicians is generally the hospice medical director, while the other is the patient's referring physician and can include but is not limited to a primary care physician, oncologist, and so on. For patients without regular medical care, it is feasible that the hospitalist will be the second physician certifying the patient for hospice. In all of these cases, the hospitalist should coordinate with the patients' other providers and communicate with the hospice medical director about who will be the patient's

Table 17.4   Checklist for Hospice Discharge

Checklist Elements	Hospice
Discharge medications	• Written schedule of medications with reason for all medications • Clear instructions about which medications have been discontinued and which medications have been started • Clear instruction for all pain medications • Confirmation with hospice formulary that discharge medications are covered • If possible, sign for the hospice emergency kit prior to discharge
Home care needs	• Determination of home care needs prior to discharge • Durable medical equipment delivered to the home prior to discharge • Home health aide information if patient needs 24 h supervision
End of life	• Include all goals of care discussions conducted with the patient and family in the discharge summary • Communicate with outpatient providers regarding discussion
Providers	Identify receiving and referring physicians: • Identify in discharge summary • Contact them and identify immediate follow-up issues • Ask outpatient provider if they would like to be attending of record while patient is on hospice

attending once they are enrolled in hospice. The responsibilities for the attending include determining the patient's initial plan of care, renewing prescriptions, and recertifying the patient's eligibility for hospice at the end of each benefit period with a face-to-face encounter. If the patient's referring physician does not want to perform these duties, this should be communicated to the hospice medical director so that he/she can take on these responsibilities.

The second consideration is medication changes. Although performing medication reconciliations prior to discharge is important for all patients, this is particularly true for patients being discharged to hospice. A discharge to hospice often means significant medication changes with chronic medications being discontinued and new medications being initiated for symptom management. Prior to discharge, the hospitalist should meet with the patient and family to determine which chronic medications should be discontinued. Medications to consider discontinuing include those that do not improve the patient's comfort such as aspirin or statins for primary prevention. Patient's symptoms should be assessed prior to discharge including anxiety, pain, dyspnea, and constipation and medications should be initiated to control these symptoms. If the patient's symptoms remain uncontrolled despite inpatient management or require frequent intravenous medications, inpatient hospice should be considered.

Once discharged, most patients will receive their medications from the hospice pharmacy. Because hospices receive a limited amount of money per day to provide care for each patient, hospice formularies have a restricted number of medications that they are able to provide to their patients. Common examples of medications that most formularies do not provide include low molecular weight heparin, donepezil, or ondansetron. Prior to discharge, the hospitalist should review the hospice formulary to ensure that all discharge medications are included on the formulary. On a more practical note, the discharge needs to include prescriptions to hold the patient over until he/she is actually enrolled in hospice and evaluated by the hospice nurse. In addition, the hospice emergency kit provided to most patients includes valuable medications for symptom management (see Table 17.5).

Finally, discharge to hospice may also mean increased self-care responsibilities for the patient as the patient may be sicker on discharge. For patients being discharged home on hospice, hospitalists should determine the patient's self-care

Table 17.5 Typical Hospice Emergency Kit Medications

Medication	Initial Dose	Symptom
Acetaminophen suppository 650 mg (6 tablets)	650 mg	Pain, fever
Haloperidol 2 mg/ml oral concentration (15 ml)	1 mg/0.5 ml	Agitation
Atropine 1% ophthalmic drops (2 ml)	2 drops	Secretions
Morphine sulfate 20 mg/ml (15 ml, needs CII prescription)	5 mg/0.25 ml	Pain, shortness of breath
Prochlorperazine 10 mg (6 tablets)	10 mg	Nausea, vomiting
Bisacodyl 10 mg suppository (2 tablets)	10 mg	Constipation

responsibilities and home needs prior to discharge. Physical and occupational therapists are excellent resources to determine home care needs. Important questions to consider include how many stairs a patient's home has, whether there is a bathroom on the first floor, and how many hours of supervision a patient will need. For patients who cannot climb stairs to the second floor, hospice should be notified so that they can have a hospital bed and commode set up on the first floor on discharge. Patients will also have a full assessment by a hospice nurse within 24 h of discharge to determine other unanticipated home needs.

The number of hours of supervision a patient needs is an important consideration that needs to be addressed to ensure a safe transition. Although hospice provides 24/7 nursing support via phone, it cannot provide continuous care for patients on home hospice. Per the MHB, "The care and services described … may be provided on a 24-h, continuous basis *only* during periods of crisis [6]." If a patient requires 24 h supervision, it should be made explicitly clear to the patient and family that hospice cannot provide this service. Options for the family include setting up a care schedule among family and friends, hiring a home health aide, or considering discharge to a long-term care facility. On average, home health aides cost $21/h, which amounts to $500/day [17]. This cost can be prohibitive for the patient and family, and therefore, other arrangements need to be made prior to discharge.

17.3 PALLIATIVE CARE

For patients with a life-altering diagnosis not interested in or eligible for hospice, discharge to palliative care is a reasonable option. A comparison of palliative and hospice services is provided in Table 17.6. Patients may choose palliative care instead of hospice if they are still interested in receiving palliative treatment related to their terminal diagnosis that is not covered by their hospice benefit such as continuous milrinone or palliative radiation. Patients may also choose a palliative care discharge if they want to pursue life-prolonging therapies such as palliative chemotherapy.

Table 17.6 Comparison of Hospice and Palliative Care

	Hospice	Palliative Care
Eligibility	Medicare A eligible Prognosis of 6 months or less	Life-limiting illness
Philosophy	Holistic noncurative care	Care focused on quality of life, pain, and symptom management
Services	Interdisciplinary team Care coordination 24/7 on-call support Bereavement services for 13 months post death	Offer more expensive palliative measure concurrent with symptom management

17.3.1 Palliative Sites of Care

There are various options for patients being discharged to palliative care programs. The first option we will discuss is outpatient palliative care clinic. These clinics are excellent options for patients with a life-altering diagnosis who are willing to travel to outpatient appointments. Palliative care clinics offer symptom management and emotional support to patients and their families facing a chronic or life-threatening illness. Studies have shown that early initiation of palliative care, even while patients are receiving life-prolonging therapies, can lead to significant improvements in patient's quality of life and mood [18]. When making appointments for outpatient palliative care clinics, hospitalists should make every attempt to coordinate all postdischarge follow-up appointments for the same day.

Nursing homes may offer a variety of palliative care services as well. Some partner with a hospice provider who is able to provide palliative care consultative services. Other nursing homes may have a "homegrown" program comprising an interdisciplinary team or nurse practitioner who focuses on the palliative care needs of the residents [19].

For patients with a high symptom burden that cannot be managed at home, admission to an inpatient palliative care unit may be an option. Patients with life-altering diagnoses, particularly advanced cancer, have a number of devastating physical and psychosocial symptoms that require active symptom management and comprehensive interdisciplinary care. If these patients are ineligible for hospice or still interested in pursuing life-prolonging therapies, inpatient palliative care units should be considered. It should be noted that inpatient palliative care units may not be available in all areas.

Finally, patients with home care needs can receive palliative care at home via 'bridge' programs or demonstration projects. These so-called "bridge" programs are intended for patients who are homebound requiring palliative care. These are often reimbursed through home care since patients usually have a skilled nursing need such as wound care, tube feedings, or rehabilitation. While on bridge programs, patients can continue to receive treatment for their life-limiting diagnosis such as palliative chemotherapy or radiation; however, they also receive special attention to symptom management with a focus on goals of care. One such example is the Penn Home Care and Hospice Program called Caring Way. The Caring Way program offers home palliative care services to those with life-limiting illness. The Caring Way patients are discussed every other week at the hospice team meetings, nursing staff are all hospice certified and additional social work or chaplain support is available. The program requires a skilled need since the payment mechanism is through home care services. A more recent demonstration example is Comprehensive Longitudinal Advanced Illness Management (CLAIM) which is funded by a CMS Healthcare Innovations Award. The CLAIM Program offers comprehensive home care services to those with advanced cancer receiving skilled home care and having essential palliative care needs but who are not yet eligible for hospice [20].

17.3.2 Discharging a Patient to Palliative Care

For all patients being discharged to palliative care, the hospital team should ideally have a family meeting prior to discharge to establish goals of care. Important issues to discuss during family meetings include resuscitation status and pertinent end-of-life issues such as intubation, future hospitalizations, ICU transfers, and artificial feeding. During the family meeting, it is also important to determine who will be the patient's health-care proxy. If there is no next of kin or the patient has identified someone other than the next of kin such as an ex-wife or friend as their health-care proxy, the patient should be encouraged to sign durable medical power of attorney paperwork. Social work can help patients with this paperwork.

The results of all family meetings and advanced care planning discussions should be communicated to the patient's outpatient providers and explicitly documented in the discharge summary. In addition to the discharge summary, options for documenting patients' end-of-life preferences include advanced directives, out-of-hospital do-not-resuscitate (DNR) forms, and physician orders for life-sustaining treatments (POLST) [21]. Advanced directives allow patients to spell out decisions about end-of-life care, such as resuscitation, intubation, tube feedings, dialysis, if they were permanently unconscious or dying and to appoint a legal health-care representative. All patients, especially those with life-altering diagnoses, should be encouraged to have advanced directives.

In some states, POLST may also be an option for seriously ill patients for whom their physicians would not be surprised if they died in the next year. POLST is not intended to replace an advanced directive but rather to complement it. POLST translates treatment preferences into medical orders, including cardiopulmonary resuscitation, artificial nutrition and in some states antibiotic use and can help guide the actions of emergency medical personnel when available. It is important to know your state laws regarding POLST. POLST programs exist or are in development in 34 states.

Another option may be an out-of-hospital DNR form. This may be required if the patient is being transported to hospice or a long-term care facility via a private ambulance company. Like the POLST, it can guide the actions of emergency medical personnel. As of 2002, it was available in 42 states.

17.4 CONCLUSION

Hospitalists are often on the front line in discharging patients to hospice and palliative care. Discharge to hospice and palliative care posthospitalization offers patients with life-limiting diagnoses access to interdisciplinary team care and excellent symptom management. Additional resources can be found in Table 17.7 to meet the needs of patients who are eligible to receive care in a wide array of settings depending on their goals of care. Hospice services should be considered for all patients with a life-limiting diagnosis interested in shifting their focus to comfort care, while palliative care should be offered to patients pursuing life-prolonging therapies.

Table 17.7 Web Resources and Applications

Web Resources

National Hospice and Palliative Care Organization—http://www.nhpco.org/

American Academy of Hospice and Palliative Medicine—http://www.aahpm.org/

Center for Medicare and Medicaid—http://www.cms.gov/Medicare/Medicare-Fee-for-Service-Payment/Hospice/index.html?redirect=/hospice/

Medicare Home Healthcare Compare—http://www.medicare.gov/homehealthcompare/search.html

POLST

www.polst.org

Applications

PalliMed

REFERENCES

1. Fischer SM, Gozansky WS, Sauaia A, Min SJ, Kutner JS, Kramer A, A practical tool to identify patients who may benefit from a palliative approach: the CARING criteria, *J Pain Symptom Manage* 2006;**31**(4):285–292.
2. Lynn J, Perspectives on care at the close of life. Serving patients who may die soon and their families: the role of hospice and other services, *JAMA* 2001;**285**(7):925–932.
3. Wald FS, Hospice care in the United States: a conversation with Florence S. Wald. Interview by M. J. Friedrich, *JAMA* 1999 May 12;**281**(18):1683–1685.
4. National Hospice and Palliative Care Organization. *NHPCO Facts and Figures: Hospice Care in America.*2011 Edition. 2012. Available at http://www.nhpco.org/sites/default/files/public/Statistics_Research/2011_Facts_Figures.pdf. Accessed on August 26, 2014.
5. Centers for Medicare and Medicaid. Medicare Benefit Policy Manual Chapter 9—Coverage of Hospice Services Under Hospital Insurance. 2012. Available at http://www.cms.gov/Regulations-and-Guidance/Guidance/Manuals/Downloads/bp102c09.pdf. Accessed on August 26, 2014.
6. Centers for Medicare and Medicaid Services. Payment System Fact Sheet: Hospice Payment System, 2012. Available at: http://www.cms.gov/Outreach-and-Education/Medicare-Learning-Network-MLN/MLNProducts/downloads/hospice_pay_sys_fs.pdf. Accessed on November 30, 2013.
7. Hospice Association of America. Hospice Facts & Statistics, February 2007. Available at http://www.nahc.org/haa/2007HospiceFactsStatistics.pdf. Accessed on November 10, 2007.
8. Department of Health and Human Services: Office of the Inspector General. *Medicare Hospice Care for Beneficiaries in Nursing Facilities: Compliance with Medicare Coverage Requirements.* 2009; September (OEI-02-06-00221). Available at http://oig.hhs.gov/oei/reports/oei-02-06-00221.pdf. Accessed on August 26, 2014.
9. Miller SC, Nursing Home/Hospice Partnerships: A Model for Collaborative Success–Through Collaborative Solutions, 2007; A Robert Wood Johnson Funded Project. Available at http://www.cms.gov/Regulations-and-Guidance/Guidance/Manuals/Downloads/bp102c09.pdf. Accessed on August 26, 2014.
10. Miller SC, Teno JM, Mor V, Hospice and palliative care in nursing homes, *Clin Geriatr Med* 2004 Nov;**20**(4):717–734, vii.
11. White P, White S, Edmonds P, et al. Palliative care of end-of-life care in advanced chronic obstruction pulmonary disease: a prospective community survey. *Br J Gen Pract* 2011;**61**:e362–e370.
12. Perley M, Dahlin C, *Core Curriculum for the Advanced Practice Hospice and Palliative Nurse.* Dubuque: Kendall Hunt, 2007.
13. Hunt SA, Baker DW, Chin MD, et al., ACC/AHA guidelines for the evaluation and management of chronic heart failure in the adult: executive summary, *Circulation* 2001;**104**:2996–3007.

14. Johnson MJ, Booth C, Palliative and end-of-life care for patients with chronic heart failure and chronic lung disease. *Clin Med* 2010;**10**:286–289.
15. Luchins DJ, Hanrahan P, Murphy K, Criteria for enrolling dementia patients in hospice. *J Am Geriatr Soc* 1997;**45**:1054–1059.
16. Halasyamani L, Kripalani S, Coleman E, et al., Transition of care for hospitalized elderly patients—development of a discharge checklist for hospitalists, *J Hosp Med* 2006;**1**(6):354–360.
17. Massachusetts Mutual Life Insurance Company. United States Home Health Aide Costs 2012. Available at https://www.massmutual.com/mmfg/pdf/Home_Health_Aide_Costs.pdfb. Accessed on August 26, 2014.
18. Temel JS, Greer JA, Muzikansky A, et al., Early palliative care for patients with metastatic non–small-cell lung cancer, *NEJM* 2010;**363**(8):733–742.
19. Carlson MD, Lim B, Meier DE, Strategies and innovative models for delivering palliative care in nursing homes, *J Am Med Dir Assoc* 2011;**12**(2):91–98.
20. Penn Medicine. University of Pennsylvania Health System Receives Two National Health Care Innovation Awards. June 18, 2012. Available at http://www.uphs.upenn.edu/news/News_Releases/2012/06/cms/. Accessed October 10, 2013.
21. Schmidt TA, Hickman SE, Tolle SW. Honoring treatment preferences near the end of life: the Oregon physician orders for life-sustaining treatment (POLST) program. *Adv Exp Med Biol* 2004;**550**:255–262.

Chapter 18

Interdisciplinary Team Care of Seriously Ill Hospitalized Patients

Dawn M. Gross and Jane Hawgood

The practice of palliative care is in its very nature multidisciplinary. It requires the expertise of multiple disciplines working together in a highly functioning team in order to accomplish the goal of providing an extra layer of support for those patients and families coping with a life-altering illness. Teams are essential to the successful implementation of both generalist palliative care, which is provided by all clinicians in the hospital, and specialist palliative care.

At the heart of any high-functioning team are shared core values and mission. In this review, we will define and expand upon the core values of teamwork and then create a foundation which any healthcare professional may use to assess their current team's level of functionality. We will also describe the contributions of different disciplines and describe how teams can leverage each discipline to work best together.

18.1 DEFINITION OF A TEAM

So what makes a team a team? Anytime you are working with one or more people focused on achieving a specific result, you are working in the context of a team. In healthcare, generally, it is the rule for providers to be working within a team. In fact, it may even be impossible for providers to find oneself alone, except for in isolated moments of silent reflection. In many settings, teams are created without intentionality, and teamwork just "happens." This lack of deliberate formation of a team often leads to lost opportunities for transformative collaboration. Recognition and definition of a team, its purpose, and the roles within it harness the full potential of professional, multidisciplinary collaboration.

Hospital-Based Palliative Medicine: A Practical, Evidence-Based Approach, First Edition.
Edited by Steven Pantilat, Wendy Anderson, Matthew Gonzales, and Eric Widera.
© 2015 John Wiley & Sons, Inc. Published 2015 by John Wiley & Sons, Inc.

18.2   CORE VALUES

Part of recognition and definition of a team is the intentional aligning of values. We represent the core values essential to a high-functioning team with the acronym TEAM:

Trust

Expertise

Agility

Multiplicity

18.2.1   Trust

Fundamental to building a team is the quality of trust. Everyone on a team must be able to trust and be trusted by each member. This trust is not based on a resume of documented skills, though a track record of productivity is supportive of garnering a basis for trust. What cultivates trust among team members is the consistency of communication and action that forward the agreed-upon common goal. If you are playing on a football team, the quarterback has to trust the receiver to catch the ball or he will never release it. Likewise, the receiver has to move into position and trust the quarterback to make the throw. The consequences of any team member not trust-ing the others to play their positions to the best of their ability will result in a failed play. In other words, trust creates the foundation of team interdependence, which is the basis of its functionality. If one team member says one thing but does another, trust will be jeopardized, and the interdependence of the team is lost. Trust is not granted in a moment but can be lost in one. It is important to constantly monitor one's own behavior and its impact on other team members. By definition, when working in the context of a team, no singular action is isolated; everything one does will have a ripple effect on each of the team members.

18.2.2   Expertise

Having team members with a variety of areas of expertise deepens and broadens the overall perspective and insight of the team. Yet breadth of expertise is advantageous only to the extent that communication within a team facilitates equal expression by all members [1]. Respect for each member's role as integral and unique is essential. Open communication allows the nuanced expertise of every member to help shape the efforts of the team.

A high-functioning team will have the value of continually educating oneself. This is not only so that each member's expert skill set is continually enhanced, but also so that each member understands and appreciates the cross-disciplinary exper-tise of the others. The expectation is that new lessons learned are shared with other team members. Each professional discipline has its own culture, set of values, and ways of framing information [2]. Cross-disciplinary communication can empower cross-disciplinary insight into each other's approach. A high-functioning team has members who are essentially multilingual and can communicate confidently and capably in the language of each other's disciplines.

Changing sport analogies to the game of baseball, sometimes the nuanced input from another player is what allows the strength of another to flourish. When supporting a pitcher who might be struggling during a game, often the catcher will approach the mound to offer insight that the pitcher cannot see.

18.2.3   Agility

In addition to being an expert in their individual roles, team members must also be sufficiently able to "pinch hit" for each other. How the team engages both internally and externally with patients, families, and other providers, requires flexibility and agility. Team members must be nimble, able to recognize when more action is required of them, even if it stretches beyond the boundary of their professional skill set. The interdisciplinary expertise of the team enables and empowers team members to step up for each other when needed. Team members who are empowered by and trusting in the interdependence of the team will hold themselves accountable when such circumstances arise. Thinking in terms of our sport analogies, zone defenses don't always work and fly balls drift unexpectedly. If each player stayed in their "designated" zones, tackles would be missed and balls dropped. Areas of overlap when appreciated, trusted, and empowered become areas of strength, not redundancy. For example, a social worker, well versed in the process of receiving a request for a new consult, including obtaining relevant medical details to assist with triaging cases, can empower the team to take on other responsibilities or even activities of self-care that might not otherwise be possible. Similarly, physicians can be educated in the key community support services that can be considered when exploring discharge options for complex family care scenarios.

18.2.4   Multiplicity

While "the more, the merrier" may not always hold true, having a variety of skills and perspectives to draw upon is highly advantageous in the complex environment of healthcare. Multiplicity of team members allows for a 360 degree view surrounding the patient and family. It also provides opportunity for the creation of interrelated support systems to meet these needs. Having multiple faces and multiple personalities with which a family may interact broadens the potential scope of communication. Multiplicity of a team also highlights the need for adequate resources. Multiplicity enables a team's agility and interdependence, and enables team members to build trust with each other. While it is difficult to play baseball with fewer than nine players on the field, the optimum number of people on a palliative care team has many variables. Matching multiplicity to the need within a healthcare context is not just a function of numbers; it is a function of the efficacy of teamwork. In the next section, we elaborate on the specific and essential roles within a palliative care team.

18.3   KEY TEAM MEMBERS FOR PALLIATIVE CARE

The specific team members can be variable, but often aim to model themselves after the Medicare-mandated hospice format comprised of the following: physician, nurse, social worker, and chaplain. This team composition is supported by many national organizations and should be leveraged at both the level of specialist palliative care and hospitalist working to provide generalist palliative care [3, 4]. Although volunteers are required to be part of a Medicare-certified hospice program, they are yet to become mainstream in most palliative care programs.

Though most hospitals with 300 or more beds have formal palliative care teams, their composition is far from uniform [5, 6]. Research is still needed to determine what composition of team members in which situations offers the most effective service. What is clear is that a formal palliative care service harnesses the advantages of multiple disciplines. In hospitals where no formal palliative care team is available, we suggest leveraging the following disciplines.

18.3.1   Physician

Captured within the Hippocratic Oath, the focus of medical training is to acquire the skills of diagnosis and treatment with the expectation of teaching this art and science as integral to its practice. For patients who would benefit from palliative care support, the first and foremost responsibility of the physician is to provide high-quality symptom management. Conversations about goals of care, advance care or discharge planning are severely constrained if a patient is experiencing any poorly controlled symptom. If trained palliative medicine practitioners are not available to aid with symptom management, consideration should be given to consultation of other subspecialists. For example, patients with intractable nausea with cancer may benefit from a consultation with a local oncologist and/or gastroenterologist. Physicians are also responsible for providing insight into disease trajectory and prognosis. Working with other physician specialists can help team members expand their own knowledge and forward implementation of care plans.

18.3.2   Nurse

A common description of the art and science of nursing is "the use of clinical judgment in the provision of care to enable people to improve, maintain or recover health, to cope with health problems, and to achieve the best possible quality of life, whatever their disease or disability, until death" [7]. Universally, nurses have the most direct patient contact and therefore offer the greatest insight into symptom triggers and intervention effectiveness [8]. Similarly, the nurse may have a unique trust relationship with the patient and an experience of family dynamics over time. In particular, nurses who introduce the concept of palliative care to patients in a skilled way, matched to the particular needs of the patient and family, may facilitate entry of other members of the team.

18.3.3 Social Worker

Medical social workers are dedicated to empowering patients and families to identify their strengths in an effort to find creative solutions needed to meet their individual and communal needs along the dynamic continuum of an illness. The relationship with patient and families is the most important tool for a social worker. In addition to being able to provide frontline psychosocial needs assessment, the social worker plays a key role in facilitating communication between patients, families, and their extended support groups. Medical social workers have an expertise in understanding the unique communities and cultural dynamics that families are a part of and will return to after discharge. Collaboration with a social worker enables optimal discharge plan implementation for the patient and family as well as the healthcare system.

18.3.4 Chaplain

Spiritual care focuses on helping patients to define and cultivate meaning in their lives. The chaplain explores any spiritual sources of pain, anxiety, and anticipatory grief and encourages spiritual expression as a way to access internal strength and sources of healing for the patient and family members. Chaplains also model and support self-care practices for team members, promoting team sustainability and functioning. The chaplain who works on a palliative care team takes primary responsibility for assessing and addressing the emotional, relational, spiritual, and existential needs and concerns of patients and families. Typical assessment domains include hopes and fears, meaning and purpose, guilt and forgiveness, beliefs about death and dying, life review and life completion tasks, and suffering, as any of these can challenge a sense of peace, worth, and wholeness. Chaplains also identify and explore spiritual and religious beliefs that can affect decision making or treatment plans. Sources of strength and coping resources are affirmed; sources of distress are identified and addressed. Support for those in caregiving roles is also provided, as well as bereavement support as needed. Chaplains also provide culturally sensitive rituals, blessing prayers, and memorials as requested.

18.4 ADDITIONAL AD HOC TEAM MEMBERS

18.4.1 Case Managers/Discharge Planner

Background training in nursing provides the case manager with core knowledge to understand the complexities of disease trajectory and medical care coordination including treatment needs, medication use, and durable medical equipment requirements. This places them in a unique position to collaborate with team members in their effort to access community resources and discover the best fit for patient and family needs, both acutely and over time.

18.4.2   Outpatient Providers

Primary care providers as well as outpatient clinicians with ongoing longitudinal relationships (e.g., oncologist, pulmonologist, cardiologist, etc.) provide continuity of care and understanding of patient values over time. Their input can be invaluable if the patient should be unable to speak for themselves. In particular, these providers can be helpful when multiple members of the family have differing perspectives of the patient's wishes.

18.4.3   Allied Health Professionals

These providers give professional insight into a patient's functional status and ability to perform both activities of daily living and executive functions. Involving them in palliative care assessment and planning facilitates a patient-centered plan of care. For example, a physical therapist who understands that the goal of care for a patient is to improve mobility at home while receiving hospice care would be able to participate in constructing a more comprehensive home-based plan for the patient, as opposed to recommending a short-term nursing facility stay for strengthening. Similarly, mental health professionals can provide expertise in coping with serious illness and the anxiety and depression that can accompany such life-altering diagnoses.

18.4.4   Insurers

Although not typically thought of as part of the hospital-based team, insurance providers can be allies in crafting continuity of care in home-care settings. In particular, hospital-based providers may be able, with the aid of local insurers, to create systems or programs that help transition hospitalized patients with complex needs to their preferred setting of choice, such as home, by carving out particular benefits that allow for optimal care outside the acute care setting.

18.5   BECOMING A HIGH-FUNCTIONING TEAM

How does a team leader facilitate team functioning among these various professionals? In this section, we will elaborate on methods for establishing and cultivating the four qualities of a high-functioning team. These strategies may be particularly useful for clinicians interested in forming and growing new palliative care teams:

1. *Give the team a name or special designation.* This creates a natural focus with which team members can identify. It also facilitates external recognition of the team in the healthcare context and by patients and families. Having explicit titles is effective at establishing identity.
2. *Create a mission statement.* Often, when important values are clearly articulated or written, it empowers team members to focus their attention as well as

those of their colleagues on the agreed-upon tasks at hand. Having a carefully thought-out mission statement also provides team members with language to explain to others across the healthcare spectrum, and to patients, what their role is. Explanations of palliative care to patients, families, and even those external to the healthcare context should be easy and clear. Taking time in a staff meeting to role play ways of communicating the mission statement of the team to others can be very helpful.

3. *Assess the team's functioning.* Evaluate the team's strengths and weaknesses. Identify where gaps in knowledge or capacity exist and the resources available to fill them. Evaluate individual interests and strengths, and align tasks with them [9]. This, naturally, not only improves functionality and performance but also increases confidence of the individual, allowing the interdependence and trust of the team to strengthen. Team members are empowered to take on new roles and challenge themselves for the benefit of the team. Taking time to evaluate the team at regular intervals should be a function of the team leader.

4. *Provide space for communication, and listen deeply with compassion.* Having a culture of open communication within a multidisciplinary team not only accesses the breadth of expertise within the team but also unearths the depth of the issues that may arise within a team. Discovering the areas that need attention is far more important than devising solutions quickly. Albert Einstein's wise commentary on problem solving, "90% understanding it and 10% finding a solution," points to a common value of all palliative care teams: allowing a story to unfold over time. This culture, essential to the provision of palliative care, is also essential within the palliative care team. Having both designated space and time to hold conversations and also an informal culture of open communication is essential to the team [10].

18.6   CONFLICT RESOLUTION

Inherent in any team setting is the likelihood of conflict and dysfunction. For any team to continue to develop and remain high functioning, ongoing effort to identify, refine, and overcome challenges is necessary.

In his book, *The Five Dysfunctions of a Team*, Peter Lencioni offers insight into team dynamics and concretely identifies the most common stumbling blocks (Table 18.1) [11]. Whereas the manuscript was initially written for the business sector, the concepts are directly applicable to both formal and informal healthcare teams. These dysfunctions often build upon one another; therefore, a careful assessment is necessary to identify the best place to start improvement work. The author suggests mechanisms for assessment and interventions to address each area of improvement. For example, teams struggling with a lack of trust often benefit from the addition of 360 degree feedback or personality preference profiles. These exercises can help to break down barriers and allow team members to better empathize with each other.

Table 18.1   Five Dysfunctions of a Team

Dysfunction	Description
Absence of trust	Fear of individuals within the group to show vulnerability. This leads to wasted energy protecting oneself. Freeing oneself from this leads to an ability to focus on the group task at hand
Fear of conflict	Seeking artificial harmony over open constructive ideological conflict. Engaging in constructive conflict allows the team to confidently commit to a task or decision with the benefit of all team members' ideas
Lack of commitment	Struggling with ambiguity around group decisions resulting in delays
Avoidance of accountability	Avoidance of holding other team members to high standards leads to the collective holding low standards
Inattention to results	Focus on a single person's status and ego over the collective ego

Source: Adapted from Lencioni P. *The Five Dysfunctions of a Team: A Leadership Fable*. San Francisco: Jossey-Bass, A Wiley Company, 2002.

Despite the necessity for the entire team to work on these as a whole, the importance of having strong leadership to guide the team through the challenges cannot be understated. It should be noted that the hierarchical medical model with the physician at the lead may not be the best fit for the delivery of palliative care [12].

Those familiar with the concept of a multidisciplinary family meeting will note that these can be a source of tension and conflict. Many of the communication techniques that can be used for disarming conflict in a family meeting can be applied to the inner workings of a team. In our experience, often reframing a situation in a low-key, open-ended format and affirming a common goal are one of the best strategies for diffusing interteam conflict. A similar approach for supporting team dynamics may be implemented, utilizing uninvolved team members for mediation.

While much can be learned from corporate team literature, particular attention should be paid to the concept of clinician burnout when caring for patients who are seriously ill. Various resources exist to assist with identifying and working through burnout or compassion fatigue [13]. The sources of burnout in the context of palliative care are the lack of sufficient multiplicity in the team, hence overstretching of team members' resources, and inadequate interteam mechanisms to provide mental and emotional support when this overstretching occurs. Having advanced, deliberate mechanisms in place to deal with this burnout within a palliative care team will reinforce the team's functionality and sustainability. Having an overt acknowledgment that burnout is not a failure of the individual but a challenge to the team's overall functioning should frame communication and the mechanisms instilled to address it.

18.7 CONCLUSION

For those of us who work in a multidisciplinary team daily, it is clear that it is much like a family, the health and success of which needs to be nurtured and cultivated over time. It must have a central mission and all parties must feel able to participate freely. A team will inevitably struggle or falter when suffering the challenges of interteam dynamics, but these challenges may be overcome with careful analysis and skilled leadership and cultivation of the four primary values of teamwork: trust, expertise, agility, and multiplicity. As medical advances enhance the quality and quantity of life, the complexity of care delivery and coordination grows. Palliative care is designed to maintain patient-centered care where this complexity is often at its highest: in advanced, life-altering illness. Meeting the dynamic and often complex, multiplicity of needs of patients and families in this area requires particularly nuanced, delicate, and comprehensive care, best performed by a high-functioning, multidisciplinary team.

REFERENCES

1. Puntillo KA, McAdam JL, Communication between physicians and nurses as a target for improving end-of-life care in the intensive care unit: challenges and opportunities for moving forward, *Crit Care Med* 2006 Nov;**34**(11 Suppl):S332–S340.
2. Hall P, Interprofessional teamwork: professional cultures as barriers, *J Interprof Care* 2005 May;**19**(Suppl 1):188–196.
3. Dahlin C, editor. *Clinical Practice Guidelines for Quality Palliative Care*, 3rd ed. National Consensus Project for Quality Palliative Care, 2013.
4. Quill TE, Abernethy AP, Generalist plus specialist palliative care—creating a more sustainable model, *N Engl J Med* 2013 Mar 28;**368**(13):1173–1175.
5. Morrison RS, Augustin R, Souvanna P, Meier DE, America's care of serious illness: a state-by-state report card on access to palliative care in our nation's hospitals, *J Palliat Med* 2011 Oct;**14**(10):1094–1096.
6. Pantilat SZ, Kerr KM, Billings JA, Bruno KA, O'Riordan DL, Characteristics of palliative care consultation services in California hospitals, *J Palliat Med* 2012 May;**15**(5):555–560.
7. Royal College of Nursing, Defining Nursing [Internet], 2003. Available at http://www.rcn.org.uk/__data/assets/pdf_file/0008/78569/001998.pdf. Accessed on July 31, 2014.
8. Ferrell BR, Coyle N, An overview of palliative nursing care, *Am J Nurs* 2002 May;**102**(5):26–31; quiz 32.
9. Collins J, *Good to Great: Why Some Companies Make the Leap—and Others Don't*. New York: HarperBusiness, 2001.
10. Jünger S, Pestinger M, Elsner F, Krumm N, Radbruch L, Criteria for successful multiprofessional cooperation in palliative care teams, *Palliat Med* 2007 Jun;**21**(4):347–354.
11. Lencioni P. *The Five Dysfunctions of a Team: A Leadership Fable*. San Francisco: Jossey-Bass, A Wiley Company, 2002.
12. Meier DE, Beresford L, Social workers advocate for a seat at palliative care table, *J Palliat Med* 2008 Feb;**11**(1):10–14.
13. Kearney MK, Weininger RB, Vachon MLS, Harrison RL, Mount BM, Self-care of physicians caring for patients at the end of life: "Being connected … a key to my survival," *JAMA J Am Med Assoc* 2009 Mar 18;**301**(11):1155–1164, E1.

WEB RESOURCES

- CAPC Training

  http://www.capc.org/palliative-care-leadership-initiative/curriculum. Accessed on July 31, 2014.
- Society for Hospital Medicine Team Building Exercises

  http://www.hospitalmedicine.org/AM/Template.cfm?Section=Special_Interest_Areas1&Template=/CM/HTMLDisplay.cfm&ContentID=15361. Accessed on July 31, 2014.

Chapter 19

Self-Care and Resilience for Hospital Clinicians

Sarah M. Piper, B.J. Miller, and Michael W. Rabow

19.1 INTRODUCTION

In the hospital setting, clinicians frequently encounter patients with serious or life-limiting illness. The care of these patients is often complex and can be accompanied by a heightened sense of urgency and emotional intensity in the face of increased suffering of patients and their families. The provision of care for these patients and their families can be particularly rewarding, both professionally and personally, but it often also represents many unique and potentially overwhelming challenges in trying to manage a patient or family's distress or to provide support at the end of a patient's life. When combined with other work-related stressors (e.g., high patient volumes, time pressures, limited resources) and the added challenges for hospital-based clinicians (e.g., transient doctor–patient relationships), the negative impact on clinician well-being can be additive. In response to mounting stressors, clinicians may experience emotional distress characterized by grief, compassion fatigue, or burnout.

The importance of clinician well-being has been increasingly recognized, not only to sustain the professional and personal satisfaction of clinicians but also to promote high-quality patient care. This chapter explores the growing understanding of the syndromes of burnout, compassion fatigue, and clinician grief; examines the particular challenges inherent in the provision of hospital-based care for the seriously ill and dying; further characterizes the many potential rewards of caring for patients facing serious illness; and presents strategies and interventions for the management or prevention of clinician burnout.

19.2 DEFINING THE CHALLENGES

Through the practice of medicine, clinicians witness suffering firsthand. For many, a dedication to the relief of others' suffering is a core value that inspired a career in medicine. The suffering of seriously ill patients or those nearing the end of their lives is often

Hospital-Based Palliative Medicine: A Practical, Evidence-Based Approach, First Edition.
Edited by Steven Pantilat, Wendy Anderson, Matthew Gonzales, and Eric Widera.
© 2015 John Wiley & Sons, Inc. Published 2015 by John Wiley & Sons, Inc.

still more intense, with the need to bear witness to patient and family frustration, anger, resentment, and sorrow. With exposure to the intense emotional experiences of these patients, clinicians understandably encounter strong emotions of their own. These can include an increased need to rescue the patient, a sense of failure and frustration as a patient's condition worsens, feelings of helplessness, or grief [1]. Clinicians are confronted with the eventuality of their own deaths or reminded of the illness or losses of loved ones. And while clinicians have traditionally been taught to focus solely on the experience of patients, there is an increasing appreciation of the impact of a clinician's stress and emotional experience on his or her quality of life, well-being, career sustainability, and even the quality of patient care. The accumulation of unrecognized emotional stress and other workplace stressors has been linked to increased rates of clinician distress, described by syndromes such as burnout, compassion fatigue, and clinician grief.

19.2.1 Burnout

Burnout has been described as "the progressive loss of idealism, energy and purpose experienced by people in the helping professions as a result of the conditions of their work" [2]. As many as one-half of clinicians report experiencing at least one of the three defining symptoms of burnout during their careers [3], which include exhaustion, a sense of professional ineffectiveness, and cynicism or depersonalization. The first symptom, exhaustion, is characterized not only by physical and mental fatigue but also emotional weariness. The second symptom, a loss of professional efficacy, refers to the perceived inability to meet one's professional obligations, and may be linked to a chronic lack of resources or inadequate training. The third symptom, cynicism, refers to the emotional detachment or disengagement from patient care, often characterized by the loss of empathic connection with patients. These symptoms can manifest as behavioral changes that can significantly impact one's work environment, listed in Table 19.1.

Conceptually, burnout is thought to arise from conflict between a clinician and his or her work environment [4]. Six key work-related factors have been identified that most significantly increase risk of burnout. These include an excessively large or intense workload, lack of control or autonomy, lack of recognition or reward, dissonance within one's workplace culture or community, lack of a sense of fairness, and discordance with the values represented within one's work environment that may lead to moral distress [4]. An individual clinician may prioritize these factors differently, and the extent to which they are discordant with one's own priorities, needs, or capabilities informs the overall risk of burnout [2, 4].

While any combination of factors producing clinician–work environment mismatch can lead to burnout, the unique demands of caring for the seriously ill and dying in the hospital setting can potentially challenge many of these factors. For instance, providing care to seriously ill or dying patients can further impact already high volume workloads. In the care of the seriously ill or dying, the intense suffering that patients and families tend to experience during hospitalization for an acute crisis often demands increased resources from clinicians providing their care, including time and energy needed for careful communication, potential conflict resolution, the coordination of

Table 19.1   Primary Symptoms and Associated Behaviors of Burnout

Primary Symptoms:
  1. Exhaustion (physical and emotional)
  2. Sense of professional ineffectiveness
  3. Cynicism or emotional detachment
Associated Behaviors:
  Avoidance of emotionally difficult patients or clinical situations
  Diminished work efficiency
  Absenteeism
  Decreased observance of professional standards
  Interpersonal conflict
  Disengagement from social or professional groups
  Blurring of personal or professional boundaries
  Diminished adaptability/flexibility (rigid thinking, perfectionism)
  Alcohol or substance abuse
  Difficulty maintaining focus in the workplace
  Impatience or irritability
  Impaired judgment
  Questioning foundational beliefs about life or religion

Source: Adapted from Kearney MK, Weininger RB, Vachon ML, Harris RL, Mount BF. Self-care of physicians: caring for patients at the end of life, *JAMA* 2009 March 18;**301**(11):1155–1164.

complex care, and often difficult decision-making [5]. Repeated encounters or a high volume of patients in crisis can tax a clinician's endurance and ability to maintain high workloads and remain empathically engaged with his or her patients.

Clinicians may experience moral distress or discordant values with their institution or practice culture when trying to balance clinical care, costs, and the demands of efficiency. While this can arise in many different contexts, the provision of end-of-life care frequently stirs strong and disparate opinions even within the same health-care setting, and the burden of negotiating these differing views can result in a sense of compromising one's own values. In one study of five hospitals, nearly one-half of all clinicians and 70% of house staff reported acting against their conscience in providing care to terminally ill patients [6].

The extent to which a work community provides support for clinicians facing these challenges may also impact burnout risk. For instance, some clinicians report that their practice setting or work culture may not permit the expression of strong emotions related to patient care or grief after the death of a patient [7]. For clinicians who value the support of their colleagues as a strategy for well-being, these community characteristics may generate feelings of isolation.

A fourth factor, sense of control, is also particularly relevant to challenges in providing end-of-life care. The care of seriously ill patients and their families frequently requires advanced skills in communication and symptom management that may not be available within a medical community's or individual clinician's resources. In many hospitals, palliative care is a new field with a set of specialized skills that may be of limited availability. Hospital-based clinicians without sufficient training in palliative medicine may feel a sense of helplessness, ineffectiveness, or loss of control in providing care to a suffering patient, especially without institutional support to seek opportunities for further training or access to other palliative care resources (including an interdisciplinary palliative care team).

Risk Factors for Burnout. While any clinician may be at risk for developing burnout, several individual characteristics have been associated with increased risk. Clinicians seem to be at higher risk earlier in their careers, with higher rates of burnout even among medical students and residents. Females seem to be at higher risk of developing burnout than males, although this finding is inconsistent across studies. Being single is an independent risk factor, with less burnout observed among married clinicians and those with children [5]. Certain personality traits may also predispose to burnout, including high levels of motivation and professional investment, an exaggerated sense of responsibility for others, and a tendency toward self-doubt or guilt [8]. In one qualitative study of 18 academic oncologists, it was observed that the cognitive framework with which a clinician approached his or her patients may also be linked to risk for burnout [9]. For example, those who viewed the medical care they provided in a biopsychosocial context experienced greater satisfaction in providing end-of-life care than colleagues who viewed their role in a purely biomedical context. The latter group tended to experience greater emotional distance from patients, as well as a sense of failure when a terminal course of illness could not be altered with medical interventions. Of note, data suggests that clinicians providing palliative care are not at increased risk and may even have lower rates of burnout than non-palliative care clinicians [10]. This may suggest that increased training and experience in managing end-of-life care may mitigate the risks of developing burnout.

Compassion Fatigue. Compassion fatigue, while related to burnout, is a distinct potential complication of providing care for the seriously ill or dying and was once termed the "cost of caring." It has also been referred to as *secondary trauma* or *vicarious traumatization.* Whereas burnout is thought to arise specifically from one's interaction with challenges or difficult-to-meet expectations within one's work environment, compassion fatigue is conceptualized as the product of repeat exposure to the traumatic experiences or suffering of patients. The process of empathic engagement with others' suffering leads to accumulated vicarious distress, and individuals with a greater empathic sensitivity may be at increased risk of developing compassion fatigue [11]. The symptom profile is similar to posttraumatic stress disorder: hypervigilance, involuntary reexperiencing of others' reported or witnessed traumas, avoidance of situations or individuals that might invoke intense feelings or memories, and mood disturbance, such as depression or anxiety. Other reported symptoms include feelings of discouragement, emptiness, or having exhausted one's emotional reserves. Najjar and colleagues [11], in their review of compassion fatigue among oncologists, suggested that given the high emotional engagement characteristic of caring for seriously ill patients, compassion fatigue may be an expected, rather than exceptional, occurrence that warrants acknowledgement, open discussion, and the institution of preventive measures where possible.

Clinician Grief. Most clinicians can recount experiences in which the death of a patient left a lasting impact. The role of clinician grief is a relatively new focus of investigation, and as yet, the prevalence and full impact of grief reactions among clinicians remain incompletely characterized [12]. Qualitative studies describing interviews with oncologists suggest high emotional intensity around the experience of patient death, particularly for close or more long-standing patient–clinician relationships, patients with children, challenging patients, long-term patients, and unexpected patient loss [7]. For many clinicians, the medical culture seems to place constraints on the expression of grief, influenced by social stigma of death, avoidance, concern that emotional expression may be perceived as weakness, and a prevailing focus on the goal of curing patients that precludes acknowledgement of death and dying. In studies characterizing the reactions of a dying patient among physicians, particularly for those earlier in their careers, the added burden of feelings of guilt, clinical uncertainty, and isolation were prominent themes that could further compound the experience of a patient's death [13]. Insofar as grief can deplete emotional reserve, the accumulated loss of patients understandably can contribute to the development of clinician distress. Similarly, prevailing attitudes within a medical community or greater medical culture may conflict with an individual clinician's need to express or process grief over the death of a patient, potentially increasing the risk of burnout.

Grief, of course, is not limited to the experience of a dying patient. Rather, the sorrow experienced by a clinician who suffers the loss of a loved one may be reignited upon encountering a dying patient or a similarly grieving family [1].

Consequences of Burnout, Compassion Fatigue, and Clinician Grief. The effects of burnout can be significant and far-reaching [3, 14]. Not only do clinicians with burnout experience increased emotional distress, when unmanaged they may also be at higher risk of developing more pervasive psychological disorders like depression, which increases the risk of suicidal ideation or suicide attempt [15]. Burnout may lead to poorer health behaviors, such as increased alcohol consumption, and may have an adverse interpersonal effect [3], leaving clinicians feeling too depleted to maintain investment in relationships with their friends or families. Those with compassion fatigue may be more likely to consume alcohol, engage in overeating, or experience exacerbations of physical ailments such as headache or other pain [11]. In terms of professional effects, burnout is linked to poor job satisfaction and increased employee turnover. Job performance may suffer, with evidence that burnout may lead to an increase in medical errors, poorer patient outcomes, and decreased patient satisfaction [14]. Research characterizing medical trainees with burnout also links the syndrome to compromised professional standards and a diminished sense of altruism [16]. These individual effects of burnout and compassion fatigue can negatively impact a health-care system as well, as reviewed by Wallace and colleagues [14], with associations of decreased productivity among clinicians with burnout, increased absenteeism or job turnover, or compromised morale of a medical community. Given the potential impact of burnout and compassion fatigue, prevention becomes an issue of not only personal well-being and job sustainability, but also one of professionalism and quality patient care.

19.3   REWARDS OF CARING FOR THE SERIOUSLY ILL AND DYING

Despite the challenges described previously, care of the seriously ill and dying can also lead to positive or even transformative experiences for clinicians and other health-care providers. Two particular benefits for clinicians caring for seriously ill patients are compassion satisfaction and vicarious posttraumatic growth.

19.3.1   Compassion Satisfaction

The act of providing care that effects an important or meaningful change in the well-being of a patient or their family can provide significant personal and professional satisfaction. The provision of compassionate care to patients can potentially bolster resilience and workplace satisfaction, even in the face of other work-related stressors, compassion fatigue, and burnout risk factors [11].

19.3.2   Vicarious Posttraumatic Growth

The term *posttraumatic growth* refers to positive changes in a person's relationships, self-concept, and perspective on life that occurs following a traumatic experience [17]. This phenomenon has also been observed among those providing care for traumatized individuals, known as *vicarious posttraumatic growth*. For example, a clinician may find significant meaning in a patient's peaceful acceptance of an untimely death that lends greater significance to his or her own relationships, appreciation for the capacity of human beings to endure great challenges, and an evolved idea of one's own hopes for the end of life. In one study that interviewed practitioners of palliative medicine regarding their experiences of caring for dying patients, several common themes were distilled to describe the perceived impact of participating in the care of a dying patient [18]. Clinicians identified an opportunity to focus on living in the present, to recognize one's own mortality, and to reinforce the preciousness of living each day fully; an opportunity for spiritual integration, whereby clinicians are able to find meaning or new understanding about life and death; and an opportunity to witness the strength, courage, and grace of those in their care facing the end of their lives that informed a new approach to living.

19.4   CULTIVATING PHYSICIAN WELL-BEING AND RESILIENCE

Medicine as a profession requires considerable personal and professional investment. While medical education continues to evolve to increasingly address career sustainability and well-being, for most practicing clinicians the skills needed to promote resilience and ensure a sustainable, meaningful career were not cultivated in the course medical training. *Resilience* has been described as the ability to respond to

Table 19.2   Measures That Can Increase Resilience

Personal Practices	Job-Related Practices
Cultivating self-awareness	Clarification and directed pursuit of
Mindfulness practices	professional goals
Peer reflection	Maintaining manageable workload
Journaling or reflective writing	Supervision and mentoring
Clarification of personal goals and values	Protecting work-home separation
Maintaining commitment to self-care	Maintaining supportive work community
Seek personal support when needed	Engagement in quality improvement activities
	Training in communication skills
	Accessing educational activities
	Diversification of professional roles
	Recognition of professional limits
	Participation in Schwartz Center Rounds®

Source: Adapted from Kearney MK, Weininger RB, Vachon ML, Harris RL, Mount BF. Self-care of physicians: caring for patients at the end of life, *JAMA* 2009 March 18;**301**(11):1155–1164.

stressors in an adaptive way that enables the achievement of personal goals without incurring a cost to one's psychological or physical well-being and with the development of greater durability to face those stressors [19]. As the impact of clinician burnout and compassion fatigue has been appreciated, there has been an increase in research to explore methods of improving clinician well-being, professional engagement, and resilience.

Based on observational, qualitative, and quantitative research to date, both personal and professional factors have been identified to support clinicians in their pursuit of overall well-being, work engagement, and resilience (see Table 19.2).

19.4.1 Personal Practices

Self-Awareness   At the core of clinician well-being is the practice of self-awareness [1, 12]. Fostering awareness of one's own emotions and behaviors can be challenging given the many competing demands of providing patient care and fulfilling other professional roles and obligations. And yet, a focus on self-awareness provides an opportunity, perhaps most importantly, to first recognize symptoms or signs of emotional distress or burnout. With ongoing observation, clinicians can identify precipitating factors causing distress. Particularly in caring for the seriously ill or dying, recognition of intense feelings of anger, grief, or helplessness that can arise in the face of witnessing suffering is the first step to managing those reactions. Meier and colleagues [1] suggested that awareness of one's emotional state enables a clinician to identify intense emotions that may impact personal well-being or patient care, to recognize and normalize the universality of these emotions in the practice of medicine, to reflect on the possible causes of those intense feelings to seek further understanding, and, importantly, to seek support or counsel from colleagues or other associates when needed. With greater understanding of their own behaviors and emotions, clinicians can begin to take action to mitigate factors that put them at risk for worsening emotional distress or burnout, to reinforce constructive patient–clinician or work–life boundaries, and to understand the difference between constructive and potentially destructive responses to stress [19].

Strategies to improve self-awareness include contemplative practices such as mindfulness, use of peer discourse to foster understanding of complex patient–clinician interactions and relationships, and journaling or narrative writing.

Mindfulness Mindfulness refers to the ability of clinicians to remain "purposefully and nonjudgmentally attentive to their own experience, thoughts and feelings," including cognitive, emotional, and physical awareness [19]. The benefits of mindfulness practices have been explored among health-care professionals in the form of meditative practice, new approaches for improved communication [20, 21], and programs for stress reduction [22]. Recent research has shown that mindful clinicians engage in more patient-centered communication—a frequent challenge in providing care for the seriously ill or dying—and have more satisfied patients [23]. In recent years, the practice of mindfulness has been investigated as another tool to prevent burnout among clinicians. An abbreviated mindfulness training course for primary care clinicians was associated with a reduction in burnout, depression, anxiety, and stress that persisted for at least 1 year [24]. Other studies investigating benefits of mindfulness demonstrate an increase in empathy, both for oneself and for others [22], and evidence of decreasing bias in decision-making [25].

Peer Reflection The use of reflection and discussion among professional colleagues (peer reflection) to process challenging or emotionally laden patient encounters can foster a sense of clinician support, diminish feelings of isolation, and facilitate a more nuanced understanding of often complex clinician–patient interactions [7]. Clinical supervision is another alternative to informal reflection and is a supportive construct widely used in psychiatric training to foster increased awareness of one's own emotional experience in providing care and to identify barriers to compassionate care including personal biases or countertransference—strong emotions triggered by interactions with certain patients that can unwittingly impact patient care or cause distress. Supervision is a recurring process, coordinated with either an experienced mentor or a community psychotherapist. For still more personalized opportunities for reflection on one's personal or professional values, emotional experience, and potential opportunities to build resilience, pursuing individual psychotherapy or other mental health support may provide more comprehensive, personalized support.

Some medical communities offer opportunities for group reflection as well. Balint groups are one established format to discuss the personal experience and challenges of caring for patients. Frequently co-led by a clinician and mental health professional, Balint groups are a longitudinal, small group forum used to broaden self-awareness in the practice of medicine and to explore the many facets of the patient–clinician relationship. Other forums, such as Schwartz Center Rounds®—a medical community-wide monthly discussion of challenging themes in providing humanistic patient care—may similarly support a community in which the emotional experience of caring for others can be discussed openly and without judgment, in the spirit of cultivating greater understanding of the challenges of providing compassionate patient care.

Reflective Writing   The practice of reflective writing has been demonstrated in groups of patients to improve self-awareness and nonjudgmental exploration of the experience of illness. Similarly, some clinicians and medical trainees have begun to utilize various methods to chronicle experiences in their practice, focusing on recounting details of the encounter as well as allowing undirected and unedited expression of the emotional impact accompanying the experience, exploring important themes, and identifying sources of meaning [2]. With further mindful contemplation of one's experience, self-awareness and empathy are cultivated.

Self-Care   Many clinicians find it challenging to maintain a self-care practice. A tradition of inattention to personal needs during medical training, a profession characterized by often unpredictable patient care needs, and increasing administrative demands on a clinician's time can underprioritize adequate sleep, nutrition, or exercise. In qualitative studies characterizing sustaining practices among palliative care providers, physical activity and self-care were among the most commonly reported strategies [8]. The benefits of these interventions are well demonstrated to promote not only physical but also emotional well-being [26]. And while many clinicians, including those already experiencing fatigue or overwhelm accompanying burnout or depression, may be daunted by the prospect of implementing a self-care routine, experienced clinicians highlight the importance of capitalizing on even brief opportunities throughout the day to promote individual health, such as taking the stairs between patient visits, keeping a stock of healthy snacks readily available, and honoring any recognized need for a break throughout the workday [2, 27].

Self-care also includes attention to one's own medical and psychological well-being. As with all new health concerns, allowing oneself to receive prompt care is important. Particularly if symptoms of emotional distress, burnout, grief, or depression become unmanageable, seeking mental health support is a priority.

Exquisite Empathy   It is a commonly held belief that the exercise of empathy has a depleting effect, over time, inevitably leading to compassion fatigue or emotional distress. However, examination of techniques used by experienced psychotherapists engaging in treatment of traumatized patients suggests that there is a way of applying one's empathy that generates great personal and professional reward without personal cost [16]. This has been termed *exquisite empathy*, further defined as a "highly present, sensitively attuned, well-boundaried, heartfelt empathic engagement" with patients [2]. The practice of exquisite empathy enables avoidance of *emotional contagion*, whereby clinicians internalize the sadness, pain, or suffering of patients or families they encounter, which can compromise clinical effectiveness and over time erode the empathic connection in the clinician–patient relationship. Exquisite empathy may be the product of strong self-awareness and self-knowledge that enables recognition of the scope and limits of one's professional role and the ability to avoid overidentification with a patient's suffering. With these boundaries intact, the rewards of witnessing the healing properties of an empathic connection remain prominent [28].

19.4.2 Professional Strategies

Burnout, as discussed earlier, is closely linked with factors within one's work environment. For those experiencing severe burnout symptoms, some clinicians may elect to cut back on their professional roles to provide more time for reflection, renewal, and implementation of the personal strategies discussed previously to cultivate resilience. Others may consider switching jobs altogether. Prior to considering large changes in one's career, exploration of possible professional routes to improve job engagement and lessen burnout is helpful. Realistically, all health-care systems bear sources of frustration that may increase risk of burnout for an individual clinician, and acquiring the skills to reengage in one's work setting to more effectively achieve one's personal and professional goals is likely to lead to more enduring fulfillment and work satisfaction [19].

In order to foster work–life balance, Chittenden and Ritchie [27] suggest a focus on clarifying one's professional goals and narrowing the scope of professional engagement to selectively pursue those that are most consistent with one's values. Limiting participation in extraneous activities that are unlikely to contribute to one's fulfillment of those goals can prevent overextension and dilution of one's effectiveness. They also suggest capitalizing on job flexibility that meets an individual's need for balancing work and personal life. This may include periods of part-time work or creative restructuring of work activities to offset stressors encountered in certain facets of one's clinical, administrative, or academic role [27]. A recent study by Shanafelt and colleagues suggested that the time spent providing direct patient care was a dominant predictor of burnout among oncologists [29], which suggests the possible benefit for some people of diversifying professional roles to improve work engagement and job satisfaction. The importance of prioritizing family relationships and working within one's practice setting to realize that priority, where possible, can support clinician resilience. Some clinicians have suggested the practice of maintaining contact with loved ones throughout the day. Others create a "role shedding ritual" at the end of each day, such as mindfully hanging up one's white coat or stethoscope, to demarcate the transition from work to home to minimize the impact of work stress on one's home life [2].

Surveys of palliative care providers also support the strategies of deriving support from professional relationships and colleagues, the cultivation of clinical or professional variety in one's career to offset the intensity of clinical work for challenging patient populations, and maintaining personal boundaries in their work [8]. In particular, engaging a mentor can provide a useful forum to discuss challenging clinical, academic or administrative concerns, or challenges within a work culture, and can decrease clinician isolation and the resulting increased risk for burnout. Capitalizing on opportunities for skill development can also improve clinician resilience. Especially for those providing care for the seriously ill or dying, additional training to build communication skills for end-of-life discussions or to manage symptoms can bolster clinician confidence and improve burnout symptoms. For example, a recent study evaluating strategies to decrease burnout among health-care professionals working in an ICU setting demonstrated a significant improvement in the severity of burnout symptoms after implementing an intensive communication course that focused on discussing principles of palliative care [30].

Burnout symptoms can lead clinicians to withdraw from their work settings, often to preserve energy and avoid further stressors. However, evidence suggests that productive engagement in one's work setting may, in itself, be protective. One recent study demonstrated an association between participation in quality improvement projects and a reduction in feelings of isolation and work dissatisfaction [31].

With increased appreciation of the scope and impact of burnout across health-care settings, improving clinician resilience is increasingly viewed as a joint venture between clinicians and health-care systems [19]. Proposals also exist to promote change within a medical center or organization that would mitigate the risk of clinician burnout. These include the promotion of clinician autonomy, the provision of adequate resources for support, investment in cultivating a collegial work environment, the integration of a value-oriented perspective that can inspire and motivate clinicians, the protection of work–home separation, and the infusion of principles and practices of work–life balance into clinician work structure [32]. Active participation in developing these strategies in the hospital setting is a worthwhile pursuit for hospitalist groups and can continue the trend toward a changing culture in medicine that supports clinicians in building resilience to optimize personal and professional fulfillment.

19.5   CONCLUSIONS

For many clinicians, shifting from a sole focus on patient care to one that incorporates one's own well-being can be challenging. Increasingly, investment in clinician well-being is viewed not only as a practice that is critical to achieving a meaningful, sustainable, and satisfying practice of medicine but also to the maintenance of standards of medical professionalism and quality patient care. Improved self-care, particularly in the setting of caring for seriously ill or dying patients, can improve one's ability to be present for a patient and their family, to withstand the emotional intensity of witnessing suffering firsthand, and to create meaning from these experiences that further fuels compassion for oneself and for others.

REFERENCES

1. Meier DE, Back AL, Morrison RS. The inner life of physicians and care of the seriously ill, *JAMA* 2001 December 19; **286**(23): 3007–3014.
2. Kearney MK, Weininger RB, Vachon ML, Harris RL, Mount BF. Self-care of physicians: caring for patients at the end of life, *JAMA* 2009 March 18;**301**(11):1155–1164.
3. Shanafelt TD, Boone S, Tan L, et al., Burnout and satisfaction with work-life balance among US physicians relative to the general US population, *Arch Intern Med* 2012;**172**(18):1377–1385.
4. Maslach C, Schaufeli WB, Leiter MP, Job burnout, *Annu Rev Psychol* 2001;**52**:397–422.
5. Vachon M, Mueller M, Burnout and symptoms of stress in staff working in palliative care. In Harvey M, Chochinov WB, editors. *Handbook of Psychiatry in Palliative Medicine*. New York: Oxford University Press, 2009. pp. 236–264.
6. Solomon M, O'Donnell L, Jennings B, et al., Decisions near the end of life: professional views on life-sustaining treatments, *Am J Public Health* 1993 Jan;**83**(1):14–23.
7. Granek L, Krzyzanowska MK, Tozer R, Mazzotta P, Difficult patient loss and physician culture for oncologists grieving patient loss, *J Palliat Med* 2012;**15**(11):1254–1260.
8. Swetz KM, Harrington SE, Matsuyama RK, Shanafelt TD, Lyckholm LJ, Strategies for avoiding burnout in hospice and palliative medicine: peer advice for physicians on achieving longevity and fulfillment, *J Palliat Med* 2009;**12**:773–777.
9. Jackson VA, Mack J, Matsuyama R, et al., A qualitative study of oncologists' approaches to end-of-life care, *J Palliat Med* 2008;**11**(6):893–906.
10. Pereira SM, Fonseca AM, Carvalho AS, Burnout in palliative care: a systematic review, *Nurs Ethics* 2011 May;**18**(3):317–326.
11. Najjar N, Davis LW, Beck-Coon K, Doebbeling CC, Compassion fatigue: a review of the research to date and relevance to cancer-care providers, *J Health Psychol* 2009;**14**(2):267–277.
12. Sansone RA, Sansone LA, Physician grief with patient death, *Innov Clin Neurosci* 2012 April 9;**9**(4):22–26.
13. Jackson VA, Sullivan AM, Gadmer NM, et al., "It was haunting…": Physicians' descriptions of emotionally powerful patient deaths, *Acad Med* 2005 July;**80**(7):648–656.
14. Wallace JE, Lemaire JB, Ghali WA, Physician wellness: a missing indicator, *Lancet* 2009; **374**:1714–1721.
15. Zwack J, Schweitzer J, If every fifth physician is affected by burnout, what about the other four? Resilience strategies of experienced physicians, *Acad Med* 2013;**88**(3):382–389.
16. Dyrbye LN, Massie FS Jr, Eacker A, et al., Relationship between burnout and professional conduct and attitudes among US medical students, *JAMA* 2010;**304**(11):1173–1180.
17. Harrison R, Westwood M, Preventing vicarious traumatization of mental health therapists: identifying protective practices, *Psychother Theory* 2009;**46**(2):203–219.
18. Sinclair S, Impact of death and dying on the personal lives and practices of palliative and hospice care professionals, *CMAJ* 2011;**183**(2):180–187.
19. Epstein RM, Krasner MS, Physician resilience: what it means, why it matters, and how to promote it, *Acad Med* 2013;**88**(3):301–303.
20. Beckman HB, Wendland M, Mooney C, et al., The impact of mindful communication on primary care physicians, *Acad Med* 2012 June;**87**(6):815–819.
21. Krasner MS, Epstein RM, Beckman H, et al., Association of an educational program in mindful communication with burnout, empathy, and attitudes among primary care physicians, *JAMA* 2009 Sept;**302**(12):1284–1293.
22. Shapiro SL, Astin JA, Bishop SR, Cordova M, Mindfulness-based stress reduction for health care professionals: results from a randomized trial, *Int J Stress Manag* 2005;**12**(2):164–176.
23. Beach MC, Roter D, Korthuis PT, et al., A multicenter study of physician mindfulness and health care quality, *Ann Fam Med* 2013 Sept–Oct;**11**(5):421–428.
24. Fortney L, Luchterhand C, Zakletskaia L, Zgierska A, Rakel D, Abbreviated mindfulness intervention for job satisfaction, quality of life, and compassion in primary care clinicians: a pilot study, *Ann Fam Med* 2013 Sep–Oct;**11**(5):412–420.

25. Hafenbrack AC, Zinias Z, Barsade SG, Debiasing the mind through meditation: mindfulness and the sunk-cost bias, *Psychol Sci* 2014 Feb;**25**(2):369–376.
26. Warburton DE, Nicol CW, Bredin SS, Health benefits of physical activity: the evidence, *CMAJ* 2006;**174**:801–809.
27. Chittenden EH, Ritchie CS, Work-life balancing: challenges and strategies, *J Palliat Med* 2011;**14**(7):870–874.
28. Harrison R, Westwood M, Preventing vicarious traumatization of mental health therapists: identifying protective practices, *Psychother Theory* 2009;**46**(2):203–219.
29. Shanafelt TD, Gradishar WJ, Kosty M, et al., Burnout and career satisfaction among US oncologists, *J Clin Oncol* 2014 Mar 1;**32**(7):678–686.
30. Quenot JP, Rigaud JP, Prin S, et al., Suffering among carers working in critical care can be reduced by an intensive communication strategy on end-of-life practices, *Intensive Care Med* 2012 Jan;**38**(1):55–61.
31. Quinn MA, Wilcox A, Orav EJ, Bates DW, Simon SR, The relationship between perceived practice quality and quality improvement activities and physician practice dissatisfaction, professional isolation, and work-life stress, *Med Care* 2009 Aug;**47**(8):924–928.
32. Maslach C, Burnout and engagement in the workplace: new perspectives, *Eur Health Psychol* 2011;**13**(3):44–47.

WEB-BASED RESOURCES

www.fammed.wisc.edu/mindfulness	Mindfulness in Medicine is a site maintained by the University of Wisconsin providing resources for developing a practice of mindfulness and accessing further research on the benefits of mindful practice
acpinternist.org	"Five strategies for physicians to overcome burnout" "Write this down: ways to overcome burnout"
thehappymd.com	Article series about the causes and effects of burnout for clinicians, including resources and strategies for prevention
compassionfatigue.org	A website dedicated to educating health care providers about compassion fatigue, including online assessments of professional quality of life, compassion fatigue, and life stress
www.helpguide.org/mental/burnout_signs_symptoms.htm	An online resource for support in assessing and managing burnout symptoms
americanbalintsociety.org	Information to guide the formation of new Balint groups within your organization
theschwartzcenter.org	Strategies to implement Schwartz Center Rounds® in your setting of practice, with the aim to increase insight into psychosocial aspects of patient care, to cultivate compassion, to improve teamwork and communication, and to decrease feelings of isolation in clinical practice

Index

Note: Page references in *italics* refer to Figures; those in **bold** refer to Tables.

acupuncture /acupressure 209
  in anxiety 88
  in nausea and vomiting 51
  in pain relief 30
acute pain 13
adjustment disorder 74, 77, 78
advance care planning forms 134–5,
    135, 136
advance care planning note 137–8
advance health-care directives 133, 134–5
  differences of family from 139–40
  multiple 140
Advanced Dementia Prognostic Tool
    (ADEPT) 151
allied health professionals 255
alprazolam in anxiety 89
ALS, enteral nutrition and 210
Alzheimer's disease (see also "dementia") 242
amitriptyline 28
anger
  family 115, 166, 199, 225, 233, 261
  patient 104, 163
anticholinergics 41
anticonvulsants 28–9
antidepressants 35, 81, **84–5**
  in anxiety 88
  choice of **87**
  in delirium 62, 65
antiemetics 51, 57–8
  properties of **55–6**
anti-inflammatory drugs 26–8
antisecretory agents 58
anxiety 62, 71–90, **78**
  in addictive behaviors 34–5

assessment 73
  differential diagnosis: anxiety disorders
    and anxiety symptoms 78
  in families 108, 118, 191
  management 87–9
  nonpsychiatric causes of anxiety **79**
  prevalence 72–3
aprepitant 54
aromatherapy 88
art therapy in anxiety 88
artificial hydration only 212–13
artificial nutrition and hydration 206
  conversation tools 217–219
  cultural factors, 213–214
  decision-making 213–15
  discussion at end of life 215–16
  ethics 216–17
  law 216
  surrogates **213**, 215
Ask–Tell–Ask Technique 98–9, **99**
automatic internal defibrillator
    withdrawal 203–4
autonomy 196
autopsy 233–4

bad news, communication of 95, 102–4,
    103–4, 115
Balint groups 267–8
barbiturates 202
benzodiazepines 57, **85**
  in anxiety 88–9
  as cause of delirium 64
  in dyspnea 45
  in terminal extubation 201

Hospital-Based Palliative Medicine: A Practical, Evidence-Based Approach, First Edition.
Edited by Steven Pantilat, Wendy Anderson, Matthew Gonzales, and Eric Widera.
© 2015 John Wiley & Sons, Inc. Published 2015 by John Wiley & Sons, Inc.

bereavement 77, 118
bilevel positive airway pressure (Bi-pap)
    devices 203
Biot's respirations 228
bipolar disorder 74
bisphosphonates 28
breast cancer 147, 175, 177
bronchodilators 41
bupropion 81, **84**
burnout, clinician 257, 261–2,
    262, 263–4, 269–70

cancer
    enteral nutrition in 208
    parenteral nutrition in 211–12
    prognosis tool 147–50
    see also under specific cancer types
cancer anorexia-cachexia syndrome 208
capnography 41
carbamazepine 29
cardiopulmonary resuscitation (CPR) 173
CARING criteria 237
case managers 254
central pain syndrome 12
CES-D Boston Short Form 73
chaplain 254
chemotherapy
    nausea and vomiting induced by 54–7
Cheyne–Stokes respirations 228
children, families with 118–19
Child–Turcotte–Pugh (CTP) score 151
chlorpromazine
    in delirium 67
    in nausea and vomiting 54
chronic obstructive pulmonary disease
    (COPD)
    dyspnea in 37
    glucocorticoids in 42
    hospice care and 241–2, **242**
    prognosis 152
citalopram 81, **82**
clinician grief 264
clinician prediction of survival 144
clonazepam **85**, 89
coanalgesics 26, **27**
cognitive behavioral therapies 80
colorectal cancer 175
comfort feeding 216
communication

importance of, with seriously ill
    patients 95
of prognosis to patient or surrogate 153–5
compassion fatigue 263
compassion satisfaction 265
complex regional pain syndrome (CRPS) 12
conflict over treatment decisions 160–7
    clinical examples 165–7
    management 160–5
conflict resolution in interdisciplinary
    team care 256–7
Confusion Assessment Method (CAM) 64, 65
congestive heart failure (CHF), hospice care
    and 241–2, **242**
continuous pump feeding 210
corticosteroids 57–8, 59
countertransference 267
crisis prevention plan 191
cultural factors, artificial nutrition and
    hydration (ANH) and 213–14

death
    documenting and disclosing 230–4
    impending, signs of 228–9, **229**
    pronouncing 229
    timing of 227–8
death note 230–1, **231**
death rattle 200, 228
delirium 61–9, 77
    algorithm *68*
    assessment 64–5
    causes 63–4
    clinical features 61–2
    differential diagnosis 62–3, **63**
    hydration in 67–8
    hyperactive 62
    hypoactive 62
    nonpharmacologic treatment 68–9
    palliative sedation (PS) 67
    pharmacologic treatment 65–8
    risk factors **64**
    terminal 64
    types 62
    vs depression 63
Delirium Rating Scale (DRS) 65
dementia, advanced 62, 77
    enteral nutrition in 209
    parenteral nutrition in 212
    prognosis 150–1

demoralization syndrome 74, 77
denial 163
depression 62, 71–73
    in addictive behaviors 34–5
    differential diagnosis: depression
        74–7, **75–6**
    families and 108, 118, 191
    management of 80–1, **82–6**
    pharmacotherapy 81–7
    prevalence 72–3
    psychotherapy 80
dexamethasone 26, 54, 57, 59
    in elevated intracrainal pressure 178
dialysis withdrawal 203
dignity therapy in depression 80
discharge planning 254
    dyspnea and 44
    for pain management 31–2
diuretics in dyspnea 42
do not intubate (DNI) order 137
do not resuscitate (DNR) order 137, 247
doctrine of double effect 196
duloxetine 28, 81, **83**
dysphagic stroke, enteral nutrition
        and 209, *210*
dyspnea 37–38
    differential diagnosis 38–40
    diagnostic procedures 40–1
    treatment 41–6
dysthymia 74

education, addiction and diversion and 34
EFFECT model 150
electroconvulsive therapy (ECT) 80
elevated intracranial pressure 177–9
emergencies, palliative care 171–92
    acute massive hemorrhage 185–7
    acute respiratory depressiondue to
        IV opioids 187–8
    definition 171–5, **172**
    factors influencing response to 172, **173**
    family emergencies on general medical
        floor 190–2
    oncologic 175–85
emotional contagion 269
empathy, expressing 99–100
endotracheal tube 200
end-stage renal disease (ESRD) 152–3, 203
enteral nutrition 206–210

disease-specific evidence 208–10
    advanced dementia 209
    ALS 210
    cancer 208
    dysphagic stroke 209, *210*
    head and neck cancer 208
    metastatic cancer 208
ePrognosis 146, 151
equal analgesia concept 21, **21**
    incomplete cross-tolerance adjustment 22, **22**
escitalopram **82**
ethics
    of allowing natural death 195–6
    artificial nutrition and hydration
        (ANH) 216–17
    withdrawal of life-sustaining treatment
        195–6
exercise programs as pain relief 30
exquisite empathy 268–9
eye contact 97

families
    comfort measures to 225–6
    communication with 109–17
    decision-making 225
    empathic communication with 226
    families with children 118–19
    interprofessional support for 117–19, **119**
    opportunities to ask questions/
        clarification 118
    psychosocial support 118–19
    spiritual and religious care 118
    surrogate decision-making 109–11, **111**
    withdrawal of life-sustaining treatment
        and 196–8, **197**
family emergencies on general medical
        floor 190–2
family meetings **109, 110,** 111–17
FAST tool 242
fentanyl **16,** 17, 23, 31
    transdermal, vs IV/SC opioids **17**
    in dyspnea 44
FICA tool 125
fluoxetine 81, **82**
force feeding 217
fracture
    pathological, of long bones 181–2
Functional Assessment Staging (FAST)
        151, **151**

gabapentin 28–9, **85**
in anxiety 89
gastric motility, impaired 54
gastric outlet obstruction 58
gastric tubes (G-tubes) 206, 207
problems with placement **207**
see also enteral nutrition
gastrostomy 208
Generalized Anxiety Disorder Screener
(GAD–7) 73
glucocorticoids 26, 42
goals of care (GOC) 121–31
assessing goals and values 124–5, **125**
case study 122, 123, 126, 128, 130
confirming, and develop treatment
plan 125–6, **127**
discussion road map 122–3
lack of 188–90
surrogate decison-makers 130–1, **131**
use of interpreters 128, **129**
goals of care, documentation 133–42
in-hospital 133–9
advance care planning forms 134–5, **135**
resources **142**
troubleshooting 139–41
multiple advance health-care
directives 140
preferences differ from advance
directive 139–40
surrogate decision-makers' preferences
differ from patient documentation 140–1
grief 74, 77
clinician 264
guided imagery 30
guilt 163

haloperidol
in delirium 65–6
nausea and vomiting and 54
in terminal extubation 201
head and neck cancer, enteral nutrition in 208
healthcare proxy document 135
heart failure (see also congestive heart
failure)
dyspnea in 37
prognosis 150
hemorrhage, acute massive hemorrhage 185–7
hepatocellular carcinoma (HCC) 151
hepatopulmonary syndrome 151

HIV, parenteral nutrition in 212
home palliative care
bridge programs 246
pain management 31
hope, truthtelling vs. 105, **105**
hospice 238–9
discharging patient to 243–5, **243**, **244**
levels of care 240–1, **240**
for specific diagnoses 241–2
for those in nursing homes 241
vs palliative care **245**
Hospital Anxiety and Depression Scale
(HADS) 73
hospital clinicians, self-care and resilience
for 260–70
challenges 260–1
cultivating physical well-being and
resilience 265–6, **266**
personal practices 266–7
professional strategies 269–70
hydromorphone (Dilaudid) 15, **16**
in dyspnea 44
hyoscine butylbromide 58
hyperactive delirium 62
hypercalcemia of malignancy 184–5
hyperthyroidism 79
hypnotherapy 88
hypoactive delirium 62
hypodermoclysis 212
hypomania 74

'I Wish' statements 101, 104, 105
ibuprofen 26
imipramine 28
incomplete cross-tolerance
adjustment 22, **22**
inflammatory pain 12
instructional directive 135–6
insurers 255
interdisciplinary team care 250–8
definition of team 250
conflict resolution in 256–7
dysfunctions **257**
high-functional team qualities 255–6
key team members 253–4
mission statement, team 255–6
intrathecal analgesia 13

jejunal tubes (J-tubes) 206

Karnofsky Performance Status Scale (KPS)
    146, **146**
ketamine 13, 29, 34
    in depression **85**, 87
    in terminal extubation 202
ketorolac 26
kidney cancer 175
kinesiology 30

last days of life 223–36
    breathing patterns 228
    care during 223–6
    documenting and disclosing
        death 230–4
    pronouncing death 229
    signposting and symptom
        management 226–9
    signs of impending death 228–9, **229**
    timing of dying 227–8
law
    artificial nutrition and hydration (ANH)
        and 216
    withdrawal of life-sustaining treatment
        and 196
lidocaine 13, 29
liver disease, chronic, prognosis of 151
Local Coverage Determination (LCD) 241
lorazepam 45, 57
    in anxiety 89
    in delirium 66
    in depression **85**
lung cancer 147, 175
    primary and secondary, dyspnea in 37

major airway obstruction 182–3
major depressive disorder (MDD) 72, 74–7
malignant bowel obstruction 57–8, **58**
mandibular breathing 228
mania 62, 74
massage 30, 88
meaning-centered psychotherapy in
        depression 80
mechanical ventilation 41
    withdrawal of 198–202
Medicaid 241
Medical Orders for Life-Sustaining
        Treatment (MOLST) 128,
        135 Medicare Hospice Benefit 238–9,
        238, 240, 241

Memorial Delirium Assessment Scale
        (MDAS) 64–5
mentoring 270
metastatic cancer, enteral nutrition in 208
methadone **16**, 17–19, 20
    in dyspnea 44
    to morphine conversion **18**
    opioid addiction and 35
methotrimeprazine in delirium 66
methylphenidate **84**
metoclopramide 54, 57
mexiletine 29
midazolam 67
mindfulness 88, 267
miracles, beliefs in 166–7, **167**
mirtazapine 59, 81, **84**
mission statement, team 255–6
mixed delirium 62
Model for End-Stage Liver Disease
        (MELD) 151
morphine 15, **16**
    discharge and 31
    in dyspnea 44
    to methadone conversion **18**
    pharmacokinetics **31**
    in terminal extubation 201
morphine titration plan 45
multiple myeloma 175
music therapy 30, 88

naloxone **189**
naproxen 26
nasogastric tubes (NGTs) 207
National Hospice and Palliative Care
        Organization (NHPCO) 238
nausea and vomiting 49–59
    common causes 51–8, **52–3**
    management 49–52
    pathophysiology 49
    reversible causes **51**
neuroleptics in delirium **66**
neuropathic pain 12
neuropathic pain agents 28–9
nitrates 26
nociceptive pain 12
non-Hodgkin's lymphoma 175
noninvasive ventilation (NIV) 46
    withdrawal of 203–4
nonmaleficence 196

nonopioid classes of medications for pain 26–9
nonpharmacological interventions for
pain 29–31
nortriptyline
side effects 28
nurse 253
N-U-R-S-E acronym 100–1, **100**, 104,
105, 114, 162, **163**
nursing homes 246

occupational therapy 30
octreotide 58
olanzapine 59
in delirium 66
oncologic emergencies 175–85
elevated intracranial pressure 177–9
hypercalcemia of malignancy 184–5
major airway obstruction 182–3
pathological fractures of long bones 181–2
spinal cord compression 175–7
status epilepticus 179–81
superior vena cava obstruction 182–3
ondansetron 54, 57
open-ended questions 114–16
opioid
addiction 34
adverse effects 19–20, **19**, 54, 64
analgesics 15–26, **16**, 32
conversion 21–3, **22**, **24**
equivalency 19
in dyspnea 44–5
in terminal extubation 201
risk evaluation and mitigation strategies 32–3
titration 20–1
transition from IV to long-acting, for
discharge 31
oral feeding 215–16
organ procurement organization 233
out-of-hospital do not resuscitate form 136
outpatient providers 255
overnarcotization 187–8
oximetry 41
oxycodone 15, **16**
oxygen in dyspnea 43–4
oxymorphone **16**

pain
addiction and diversion 34–5
biopsychosocial model of *12*

complications of 13
consequences of 13
etiology and types 11–13
interdisciplinary approach to 13
medication reconciliation 15
nonopioid classes of medications 26–9, 32
nonpharmacological interventions 29–31
opioid analgesics 15–26, **16**, 32
practical general approach 13–14
scales 13–14
transition to outpatient 31–3
pain psychology 30–1
palliative care 3, 245
benefits of 4
case study 1, 7–8
concurrent model 5
patients appropriate for **4**
role of hospital-based clinician in 5–6
sites of care 246
vs hospice care **245**
palliative care clinic 246
Palliative Performance Scale (PPS) 146,
147, **148–9**, 150
paradoxical pain 12
paralytics in terminal extubation 202
parenteral nutrition 206, 211–13
disease-specific evidence 211–12
surrogate decision-making **213**
timing 211, **212**
paroxetine **82**
patient-clinician interaction
emotional cues: expressing empathy
99–100
informational concerns: *"Ask–Tell–Ask"*
Technique. 98–9, **99**
key skills 98–101
opening 97–8
resources **106**
responding to concerns and cues 98–9
see also communication
patient-controlled analgesia (PCA) 23–6
responding to concerns and cues 98–9
indications to contraindications **25**
opioid starting doses **25**
responding to concerns and cues 98–9
Patient Health Questionnaire (PHQ-9), the 73
peer reflection 267–8
percutaneous endoscopic gastrostomy
(PEG) tube 58

personality disorders
  in addictive behaviors 34–5
physical therapy 30
physician 253
physician orders for life-sustaining
    treatment (POLST) **135**, 136, 247
posttraumatic growth 265
posttraumatic stress disorder (PTSD),
    families and 118
pregabalin 29
prescription drug monitoring programs
    (PDMP) 15, 34
pressure ulcers, enteral nutrition and 209
prochlorperazine 54
proctoclysis 212
Profile of Mood States 73
prognostic indices 145, 146, 147,
    148–9, 150
prognostication 143–58, 224
  communication of prognosis to patient
      or surrogate 153–5
  disease-specific prognosis tools 147–53
  prognostic estimates, delivery of 156–7
progress note 137–8
propofol 202
prostate cancer 147, 175
proton pump inhibitors (PPI) 26
pseudoaddiction 34
psychosis 62
psychosocial components of pain 30–1
psychosocial support 118–19
psychostimulants 81–2, **84–5**

quality of life (QOL) 4, 208
quetiapine in delirium 66
Quinlan case 195

ranitidine 58
rapport 97
reflective writing 268
reflex sympathetic dystrophy 12
rehabilitation techniques as pain relief 30
relaxation training, anxiety and 88
religious belief 118, 167
  artificial nutrition and hydration (ANH)
      and 213–14
requests to 'do everything' 165–6
respiratory depression, acute, due to
    intravenous opioids 187–8

Respiratory Distress Observation Scale
    (RDOS) 38, **39**
respiratory therapy 30
Richmond Agitation Sedation Scale (RASS) 67
Risk Evaluation and Mitigation Strategies
    (REMS) 32–3, **32**, **33**
Risperidone 66
role shedding ritual 269

Schwartz Rounds 268
Seattle Heart Failure Model 150
secondary trauma 263
selective serotonin reuptake inhibitors
    (SSRIs)
  in anxiety 88
  in depression 81
self-awareness 266–7
self-care 268
serious illness, definition 3
serotonin/norepinephrine reuptake
    inhibitors (SNRIs) 28, 35, 81, **83**
  in anxiety 88
sertraline 81, **83**
shame 163
sign-out 139
social worker 254
sodium channel blocker 29
S-O-L-E-R acronym 100, **100**, 104
somatic pain 12
speech therapy 30
SPIKES protocol 102–4, **103–4**, 154, **155–6**
spinal cord compression 175–7
spiritual and religious support 30, 118, 124–5
status epilepticus (SE) 179–81
steroids, as causes of delirium 64
Stevens-Johnson syndrome 180
subacute pain 13
suicidal thoughts, families 191
superior vena cava obstruction 182–3
supportive–expressive group therapy in
    depression 80
surrogate decision-making
  expectations 215
  family meetings and 109–11, **111**
  goals of care and 130–1, **131**
  preferences differing from patient
      documentation 140–1
  artificial hydration nutrition and 213, 215
symptoms, relief of 3

Tai Chi 30
terminal delirium 62, 64
trazodone **86**, 89
treatment preference orders 137
tricyclic antidepressants (TCAs) 28, 81
truth telling vs. hope 105, **105**

valproic acid 29, **86**, 89
VALUE mnemonic **197**
venlafaxine 28, 81, **83**
ventilator withdrawal 198–202
vicarious posttraumatic growth 265
vicarious traumatization 263
visceral pain 12
vomiting *see* nausea and vomiting

Walter Index 146
withdrawal of life-sustaining treatment
    195–204, 224
  communication and critical role of family
    196–8, **197**
  ethical consideration 195–6
  medical-legal considerations 196
  medication protocols 202
  ventilator withdrawal 198–202
  ICU policies to support
    families 202–3
withholding life-sustaining
    treatment 195
Wong-Baker FACES scale 13
work–life balance 269